Human Well-Being Research and Policy Making

This series includes policy-focused books on the role of the public and private sectors in advancing quality of life and well-being. It creates a dialogue between well-being scholars and public policy makers. Well-being theory, research and practice are essentially interdisciplinary in nature and embrace contributions from all disciplines within the social sciences. With the exception of leading economists, the policy relevant contributions of social scientists are widely scattered and lack the coherence and integration needed to more effectively inform the actions of policy makers. Contributions in the series focus on one more of the following four aspects of well-being and public policy:

- Discussions of the public policy and well-being focused on particular nations and worldwide regions
- Discussions of the public policy and well-being in specialized sectors of policy making such as health, education, work, social welfare, housing, transportation, use of leisure time
- Discussions of public policy and well-being associated with particular population groups such as women, children and youth, the aged, persons with disabilities and vulnerable populations
- Special topics in well-being and public policy such as technology and well-being, terrorism and well-being, infrastructure and well-being.

This series was initiated, in part, through funds provided by the Halloran Philanthropies of West Conshohocken, Pennsylvania, USA. The commitment of the Halloran Philanthropies is to "inspire, innovate and accelerate sustainable social interventions that promote human well-being." The series editors and Springer acknowledge Harry Halloran, Tony Carr and Audrey Selian for their contributions in helping to make the series a reality.

More information about this series at https://link.springer.com/bookseries/15692

Josef Kuo-Hsun Ma · Simon Cheng

Adolescent Well-Being and ICT Use

Social and Policy Implications

Springer

Josef Kuo-Hsun Ma
Department of Sociology
National Taipei University
New Taipei City, Taiwan

Simon Cheng
Department of Sociology
University of Connecticut
Storrs, CT, USA

ISSN 2522-5367 ISSN 2522-5375 (electronic)
Human Well-Being Research and Policy Making
ISBN 978-3-031-04411-3 ISBN 978-3-031-04412-0 (eBook)
https://doi.org/10.1007/978-3-031-04412-0

This Springer imprint is published by the registered company Springer Nature Switzerland AG
The registered company address is: Gewerbestrasse 11, 6330 Cham, Switzerland

To my wife Tammy. Thanks for her help with tirelessly taking care of our little ones, Rita and Baby Ray.

—Josef Kuo-Hsun Ma

To my family.

—Simon Cheng

Preface

Many of us remember the truly remarkable development of digital technologies from the twentieth to the early twenty-first century. The internet started in the 1960s, long before today's "digital natives" were born. Microsoft introduced the Windows operating system in 1983. Around the same time, Apple produced the first Macintosh computers. In the 1990s, when we were attending school in the U.S. and Taiwan, email became a standard means of communication among academics, and quickly entered popular use. Smartphones began to dominate the consumer market after 2000. Apple released the first iPad in 2010. Tablets from other companies quickly followed. Since then, the developed world has been immersed in digital devices, internet connections, and information technologies.

Concerns over digital inequalities emerged in the early 2000s once digital technologies had permeated daily life. Educators and researchers warned that unequal access to digital technologies in homes, schools, and workplaces would push people and families who were already disadvantaged even further behind. Despite the belief by some that this new form of social inequality would be short-lived, disparities in access to the internet and digital devices not only continued but extended to the quality of involvement with computing and use of information technologies.

From 2020, the lockdowns and school closings caused by the coronavirus pandemic took digital inequality to an unprecedented level. The urgency brought attention to the clear and present educational problem:Without a strong ICT infrastructure, many less developed countries had no remote learning platforms, making it impossible to offer even basic education to their students. In some developing countries, students used radio, television, or personally collected learning packets from their teacher's house. In developed countries, poor internet access and the lack of computers at home limited the learning opportunities of disadvantaged students. Even among students with internet-enabled computers at home, digital literacy, adult supervision, and other family factors compounded with unequal school resources to drive another wedge between disadvantaged and advantaged students. Teachers were underprepared for remote teaching. All students had to adapt quickly to unfamiliar virtual learning modalities. Many were not able to adapt. The digital divide therefore played a central role in the global education crisis and affected *all* students.

As teachers, we have seen the impact of the digital divide on our students.

Our book sheds additional light on the use of ICT in schools as a solution to the present educational crisis and, ironically, also as a source of the crisis when digital divides are considered. This book focuses on the intersection between educational inequality and the digital divide. We ask the following research questions: How does the use of digital technology influence the well-being of secondary students, including their academic performance, learning attitudes, mental health, and digital competence? Who is being excluded from digital learning? How large are the socioeconomic gaps in digital access and ICT use? Although these questions are not new, previous studies have produced inconclusive results on the relationship between adolescents' ICT use and their well-being. Our systematic meta-analytic review of the research literature and cross-national comparative examination of adolescents across a wide range of developed societies allow us to understand the inconsistent findings of previous studies and to articulate the relationships between adolescents' ICT use and their well-being. However, there are no simple answers to our research questions. By analyzing data from 28 developed countries—which represent the most affluent regions of the world—we offer a clear and comprehensive sketch of the effects of the digital divide on adolescent students.

Our analyses found that the relationships between ICT use and well-being are sometimes stronger for socioeconomically advantaged students, and sometimes stronger for their disadvantaged counterparts. The effects depend on whether ICT is used at home or in school, how it is used, student outcomes, and the societies in the analysis. These variations are not random. In each empirical chapter, we explain the patterns of the variations. The concluding chapter explains the implications of these patterns.

Many schools were closed, reopened, and closed again during the pandemic. In the two years since COVID-19 struck, we learned that some students prefer online learning to in-person instruction. Some subjects are easier than others to teach online. Variations among individual students and subjects, in light of our empirical findings, have important policy implications: Curriculum design is not a binary choice between online and in-person instruction, but should maximize the strengths and minimize the weaknesses of e-learning. Accommodations for different learning styles can help students learn in the most effective way, and educators should factor subject areas into curriculum designs. In this book, we explore these policy directions and the challenges educators may face.

Taipei, Taiwan Josef Kuo-Hsun Ma
Storrs, USA Simon Cheng

Acknowledgments

We thank Series Editors Dr. M. Joseph Sirgy and Dr. Richard J. Estes who invited us to work on this book project.

We also acknowledge the assistance of National Taipei University (NTPU) research assistants Yong-Jian Wu, Chia-Yu Yao, Yuan-Yuan Chuang, and Yu-Shan Chen who helped with earlier versions of the book. We are grateful for the much-needed encouragement by colleagues Dr. Heng-Hao Chang, Dr. Yi-Fu Chen, Dr. Ming-Chang Tsai, Dr. Tsui-O Tai, and Dr. Yu-Hsiang Chen from NTPU and many others who provided useful suggestions on finding additional resources to support this book project. In relation to this book, Josef's recent research on adolescent ICT use is supported by NTPU Flagship Project 2021–2022 (granted by the Ministry of Education).

We offer special thanks to the Springer Nature editorial team, especially to Karthika Purushothaman, Banu Dhayalan, Mythili Settu, and Shinjini Chatterjee who helped us through the entire process.

Contents

About the Authors

Josef Kuo-Hsun Ma, Ph.D. is Assistant Professor in the Department of Sociology at National Taipei University. He also serves as Director of International Education and Engagement Division, Office of International Affairs at National Taipei University. His primary areas of research interests are social stratification and inequality, the sociology of education, the sociology of the family, comparative/global sociology, and teens and social media. His past research has centered on how macro-structural forces such as human capital investment and income inequality influence the role of digital technology and the life chances of adolescent students. Other work has focused on the family formation (e.g., transition into parenthood and entry into marriage) among East Asian young adults. Recently, he has been gathering quantitative and qualitative data to examine the effect of COVID-19 on adolescent students' learning. A goal of this research is to understand how the coronavirus pandemic has exacerbated the digital divide, which has created a new form of the (e)learning gap and worsened educational disparities. His new line of research on teens and social media examines the causes and consequences of cyberbullying among teenagers. He has published articles in *Social Forces, Sociological Forum, Social Indicators Research, International Journal of Comparative Sociology, International Sociology, Journal of Family Issues*, and *Journal of Population Studies.*

Simon Cheng, Ph.D. is Professor of Sociology at the University of Connecticut. His research and teaching interests include sociology of education, sociology of family, sociology of sexuality, race/ethnicity, and quantitative methodology. His research addresses a combination of traditional and emerging problems in the discipline and represents a diverse yet coherent set of topics and projects, connected by common threads of interest—in family change and family forms, in gender, race, and sexuality issues in the family and education, in the importance of classification and measurement, and in documenting contexts that condition education and inequalities. His articles are consistently placed in the top journals in his discipline including the *American Sociological Review, American Journal of Sociology, Social Forces, Social Science Research,* and the *Annual Review of Sociology* as well as the leading journals in his sub-specialties like *Sociology of Education, Journal of Marriage and*

Family, and *Sociological Methods and Research*. His article on the effects of same-sex parents received the Sociology of Sexualities Distinguished Article Award in 2017. His research on social media and adolescents appeared in *International Sociology* (Cheng, Ma, and Missari, 2014) and *Social Indicators Research* (Ma, Vachon, and Cheng, 2019).

List of Figures

List of Tables

Chapter 1
Introduction

Abstract Information and Communication Technology (ICT) has become an indispensable component of education around the world. Taking a comparative approach, *Adolescent Well-Being and ICT Use: Social and Policy Implications* examines the relationships among ICT usage, well-being, and social class background of adolescent students in 28 developed countries and societies. This chapter provides an overview of the research background, study design, and analytical framework. The introduction begins with a description of ICT's role in education both before and during the COVID-19 pandemic, followed by a review of the four phases of the digital learning divide from the early 1990s to the 2020s. After an overview of the social and policy contexts of ICT use in education in affluent countries, the chapter ends with research questions, empirical data, and measures of key variables, as well as an outline of the organization of the book.

Keywords COVID-19 · Remote education · Digital learning · Digital divide · Digital natives · Secondary school students · Affluent countries

INFORMATION and Communication Technology (ICT) has become an indispensable component of education around the world. Taking a comparative approach, this book examines the relationships between ICT usage, well-being, and social class background of adolescent students in 28 developed countries/societies. In this introductory chapter, we provide an overview of the research background, study design, and analytical framework. In the following section, we highlight the increasingly important role that ICT has played in education both before and after the COVID-19 pandemic, review the development of the digital learning divide from the early 1990s to the 2020s, and outline the social and policy contexts of ICT use in education in developed societies.

J. K.-H. Ma and S. Cheng, *Adolescent Well-being and ICT UseX*,
Human Well-Being Research and Policy Making,
https://doi.org/10.1007/978-3-031-04412-0_1

1.1 Adolescent ICT Use in Education Before and Since the COVID-19 Pandemic

1.1.1 Why Studying ICT Use in Education Is Important

ICT has changed the daily activity patterns of millennials and young people. It has also altered the educational landscape in the twenty-first century, influencing how young people are taught in the classroom, how they work on school assignments at home, and how they acquire and learn new skills and knowledge. From 2000 to 2010, the use of ICT in educational settings was supplementary and often seemed optional. E-learning was encouraged in schools and by educators but was rarely required. Although e-learning materials and digital technology were readily available, many teachers did not have a strong desire to adopt them; parents were not pressured to upgrade their computers or acquire high-speed internet; and most children did not feel an urgent need to use digital screens or an internet search engine for their schoolwork.

Things are different now. With the rapid development of ICT and the growth of the global knowledge society (ITU, 2018; Ragnedda & Muschert, 2013; Sefton-Green et al., 2016), e-learning technology has matured. Familiarity with a variety of ICT devices (e.g., computers, smartboards, and e-tablets), office processing software (e.g., Microsoft Office, LibreOffice, and Adobe), web-related resources (e.g., Apple iCloud, Google Workplace, and Dropbox), and e-learning platforms/sites (e.g., Blackboard, Wikipedia, Zoom, academic search engines, and online libraries) has become popular. In most countries, e-learning has not replaced traditional teaching and learning methods, nor can it replace a physical classroom. However, the COVID-19 outbreak unexpectedly closed schools and forced educational activities online. Fast adoption of e-learning during the pandemic would not have been possible without the prior development of forms of ICT that can be used in curricula and for student learning—at least among more affluent societies with a mature ICT infrastructure.

In this context, *Adolescent Well-Being and ICT Use: Social and Policy Implications* examines the causes and consequences of digital inclusion and exclusion among secondary school students. We discuss how ICT use affects adolescent academic and psychological outcomes, and evaluate how it is shaped by students' digital experiences at home. We suggest the importance of considering the family context when we study the benefits and outcomes of ICT use. Although adolescents may participate in digital activities in school and at home, we argue that home environments are more influential than schools in shaping adolescents' (e)learning experiences and digital competencies. Therefore, a goal of this book is to analyze how family socioeconomic status (SES) may affect the number of ICT resources that students possess for education, the types of online activities in which students engage, and whether parents are involved in children's online activities and (e)learning processes at home. Focusing on students in secondary education, we discuss how inequalities in access, skills, and uses of digital technologies—commonly known as the "digital divide"—perpetuate educational inequality, and we also describe patterns of social inclusion and exclusion regarding technology and education. By answering the classic question "how does technology generate new forms of social exclusion?" we investigate whether and how the potential benefits accruing from digital inclusion differ between higher- and lower-SES students, which are in part due to variations in home learning environment.

We analyze data from 28 developed countries and societies to examine differences in relationships between students' social class background, ICT usage, and well-being across countries. A clear advantage of cross-national research is that it can help us to see similarities and differences among countries included in our analyses, thereby helping us to know whether specific theoretical concepts and/or policy implications can be applied to different national and social settings. Large cross-national variations in ICT policies in education suggest that researchers and policymakers have much to learn from a comparative analysis of this topic. We focus on more affluent countries or societies where the development of ICT, internet infrastructure, and advanced forms of ICT are ubiquitous, which facilitate the integration of ICT into the learning process. Students in these countries/societies have more e-learning opportunities, both formally within a classroom and informally outside the school system. Despite high levels of ICT development in affluent countries, a digital divide both within and across those countries remains (see our research findings from Chaps. 4 to 7).

The digital divide in less-developed countries is qualitatively different from the digital divide in developed countries. However, developing and less-developed countries may soon experience similar benefits and challenges regarding ICT use in education. Although our analyses are based on empirical findings from data on developed countries, the policy implications derived in this study also may inform policy recommendations for developing and less-developed countries.

In short, in this book, we examine the connection between the digital divide and educational inequality—what we call the digital learning divide. We describe the patterns of social exclusion from technology and education, and discuss related social implications and policies concerned with the role of ICT in education.

1.1.2 The Digital Learning Divide as a Global Social Problem: The First Phase

At the turn of the twenty-first century, many believed that the digital divide would increasingly shrink and eventually disappear as ICT development and adoption became more widespread. But despite a surge in rates of internet acquisition, computer ownership, and smartphone use all over the world during the last decade (ITU, 2011, 2015, 2018), the digital divide has become more pronounced than before. Today, few will attempt to predict the end of digital inequality.

There are four phases of the digital learning divide. The first phase began in the 1990s, and the fourth began with the spread of COVID-19 in 2020. As shown in

Table 1.1 Four phases of the digital learning divide

<table>
<tr><th>Phase</th><th>Years</th><th>Role of ICT in education</th><th>Sources of the digital divide (research foci)</th></tr>
<tr><td>1</td><td>1990–early 2000</td><td>Many schools and homes did not have computers or internet access</td><td>• Inequality of digital access (1st level digital learning divide)</td></tr>
<tr><td>2</td><td>2000–2010</td><td>The adoption of ICT in schools and learning fields increased steadily, while the role of ICT in education remained questionable and debatable</td><td>• Inequality of digital use and digital skills (2nd level digital learning divide)
• Differential outcomes and benefits of educational technology (3rd level digital learning divide)</td></tr>
<tr><td>3</td><td>2010–early 2020</td><td>Most teachers and students adopted ICT; but believed that ICT should only play a supplementary role in the learning and teaching process</td><td rowspan="2">• The resurgence of inequality in digital access (1st level digital learning divide)
• Inequality of digital use and digital skills (2nd level digital learning divide)
• Differential outcomes and benefits of educational technology (3rd level digital learning divide)</td></tr>
<tr><td>4</td><td>2020–present</td><td>Due to the COVID-19 outbreak, the full integration of ICT and online networked technologies in educational settings became a requirement</td></tr>
</table>

Table 1.1, although these phases overlap, each phase is unique in how educators and students utilized digital technologies and their roles in the learning process.

The first phase of the digital learning divide emerged before the millennium, when scholars began to notice that even in developed societies, access to computers and the internet was highly restricted within most schools, and the availability of digital technology and internet access varied dramatically across households of different socioeconomic status (e.g., DeBell & Chapman, 2006; Wells & Lewis, 2006). Scholars focused then on disparities that are associated with sociodemographic characteristics (for instance, see DiMaggio et al., 2004). In this phase of the digital divide—the "first-level digital divide" (Attewell, 2001; Attewell & Battle, 1999; Davison & Cotten, 2003)—much attention was devoted to institutional educational policies and initiatives designed to expand internet access in schools, to increase ICT resources in classrooms, and to promote the rate of ICT adoption in households as much as possible (Culp et al., 2003; DiMaggio et al., 2001; Selwyn et al., 2001; Warschauer et al., 2004; Wells & Lewis, 2006). To achieve these goals, schools increased expenditures on new computer equipment, installed broadband internet infrastructure, and set up computer labs with an aim to enhance students' basic computer knowledge.

Also during this phase, many scholars and educators questioned whether ICT use in schools would yield the benefits for students and teachers that some claimed, and whether educational reforms might be more effective if resources were invested elsewhere. The extent to which technology enhanced students' learning experiences in different subjects, such as reading and math, was unclear. It also was not clear how e-learning could be best integrated into curriculum design. In addition, most classrooms were not designed for user-friendly access to classroom technology, and many teachers were not prepared to adopt ICT in their teaching due to their insufficient computer competency. Because online texts had not yet become widely available, students learned subjects mostly from printed materials. At most, ICT was used as a means to supplement education.

1.1.3 The Second Phase of the Digital Learning Divide

The second period of the divide entailed a different form of digital inequality—the "second-level digital divide" (Hargittai, 2002). The main argument relating to this form of inequality is that, even if equality of digital access could be fully achieved, digital learning inequalities would persist, which are associated with how people use computers, the types of online activities in which they participate, and the degree of ICT skills that they possess (Attewell, 2001; Hargittai & Hinnant, 2008; Natriello, 2001).

In this second phase, both the quality and quantity of e-learning opportunities increased steadily within and outside of schools in developed countries. Overall, learners and educators also increasingly relied on digital and online-networked devices. However, researchers noticed a stark division between students who frequently used ICT for learning and knowledge-seeking purposes versus those who mainly used ICT for non-academic activities, such as gaming and social networking (Hargittai & Hinnant, 2008). Researchers reported that students from affluent and highly educated families were more likely to use computers for educational purposes than students from socially disadvantaged backgrounds (Attewell, 2003; Leu et al., 2015). In relation to this finding, a debate emerged regarding whether existing or newly invented technologies provided beneficial or detrimental effects on academic learning. Critics suggested that underperforming students, especially those from socially disadvantaged families, tended to receive fewer benefits from e-learning. In this phase, ICT was used most often for remedial purposes, to help underperforming students meet course requirements and pass to the next grade (Banerjee et al., 2007; Natriello, 2001; Warschauer et al., 2004).

Witnessing these new developments in ICT uses and the new forms of digital inequality, scholars focused their research on this "third-level digital divide" (Mihelj et al., 2018; Scheerder et al., 2017; van Deursen et al., 2017). Unlike the first digital divide (mainly focused on digital access) and the second digital divide (mainly focused on digital literacy, skills, and usage of ICT for educational versus non-educational purposes), research on the third-level digital divide examined the effects of internet use and the benefits that may be derived from a more comprehensive use of digital technologies (Scheerder et al., 2019; van Deursen & van Dijk, 2019). Researchers argued that the digital divide is due to social inequality, and that it generates large and significant effects on student outcomes and deepens educational inequality across geographical regions and socioeconomic categories (Scheerder et al., 2017). In education, an important yet underexplored question is how students obtain (or not) the benefits from e-learning, and whether the benefits of digital inclusion may differ across students from various social, economic, and demographic backgrounds.

1.1.4 The Third Phase of the Digital Learning Divide

The third phase emerged in the mid of 2010s. During this period, many countries and educational institutes set clear goals to enhance the next generations' e-literacy and integration of ICT in education (Eickelmann, 2018; United Nations Educational, Scientific and Cultural Organization Institute for Statistics [UNESCO-UIS], 2014, 2016). From 2010 to 2020, the number of teachers who adopted ICT for use in lectures skyrocketed. Many teachers regularly used PowerPoint and smartboards in their presentations in the classroom, integrated online platforms to monitor student progress, created internet discussion forums to encourage student interactions, and played video clips to stimulate students' learning interests. Many assignments required students to use a computer, work online, and/or submit assignments electronically, and students also frequently prepared PowerPoint slides to present their work across a wide range of subjects, including reading, the sciences, social studies, and the arts. Both in school and at home, many students became accustomed to using the internet to search for information related to their school learning activities or to deepen what they learned in class. During this period, online private tutoring services also mushroomed to meet some students' special needs (Choe, 2009; Park et al., 2016).

The digital learning divide in this phase was conceptualized as a multidimensional construct involving a complex set of inequalities relating to access, usage, skills, and literacy in digital technologies. The second-level and third-level digital divides in students' knowledge, skills, and usage of ICT for educational vs. non-educational activities continued. Simultaneously, inequality in access to digital technology—the first-level digital divide—now became more complex due to rapidly changing technologies, the availability of an even wider variety of new devices, and "the reality that not all of the materials provide the same online opportunities" (van Deursen & van Dijk, 2019, p. 355). IT companies continued to release new models of computers (e.g., laptops, e-tablets, and Smart TVs) and peripherals (e.g., scanners, printers, and smartphones) and found new ways to provide e-services, manage businesses, and make profits. E-service companies and computer software/apps began to charge subscription fees. Because not everyone could afford the monthly cost of high-speed broadband internet or upgrade digital appliances in the household, many lower-middle- and working-class families were forced to rely on lower speed internet and had to use less sophisticated or poorly functioning digital devices when surfing the internet (Gonzales et al., 2020; Rideout & Katz, 2016).

A report based on the 2016 Progress in International Reading Literacy Study (PIRLS) on fourth graders across countries suggested that students' reading achievement was associated with the availability of more digital devices at home (Mullis et al., 2017). The rates of students' access to high-speed internet and high levels of digital technologies at home varied across countries, even in the developed world. Around half of the students in Scandinavian countries lived in households with high-speed internet and a high level of digital devices (Denmark 49%, Finland 53%, and Norway 58%). Approximately one-third of the students from the Netherlands (32%), Australia (29%), Belgium (29%), and Canada (28%) had access to high-speed internet and various digital devices at home. The rates were relatively lower in other developed countries, such as Austria (17%), Germany (15%), Italy (14%), France (13%), and Taiwan (11%).

Using data from the 2013 American Community Survey, Pew Research Center reported that approximately 40% of low-income households with school-aged children did not have a high-speed internet connection at home. In contrast, less than 10% of high-income families did not have high-speed internet access (Horrigan, 2015).

More recently, in 2018 a survey conducted by Pew Research Center reported that 24% of American teens from lower-income households were unable to complete their homework due to the lack of a reliable computer or internet access, compared to only 9% of teens from higher-income households that reported the same problem. Nearly 25% of lower-income teenagers still did not have computer access at home and had to use public Wi-Fi to complete homework (Anderson & Perrin, 2018).

Using data from the 2018 Programme for International Student Assessment (PISA) survey to analyze digital access for 15-year-old students across the world, OECD reported that although more than 90% of students had internet access at home in most OECD nations, households differed in the speed of internet access and types of digital devices that were connected to the internet (computers vs. mobile phones) (OECD, 2019b). Some students used only mobile devices to access the internet at home because their families did not have a desktop or laptop computers to be used for educational purposes. Even among these more affluent nations, moreover, less than 70% of socioeconomically disadvantaged students had both a quiet place to study and at least a computer that can be used for schoolwork at home (OECD, 2019a).

More than ever before, students in developed societies rely on digital access outside of schools as the primary means of learning ICT skills and digital literacy (van Dijk & van Deursen, 2014). However, students who are socioeconomically disadvantaged are more likely to rely on cheap, less sophisticated, or low-end digital devices to access resources via the internet than socially advantaged students (Gonzales et al., 2020). Even in the developed world, low-SES students are experiencing a digital learning crisis. The problem only got worse during the coronavirus pandemic.

1.1.5 *The Fourth Phase: The Digital Learning Divide Since the COVID-19*

The global coronavirus pandemic marked the fourth phase of the digital learning divide. Before the outbreak, remote/online classes were offered only to a small group of students who had special needs or lived far from their schools. Most teachers had never received formal training for online teaching (Ellis, 2020; Yu, 2020) and felt uncomfortable or awkward recording their own voices on computers, let alone virtually interacting with learners. Teachers in primary and secondary education had even less experience teaching online courses, compared to teachers in higher education. Many of them had only used online materials to supplement their teaching in physical classrooms. Until the COVID-19 pandemic, courses had never been moved entirely online (OECD, 2020a).

The COVID-19 pandemic forced schools to move classes online. With little to no formal training, teachers had to learn to teach online classes "on the job" and learned through trial and error. By April 2020—a month after the coronavirus pandemic began—188 countries had reported school closures due to the need to maintain physical distancing; this affected over 1.5 billion students and 60 million teachers worldwide (UNESCO-UIS, 2020). A few months later, some governments attempted to re-open campuses and allow students to return to schools. But though school administrations expended great effort to clean their campuses, to adequately space the distances between students, and to implement many policies to keep faculty and students safe, the risk of spreading the infection was still too high. Many schools closed again due to a resurgence of coronavirus cases.

It is difficult to overstate the impact of COVID-19. In education, the global crisis has led to many adverse consequences. For example, schools have been forced to close, at least two-thirds of students across the globe subsequently have been unable to return to their classrooms (UNESCO, 2020b), traditional schooling has been replaced by e-learning and remote education, and working parents who are struggling with low income and job losses have felt worn out by their required effort to facilitate distance learning and home-schooling for their children who also struggle to keep up with their schoolwork (UNESCO, 2020a).

COVID-19 has worsened the problem of the digital learning divides in digital access (the first-level digital divide), in the skills, literacy, and usage of ICT (the second-level digital divide), and the effects of ICT use (the third-level digital divide). Without a doubt, COVID-19 has severely challenged current information and communication technologies (UN's Committee for the Coordination of Statistical Activities [CCSA], 2020). The crises faced by less-developed countries and poor societies during the pandemic are huge: political instability, social unrest, economic downturns, and shortages of basics (including food, healthcare, and energy) (CCSA, 2020; United Nations Conference on Trade and Development [UNCTAD], 2020). Families in many poor villages lack basic internet infrastructure. Their children do not have a desk at which to study or any access to technology at home (Iivari et al., 2020; Li & Lalani, 2020). These difficult conditions explain why more than two-thirds of low-income countries and approximately one-third of mid-income countries cannot provide any type of remote learning platforms to students and are unable to continue basic education for their children (Vegas, 2020). In Nigeria, some teachers are using radio stations to deliver lessons to teach youngsters. In remote areas of Uganda, teachers have asked the local government to make public announcements so that students know they can stop by their teacher's house to pick up learning packets (OECD Education & Skills TopClass Podcast, 2020). In Peru, students without internet access use televisions and radios to participate in school activities (Teacher Task Force, 2020).

COVID-19 also has negatively affected affluent/developed countries, which have faced a number of crises. However, developed countries are able to mobilize and integrate more resources to make fully remote education possible (NSW, 2020b; OECD, 2020a). Despite school lockdowns, nearly 90% of developed countries have continued to offer basic education by adopting different forms of online platforms (Vegas, 2020). This is due to their provision of online educational opportunities offered by schools and supported by governments. In Finland (Iivari et al., 2020), New South Wales, Australia (NSW, 2020a), and South Korea (Bicker, 2020), the governments either have helped to pay internet bills for low-income families or have loaned them digital devices, such as laptops and e-tablets, so that needy students can continue their education at home. For developed countries, the major remaining issues are the quality of e-instruction and whether parents and children can quickly adjust to the new, online learning styles that are quite different from the past.

This said, developed countries are not exempt from digital inequalities in access and usage of online education, which can affect the quality of education and also deepen the existing educational inequality between socially advantaged and disadvantaged students. Puckett and Rafalow (2020) highlighted three questions that should be addressed amidst the pandemic. First, how robust is the technological infrastructure? Even in developed countries, a significant proportion of under-resourced students still lack internet access at home. Second, how prepared are educators and students for online education? It is likely that many schools are not well prepared for remote education, especially low-performing schools and those with large numbers of low-income and racial minority students. Compared to their more affluent peers, students from low-income families are less likely to seek help or receive proper assistance with technology issues at home. Third, a critical question is how students might be unequally rewarded for ICT usage. Even if students have the requisite digital skills, it is likely that teachers will reward and evaluate their performance differently, depending on their social class and racial backgrounds. As a result, the full adoption of online e-learning platforms may exacerbate the already existent educational inequality.

Several reports have provided evidence of adverse effects from online/virtual education during the pandemic. In South Korea, where digital technologies are relatively advanced, more than 200,000 students reported not having the needed ICT access to engage in online education during school lockdowns (Bicker, 2020). In the Netherlands, the cancellation of central exams at the end of primary education potentially might increase inequality, because without further intervention many students from immigrant families and families of lower parental educational attainment will miss advice concerning their decisions about secondary education (CPB Economic Policy Analysis, 2020). In France and Norway, the absence of traditional schooling is associated with school disengagement and low educational aspirations among underprivileged students (OECD, 2020b). A recent survey of 330 educators and school personnel across 98 countries reported that approximately 87% of the respondents were worried about technological infrastructure for online education during the pandemic. The respondents were also concerned that parents or guardians might not be available at home to support children's learning during the pandemic (Reimers & Schleicher, 2020).

The use of online/virtual schooling to replace traditional classrooms is likely to make the family's role in educational inequality even more significant. A South Korean teacher stated that, "For many low-income, single-parent, or grandparent families, the biggest concern is about having to leave their children at home when they have to go to work. We try to help these families by either calling the children by phone to check up on them or by checking in by sending these food packages, and asking if they need any help" (Bicker, 2020). A new "digital homework divide" along the lines of family income and social class has emerged during the coronavirus outbreak. In Finland, scholars found that some parents are able to take an active role in supporting their children's education at home, whereas others clearly have difficulties assisting their children due to the lack of time or well-equipped devices at home (Iivari et al., 2020). Pew Research Center (2020) reported that less than 10% of higher-income parents in the United States and approximately 40% of lower-income parents face digital obstacles when trying to help with children's assignments (Vogels et al., 2020). Like other parents, lower-income parents try to provide more home resources to support their children's education, while they are forced to work excessively long hours, or are laid off or furloughed. But a higher percentage of low-income parents than high-income parents (41% versus 17%) are worried about the possibility that their children may fall behind in education during school lockdowns caused by the pandemic (Horowitz, 2020). The digital homework divide may be more serious, with greater negative impacts on learning amidst the COVID-19 outbreak, even in the most affluent countries and societies.

1.2 Social and Policy Context Among More Affluent Countries

1.2.1 The Digital Natives

> *Digital Natives will move markets and transform industries, education, and global politics. The changes they bring about as they move into the workforce could have an immensely positive effect on the world we live in. By and large, the digital revolution has already made this world a better place. And Digital Natives have every chance of propelling society further forward in myriad ways—if we let them.*
>
> *But make no mistake: We are at a crossroads. There are two possible paths before us—one in which we destroy what is great about the Internet and about how young people use it, and one in which we make smart choices and head toward a bright future in a digital age.* (Palfrey & Gasser, 2008, p. 7)

Scholars and media commentators often use the term "digital natives" to describe the new generation of children, adolescents, and young adults who were born after 1990 and grew up in an environment that is full of digital devices and online information (Prensky, 2001). Digital natives learn how to use ICT at a very young age, and "think and process information fundamentally differently from their predecessors…[and] are all 'native speakers' of the digital language of computers, video games and the Internet" (Prensky, 2001, p. 1). They live much of their lives online—playing, maintaining social contacts, searching for information, and learning. Because of their early and high exposure to technology, they may interact with and respond to digital devices more comfortably than do people of older generations. To meet the unique learning needs of digital natives, scholars suggest curriculum designs that include digital tools which can respond immediately and interactively with the spontaneous and exploratory learning style of modern students (Bradbrook et al., 2008; Cheung & Slavin, 2013; Jaggars & Xu, 2016; Mullis et al., 2017; van Dijk & van Deursen, 2014). **Because it is difficult, if not impossible, to separate ICT use and** digital natives, policymakers and educators must consider how ICT use may affect students' learning, social, and psychological outcomes.

The theory of "digital natives" is no more than that—a theory. The concept assumes that children who were born and grew up in a digital environment are natural at using digital devices and masterful in online information searches. But the extent to which this assumption holds true has yet to be tested (Bennett et al., 2008; Dolan, 2016). Moreover, we also know little about the ways digital natives learn ICT and digital skills. Do all digital natives learn the same digital and ICT skills? If the answer is somewhat uncertain, then we should also investigate factors that may affect the digital skills and knowledge that digital natives possess.

At the international level, whether a student lives in a developed or less-developed country or society may affect the student's chance of growing up as a "digital native." **Obviously, digital technology is more ubiquitous in affluent societies, whereas many** low-income and developing countries lag behind in basic internet infrastructure and more advanced forms of ICT. As a result, a larger number of young people in affluent countries benefit from more e-resources and digital learning opportunities. Both homes and schools in affluent countries play a pivotal role (Attewell, 2001; Kim, 2011; van Dijk & van Deursen, 2014) by promoting basic ICT literacy, implementing ICT curricula, and distributing e-learning resources to students. With the support of private and public ICT investments and government educational expenditure (Eickelmann, 2018; Ottestad & Gudmundsdottir, 2018; Starkey & Finger, 2018), schools in affluent countries strive to build a foundation of ICT skills and knowledge for the upcoming generation, with a hope that this training will reduce the difference in students' ability to use the internet outside of schools (Erichsen & Salajan, 2014). To the extent that ICT more deeply penetrates individual homes in affluent countries compared to lower-income countries, this also may allow the affluent countries to reduce educational inequalities associated with family background by providing access to e-learning materials for disadvantaged students, or by offering online remedial programs. Therefore, in addition to the economic benefits that ICT may contribute to societies and the convenience it may provide for our daily lives, ICT education could potentially become a model for the educational system in modern times. Analyses of ICT usage by youths for education in developed countries may yield important policy implications for both developed and less-developed countries at present and in the very near future.

1.2.2 Two Remaining Concerns

Two concerns arise from the above portrayal of ICT education in economically more developed countries. The first concern is that, within the most affluent part of the world, both social and digital inequalities between students of different backgrounds may remain pronounced (Dolan, 2016; Rafalow, 2018; Selwyn et al., 2009; Warschauer, 2016). Regarding social inequalities, a general consensus among researchers of education and social stratification is that public education can teach basic digital skills and knowledge to both advantaged and disadvantaged students to partially equalize the inequality resulting from family resource differences. But as social inequality increases in a given society, the equalizing role played by schools might be compromised by disparities in family resources, which may result in inequalities of ultimate educational attainments for underprivileged students (Buchmann & Hannum, 2001; Hannum & Buchmann, 2005). A similar and related causal mechanism may extend to digital inequality between families (Leu et al., 2015; Scheerder et al., 2019; Yuen et al., 2018). Despite high levels of educational expenditures and ICT investments in affluent countries, and though ICT infrastructure and public e-resources are a lesser problem, family may still be a source of inequality in digital learning. Following this line of argument, we may speculate that digital learning inequality potentially might be amplified in affluent countries when digital learning techniques further mature and reliance on ICT increases. The growing disparity that derives from wider and deeper reliance on digital learning may in turn affect student outcomes and thus widen existing educational inequality in affluent countries. This problem currently may not apply to less-developed countries, where ICT education is hindered by overall poor internet infrastructure and low levels of ICT investments (Beuermann et al., 2013; Ma et al., 2019; Ragnedda & Muschert, 2013). However, as ICT continues to develop and the digital divide in these countries begins to move from the aforementioned first to the second and then the third phases, the experiences recorded and studied in developed countries may help with policymaking in the lesser-developed countries as well (i.e., they may benefit from observing the first steps of other countries, to find successful policy pathways for maximizing digital learning attainments and minimizing their own digital divides). We further illustrate more recent patterns and trends of digital learning inequalities among the selected developed countries in Chap. 7.

The second concern is that, though previous scholars have extensively explored adolescents' experiences with technology and their outcomes of ICT use (Agasisti et al., 2020; OECD, 2011; van der Schuur et al., 2020; Vigdor et al., 2014), research findings to date are mixed. As a result, the extent to which digital technologies affect students' academic achievement and well-being is still less than clear. Some studies report a positive association between ICT adoption and academic performance (e.g., Attewell & Battle, 1999; Fairlie et al., 2010), while others suggest that the relationship between ICT usage and educational outcomes is nonexistent (e.g., Fairlie & Robinson, 2013; Hunley et al., 2005) or even negative (e.g., Agasisti et al., 2020; Vigdor et al., 2014). Beyond speculations about the research designs and factors that may contextualize these findings, the starkly different research findings also lead to a fundamental question: Is the use of digital technology harmful or beneficial to adolescents' academic achievement and well-being? And what clear evidence do we have for seeing emerging digital technology as an important factor in contributing to the well-being of youth, in particular their performance in learning? We further address these issues in Chaps. 4–6.

Equally important, as remote teaching through ICT was never fully substituted for physical classrooms before COVID-19, research studies before 2020 mostly assessed the effects of digital learning on student outcomes when used as a supplementary tool in the physical classroom environment and in traditional curriculum designs. For the most part, although there has been limited research on the relationship between distance learning and students' achievement and well-being during the COVID-19 pandemic, it is highly speculated that there have been notable adverse effects of full remote teaching on the students' achievement outcomes and psychological well-being. These results suggest that digital learning cannot fully replace physical classrooms and in-person school environments. They also raise the questions regarding how educators may better use digital learning aids to improve student outcomes and how curriculum designs may be successfully balanced between in-person instruction and digital learning. Policymakers must carefully consider effective ICT investments and educational expenditures to maximize the benefits of digital learning and minimize its negative effects, such as how the increased use of e-learning in school and at home exacerbates (but does not reduces) educational inequality.

Answers to these questions are the focus of this book. In searching the literature for these questions, we have found that many previous studies examine ICT uses in education based on data from a single country. Understandably, early analyses (e.g., DeBell & Chapman, 2006; UNESCO-UIS, 2014; Wells & Lewis, 2006) also tend to rely on extensive descriptive statistics to describe levels of adopted ICT in pedagogical and curriculum designs, in classrooms, and for students' homework. Other studies consider the effects of ICT usage or online activities on student well-being (e.g., Angrist & Lavy, 2002; Biagi & Loi, 2013; Hassoun, 2015), but they typically focus on one type of ICT and limited measures of student outcomes. Together, these limitations may explain why previous studies find different and sometimes contradictory results. The fact that many studies focus on a single country or society additionally highlights the importance of national contexts, but this also suggests that, at some point, researchers must consider a more global perspective.

To partially fill these gaps, this book takes an international, comparative approach for the examination of ICT usage and its effects in different countries. The world is becoming more globalized every day. ICT further shortens the distance between individuals, both within and across countries. A global perspective allows us to look at interrelations between ICT usage in different countries, various educational policies about e-learning, and their effects on student outcomes. Our analyses incorporate a wide range of developed countries that are economically more developed and highly industrialized, in order to more precisely examine the country-specific versus more general patterns of causes and effects of ICT usage among teenagers. We also take a multidimensional perspective by examining how different forms of ICT usage and online activities affect adolescent well-being, including their academic, behavioral, and psychological outcomes. By doing so, we hope to better understand ways in which ICT usage influences learning, identify problems associated with digital exclusion, and explore solutions to bridge digital learning gaps. This may provide policymakers and future researchers with better insights regarding the roles of ICT in education.

1.2.3 The Social Landscape of More Affluent Societies

Before we further elaborate on the goals and the research framework of this study, we wish to provide readers with some general background information about the social, technological, and policy contexts of the focal affluent countries. This allows us to understand how national contexts and institutional arrangements shape young people's attitudes and values concerning ICT and their readiness to participate in ICT activities for educational purposes.

Compared to less-developed countries, young people in developed countries have more opportunities to access a wide range of ICT resources, both in and outside of school. In developed countries, nearly universal, fixed broadband internet connectivity is common. In less-developed countries, it is difficult to obtain the same digital access in all locations (in some cases because the electricity supply is unreliable). The higher the national income level, the faster the rate of technology diffusion (Cruz-Jesus et al., 2017). As national wealth increases, average life quality improves.

Individuals spend a smaller proportion of their income on necessities, such as food, shelter, and clothing. This allows people in affluent countries to allocate more money to buy luxury goods, including newer models of digital products. Because of higher standards in different areas of social life, including recreation, work, health, and most important to our study, education, developed countries also face higher pressure to expand public and private investments in digitally networked technology and infrastructure (Robison & Crenshaw, 2010). Overall, developed countries have higher rates of internet penetration and computer ownership in private households (Chinn & Fairlie, 2010; Cruz-Jesus et al., 2017; Hilbert, 2016; ITU, 2018; Norris, 2001).

Differences in ICT infrastructure between more- and less-developed countries affect adolescents' digital educational resources on several levels. On the institutional level, advanced, digitally networked technology and infrastructure enable affluent countries to establish wired schools, e-learning centers, and digitalized libraries (Cruz-Jesus et al., 2017; Norris, 2001; van Dijk & van Deursen, 2014). Less-developed countries often face multiple barriers in their attempt to provide e-learning opportunities for students due to the lack of widespread digital infrastructure and unbalanced technological progress. As a result, in less-developed countries, comprehensive adoption of ICT is often exclusively for the wealthy and socially privileged, and a substantial proportion of students have limited or no digital access (Beuermann et al., 2013; Malamud & Pop-Eleches, 2011; Ragnedda & Muschert, 2013). In contrast, a larger proportion of students in developed countries have little to no problem with digital access. They have more opportunities to learn a variety of ICT appliances, benefit from e-services, and access free and/or high-speed internet in public areas, such as schools, open-to-public campuses, libraries, and public transportation stations.

Affluent countries have multiple options to deploy digital learning resources in school: computers, interactive whiteboards, LED projectors, computer stations in school libraries, and laptops or portable digital tablets that teachers can conveniently use anywhere in school (UNESCO-UIS, 2014). Less-developed countries not only have a higher student-to-computer ratio but are also more likely to rely on a few computer laboratories for ICT instruction. Sometimes, most computers are used only for administrator purposes but not for teaching. In contrast, schools in affluent countries tend to allocate a high proportion of computers to pedagogy. Instead of traditional computer laboratories, many schools provide multifunctional ICT support services to support the effective use of computers and other digital appliances by teachers and students in classrooms.

Children in developed countries are more likely to grow up as "digital natives" than children in less-developed countries (UNESCO-UIS, 2015). They begin to use computers early, are more likely to use computers for educational purposes, and can access e-learning resources from a diverse set of digital devices (Plowman, 2015). In the United Kingdom, for example, more than one out of three children below five years old use mobile phones and touch screens to access apps and play games. Approximately 30% of children in the same age group have their e-tablets (Marsh et al., 2015). While the majority of primary school children in New Zealand (93%), the

Netherlands (87%), and Sweden (83%) use computers in reading lessons, only 12% of primary school children in Trinidad and Tobago, 8% of primary school children in South Africa, and 6% of primary school children in Morocco use computers in reading courses (Mullis et al., 2017). The IEA (International Association for the Evaluation of Educational Achievement) reports that more than 40% of fourth-grade students in Scandinavian countries have seven or more ICT devices that can be used for reading and academic learning at home, compared to considerably lower proportions of fourth-grade students in many less-developed countries, who have no computer or internet access at all in their homes, such as Morocco (47%), Azerbaijan (34%), South Africa (33%), Egypt (30%), and Iran (23%) (Mullis et al., 2017).

Most importantly, differences in ICT infrastructure may lead to divergent educational paradigms and pedagogical practices. Drori (2006, 2010) suggests that because developed countries have greater ICT innovation capacity than developing and less-developed countries, their software developers, educators, and researchers can design more educational apps and distribute their use through a wide range of online networked platforms. Often, these e-learning tools and materials are protected by intellectual property rights and blocked by IP address. These protections make it difficult for students and teachers in the developing and impoverished regions of the world to access the resources. Educational innovations are often piloted in developed countries to help the next generation keep up with new technological developments. As Heyneman and Loxley (1983) suggest, "the areas of the world with comparatively large amounts of research and development capital tend also to be the areas where educational paradigms are invented" (pp. 1183–1184). ICT access and capacity allow developed countries to initiate experiments and research projects to test existing and a new learning and instructional methods. Over time, the digital divide becomes intertwined with the innovation divide, which separates the social progress of the world's technology laggards and leaders, and affects the well-being of those living in these societies (Drori, 2010; Ma et al., 2019).

1.2.4 The Policy Landscape of More Affluent Societies

Several developed countries have a long history of formal policies to promote the application of technologies in education and the spread of e-learning (Erichsen & Salajan, 2014; U.S. Department of Education, 1996). The earliest ICT learning policy can be traced to the 1983 federal report, *A Nation at Risk*, in the United States, which regarded basic computer skills as one of the "Five New Basics" that should be covered in public schools (National Commission on Excellence in Education, 1983). 10 years later, in 1993–94, the European Union (EU) released the Bangemann report, which recommended that governments "extend advanced distance learning techniques into schools and colleges" (European Commission, 1994). In another report in 1995, *Teaching and Learning: Towards the Learning Society*, the EU further outlined the forces that propel countries to raise digitally literate populations:

> *Three major, profound and wide-ranging factors of upheaval have emerged, however, which have transformed the context of economic activity and the way our societies function in a radical and lasting manner, namely: the onset of the information society; the impact of the scientific and technological world; and the internationalisation of the economy. These events are contributing towards the development of the learning society.* (European Commission, 1995, p. 5)

As more countries and societies seek to compete in the knowledge economy (Dale, 2005; Powell & Snellman, 2004), the quantity and urgency of national-level and international-level efforts to promote ICT use in education have also increased considerably across the globe, particularly since the turn of the millennium. In 2000, two international reports were released, respectively, by the United Nations and UNESCO. Although the reports do not list concrete objectives and specific goals of ICT usage in education, both include statements about how to integrate ICT in educational settings. The Millennium Development Goals (MDGs) state that all participant countries and leading development institutions, "in cooperation with the private sector, make available the benefits of new technologies, especially information and communications" (United Nations, 2000). Another report, *The Dakar Framework for Action, Education for All*, also recommends that future educators "harness new information and communication technologies to help achieve [these] EFA goals," such as by improving all aspects of the quality of education and ensuring the excellence of learners (UNESCO, 2000, p. 9). In 2003 and 2005, the World Summit on the Information Society (WSIS) recommended that governments should "connect all secondary schools and primary schools with ICT" and "adapt all primary and secondary school curricula to meet the challenges of the information society, taking into account national circumstances" (Partnership on Measuring ICT for Development, 2011).

To date, most developed countries and societies have developed a long-standing, sector-wide plan for the adoption of ICT in education. Many have a nationwide regulatory body or institution to monitor the progress of ICT integration, and some also make formal recommendations to integrate ICT across all subjects and educational levels. These policies allow students to have more time and opportunities to use ICT for learning a variety of subjects (UNESCO-UIS, 2014). Although there are increasing commitments and government efforts to incorporate ICT in schools and education in less-developed countries, their efforts are often limited by a lack of resources and basic ICT infrastructure (Drori, 2006; UNESCO-UIS, 2015). It is also important to note that more- and less-developed countries tend to have different agendas in ICT policies for education. The ICT policies of less-developed countries prioritize poverty alleviation, such as by using ICT to improve teachers' teaching competencies and students' learning in core academic subjects, whereas the policies of developed countries tend to focus on innovations, such as the acquisition of advanced knowledge and knowledge creation (Yuen & Hew, 2018).

Moving forward, scholars suggest that at least three goals should be considered in policy agendas (Moonen, 2008; Yuen & Hew, 2018). First, schools should provide opportunities for students to learn digital literacy and ICT skills, and they should support ICT use in classroom teaching on a daily basis. Second, governments should implement policies that help to build informal support systems between school teachers, so that they can work together and help each other to enhance ICT knowledge and skills. Finally, governments should provide free and/or high-speed internet access to students, both in and outside of schools (including in homes, libraries, and sports facilities). UNESCO-UIS (2014) suggests that policymakers and educators consider both computer-assisted instruction (e.g., the use of computers to present instructional materials and to perform tasks for learning) and internet-assisted instruction (e.g., the use of the internet for pedagogical purposes) in their ICT implementation. In light of these policy guidelines, we discuss the implications of our empirical findings to offer evidence-based policy recommendations. We suggest that policymakers and practitioners assume active leadership roles in addressing challenges and obstacles in the implementation of technology for education. Educators and policymakers also should ensure that ICT benefits all students, across different backgrounds, and have plans to prevent any negative effects of new technologies. Strategic policies can provide a vision for the next generation regarding how educational systems may motivate, coordinate different layers of effort, and set clear goals for the integration of ICT in future curriculum designs (Kozma, 2008; Yuen & Hew, 2018).

1.3 Aim of the Book

1.3.1 Analyzing Data and Countries

Our analyses focus on secondary school students across 28 developed countries and societies in different geographical regions: (1) North America (America and Canada), (2) West and South Europe (Austria, Belgium, Britain, France, Germany, Ireland, Italy, Luxembourg, the Netherlands, Portugal, Spain, and Switzerland), (3) Scandinavia (Denmark, Finland, Iceland, Norway, and Sweden), (4) Pacific (Australia and New Zealand), and (5) Asia (China-Eastern Coast cities, Hong Kong, Japan, South Korea, Macao, Singapore, and Taiwan). Table 1.2 lists the countries and societies that are considered in our analyses. But among these 28 analyzing countries, six (i.e., Canada, Germany, the Netherlands, Portugal, Norway, and China) of them are excluded from many results that we present in our empirical chapters. This is because the use of key independent variables or dependent variables is not available, and therefore missing, from these countries. Secondary school students are ideal for the study of the causes and effects of ICT use in education. Because many students in this age group are raised in an environment that provides ready access to digital devices and online information flow, most directly experience the results of ICT policy implementation in education. They also represent the young population that will soon transition to tertiary education and/or the labor market.

Table 1.2 List of countries and societies that are considered in the analyses

North America	West and South Europe	Scandinavia	Pacific	Asia
America	Austria	Denmark	Australia	China[a]
Canada[a]	Belgium	Finland	NewZealand	HongKong
	Britain	Iceland		Macao
	France	Norway[a]		Japan
	Germany[a]	Sweden		Korea
	Ireland			Singapore
	Italy			Taiwan
	Luxembourg			
	Netherlands[a]			
	Portugal[a]			
	Spain			
	Switzerland			

[a]Because some of the key analyzing variables are not available from the data, results from these countries are only presented in Chap. 7

Our analyses focus on data from the 2018 wave of the Programme for International Student Assessment (PISA) survey, collected by the Organization of Economic Cooperation and Development (OECD). PISA is repeated triennially and is a nationally representative survey that collects information about ICT user experiences, problem-solving skills, and the learning performance of 15-year-old students, regardless of their grade levels. While the original PISA data included over 70 countries and societies across a wide range of economic development levels, we restricted our analyses to 28 countries and societies representing the most affluent and technologically advanced parts of the world. PISA is uniquely suited to our research objectives, because it evaluates outcomes of learning rather than outcomes of schooling—i.e., the general skills and competencies that 15-year-old students have learned, both inside and outside of the classroom throughout their lives rather than only in a specific school grade (Werfhorst & Mijs, 2010, p. 412). Equally Important, PISA's learning assessments include a variety of questions related to the students' online behaviors, familiarity with digital technology, and ICT accessibility within and outside of school. Finally, it is worth noting that the timing of the data collection of the 2018 PISA coincides with a period of increasing reliance on the internet and use of ICT in education.

1.3.2 Two Research Questions

This study presents both empirical analyses and policy explorations. An important focus is the influence of ICT usage on secondary school students. The research literature on the digital divide helps us to examine how the use of digital technology generates or regenerates forms of educational inequality that may further widen the academic learning gap between students of different sociodemographic backgrounds. We have two overarching research questions:

Question 1: How does the use of digital technology influence the well-being of secondary students, such as their educational performance, attitudes of learning, psychological health, and digital competence?

Question 2: Who is being excluded from digital learning, and in what ways? More specifically, how large are the socioeconomic gaps in digital access and ICT use?

Regarding the first question, we note that a large body of empirical research, while insightful, has provided inconclusive and mixed results about the relationship of adolescent ICT usage and well-being. For example, some scholars suggest that ICT usage positively predicts academic outcomes (for instance, see Attewell et al., 2003; Jackson et al., 2006); other researchers contend that the longer students use digital technologies, the more harmful these become to their learning process (for instance, see van der Schuur et al., 2020; Vigdor et al., 2014); still others find no apparent relationship so far between technology usage and educational outcomes (for instance, see Goolsbee & Guryan, 2006; Hunley et al., 2005). These inconsistent findings may be attributable to foci on different populations and/or uses of different variables to measure students' digital inclusion. The findings, conclusions, and explanations of how ICT influences the lives of adolescents therefore must be contextualized with the specific research design and selection of variables and samples in each study.

1.3.3 The Four Dimensions of Digital Inclusion

To build upon the research literature on this topic, we adopt a more holistic perspective and consider the following analytical approaches: We conceptualize students' ICT usage and online activities as a multidimensional construct and operationalize the concepts in a more diverse set of measures. This helps us to better understand why previous studies have found positive effects, negative effects, or no effects on students' engagement with digital technology. There are various forms of digital inclusion (Bradbrook et al., 2008). We identify at least four basic dimensions of digital inclusion that may affect students in different ways, which include:

Dimension One: Digital access to both basic and highly-functional devices.

Dimension Two: Digital uses for multitasking (e.g., using social networking sites, watching films, and gaming).

Dimension Three: E-learning or ICT use for educational purposes (e.g., the use of ICT to complete schoolwork and the engagement of e-learning platforms).

Dimension Four: Digital competence (e.g., basic computer knowledge, online literacy, and ICT-related skills).

1.3.4 The Conceptual Framework and the Organization of the Book

In order to address the first research questions, we review related literature in Chap. 2 and argue that a large body of research on the relationship between ICT and learning-related outcomes fails to distinguish the aforementioned different dimensions of ICT inclusion. To further understand how digital inclusion affects students, we analyze four outcomes: (1) academic performance, (2) learning attitudes, (3) psychological well-being, and (4) digital competence. In this book, we center on how ICT use for general schoolwork (i.e., the third dimension as indicated above) may influence these outcomes, though we believe that future scholars and educators should also elaborate and examine other dimensions of digital inclusion when they seek to know whether (and in what conditions) ICT has a positive or negative effect on students.

In addition, a long-standing debate in the social sciences concerns the role that family plays in the reproduction of educational inequality. Many studies on education and stratification suggest that in developed countries, families may occupy a more important role than schools in shaping students' learning processes and future occupational outcomes (for instance, see Lucas, 2001; Raftery & Hout, 1993). Other researchers contend that the use of ICT in schools is mainly helpful to students who are either socioeconomically underprivileged or academically underperforming. To some extent, this may help underprivileged students to reduce their educational disadvantages (Jackson et al., 2006). Still others suggest that the use of digital technology in school environment does not reduce but further aggravates social class inequality. In Chap. 3, we more formally discuss related literature, with a focus on the socioeconomic digital divide in adolescent student outcomes.

To integrate these different arguments as well as to address our first research question, we hypothesize that adolescents' experiences of ICT usage may vary by their socioeconomic background and also may depend on where they use ICT. We assess whether the relationship between ICT usage and well-being is contingent on students' usage of digital technology at school or at home. To highlight the difference between high-SES *versus* low-SES students, we also test whether the potential benefits accrued from digital involvement vary along socioeconomic lines. Figure 1.1 presents the conceptual framework of the research.

In the later part of the book, we show empirical analyses on the effects of the digital divide on adolescent well-being (i.e., the third-level digital divide): Chap. 4 focuses on students' academic performance, Chap. 5 assesses their learning attitudes, and Chap. 6 focuses on both their psychological well-being and digital competence.

Our second research question, *who is being excluded from digital learning and in what ways*, builds upon a large body of research literature on the digital divide (for instance, see Goedhart et al., 2019; Goode, 2010; Ma et al., 2019; Scheerder et al., 2019). For this research question, we are still interested in the digital divide defined by students' sociodemographic characteristics—in particular, family's SES *within* a country or society. We review evidence from literature on the digital divide

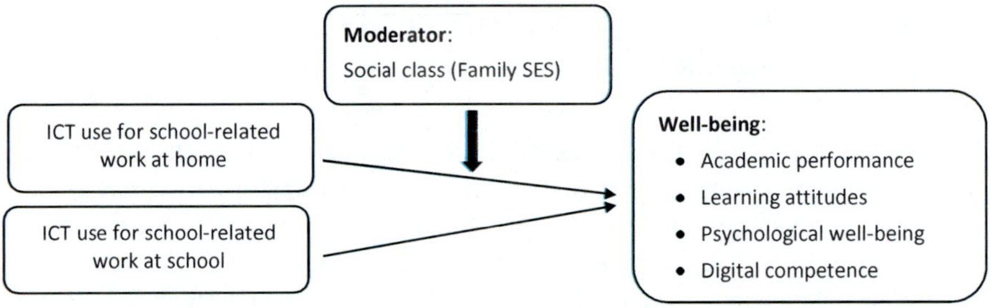

Fig. 1.1 A conceptual framework for examining the socioeconomic digital divide in adolescent student outcomes

in Chap. 3. And in Chap. 7, we show empirical analyses pertaining to the size of the first-level (e.g., differences in digital access) and second-level (e.g., variations in digital use and digital use) digital divides.

Finally, as noted, this is also a book about ICT policies and the well-being of secondary school students. In the final chapter (Chap. 8), we highlight several important policies that have been formalized and the efforts that have been made in more developed countries. Taking a comparative perspective, we also extend the discussion to identify whether and how the patterns of digital inequality may differ across cultural and geographical regions (e.g., Scandinavian countries vs. West European countries).

1.4 Summary and Conclusion

Despite the spread of ICT in education over the past few decades, a digital divide persists. The impact of this digital divide on children's education was intensified when governments were forced to shut down schools and move education online in response to the COVID-19 outbreak. In this chapter, we review the four phases of the digital learning divide from the early 1990s to the 2020s and outline the social and policy landscapes of ICT use in education in developed societies. This review provides a background for our analyses of the causes and influences of digital inclusion and exclusion among secondary school students. As soon will be discussed in the following chapters, targeted investments and ICT policymaking from the governments can effectively reduce digital inequality, improve students' learning experiences and academic achievement, and thus promote their well-being.

References

Agasisti, T., Gil-Izquierdo, M., & Han, S. W. (2020). ICT use at home for school-related tasks: What is the effect on a student's achievement? Empirical evidence from OECD PISA data. *Education Economics, 28*(6), 601–620. https://doi.org/10.1080/09645292.2020.1822787

Anderson, M., & Perrin, A. (2018, October 26). *Nearly one-in-five teens can't always finish their homework because of the digital divide.* Pew Research Center. https://www.pewresearch.org/fact-tank/2018/10/26/nearly-one-in-five-teens-cant-always-finish-their-homework-because-of-the-digital-divide/

Angrist, J., & Lavy, V. (2002). New evidence on classroom computers and pupil learning. *The Economic Journal, 112*(482), 735–765.

Attewell, P. A. (2001). The first and second digital divides. *Sociology of Education, 74*(3), 252–259.

Attewell, P. A. (2003). Beyond the digital divide. In P. A. Attewell & N. M. Seel (Eds.), *Disadvantaged teens and computer technologies* (pp. 15–34). Waxmann.

Attewell, P. A., & Battle, J. (1999). Home computers and school performance. *The Information Society, 15*(1), 1–10.

Attewell, P. A., Suazo-Garcia, B., & Battle, J. (2003). Computers and young children: Social benefit or social problem? *Social Forces, 82*(1), 277–296. https://doi.org/10.1353/sof.2003.0075

Banerjee, A. V., Cole, S., Duflo, E., & Linden, L. (2007). Remedying education: Evidence from two randomized experiments in India. *The Quarterly Journal of Economics, 122*(3), 1235–1264. https://doi.org/10.1162/qjec.122.3.1235

Bennett, S., Maton, K., & Kervin, L. (2008). The 'digital natives' debate: A critical review of the evidence. *British Journal of Educational Technology, 39*(5), 775–786. https://doi.org/10.1111/j.1467-8535.2007.00793.x

Beuermann, D., Cristia, J., Cruz-Aguayo, Y., Cueto, S., & Malamud, O. (2013). *Home computers and child outcomes: Short-term impacts from a randomized experiment in Peru.* NBER Working Paper Series, 18818. https://doi.org/10.3386/w18818

Biagi, F., & Loi, M. (2013). Measuring ICT use and learning outcomes: Evidence from recent econometric studies. *European Journal of Education, 48*, 28–42. https://onlinelibrary.wiley.com/doi/10.1111/ejed.12016

Bicker, L. (2020, April 10). Coronavirus: How South Korea is teaching empty classrooms. *BBC News.* https://www.bbc.com/news/world-asia-52230371

Bradbrook, G., Alvi, I., Fisher, J., Lloyd, H., Moore, R., Thompson, V., Brake, D., Helsper, E., & Livingstone, S. (2008). *Meeting their potential: The role of education and technology in overcoming disadvantage and disaffection in young people.* Becta. http://eprints.lse.ac.uk/4063/1/Meeting_their_potential.pdf

Buchmann, C., & Hannum, E. (2001). Education and stratification in developing countries: A review of theories and research. *Annual Review of Sociology, 27*, 77–102.

CCSA. (2020). *How COVID-19 is changing the world: A statistical perspective, volume II.* The Committee for the Coordination of Statistical Activities. https://www.un.org/development/desa/pd/news/how-covid-19-changing-world-statistical-perspective-volume-ii

Cheung, A. C. K., & Slavin, R. E. (2013). The effectiveness of educational technology applications for enhancing mathematics achievement in K-12 classrooms: A meta-analysis. *Educational Research Review, 9*, 88–113. https://doi.org/10.1016/j.edurev.2013.01.001

Chinn, M. D., & Fairlie, R. W. (2010). ICT use in the developing world: An analysis of differences in computer and Internet penetration. *Review of International Economics, 18*(1), 153–167. https://doi.org/10.1111/j.1467-9396.2009.00861.x

Choe, S.-H. (2009, June 1). Tech company helps South Korean students ace entrance tests. *The New York Times.* https://www.nytimes.com/2009/06/02/business/global/02cram.html?_r=0

CPB Economic Policy Analysis. (2020, July 6). *Schrappen eindtoets groep 8 kan ongelijkheid vergroten.* https://www.cpb.nl/en/node/160280

Cruz-Jesus, F., Oliveira, T., Bacao, F., & Irani, Z. (2017). Assessing the pattern between economic and digital development of countries. *Information Systems Frontiers, 19*(4), 835–854. https://doi.org/10.1007/s10796-016-9634-1

Culp, K. M., Honey, M., Mandinach, E., Education Development Center, & Center for Children and Technology. (2003). *A retrospective on twenty years of education technology policy*. U.S. Department of Education.

Dale, R. (2005). Globalisation, knowledge economy and comparative education. *Comparative Education, 41*(2), 117–149. https://doi.org/10.1080/03050060500150906

Davison, E., & Cotten, S. (2003). Connection discrepancies: Unmasking further layers of the digital divide. *First Monday*. https://doi.org/10.5210/fm.v8i3.1039

DeBell, M., & Chapman, C. (2006). *Computer and Internet use by students in 2003 (NCES 2006–065)*. U.S. Department of Education, National Center for Education Statistics.

DiMaggio, P., Hargittai, E., Celeste, C., & Shafer, S. (2004). Digital inequality: From unequal access to differentiated use. In K. Neckerman (Ed.), *Social inequality* (pp. 355–400). Russell Sage Foundation.

DiMaggio, P., Hargittai, E., Neuman, W. R., & Robinson, J. P. (2001). Social implications of the Internet. *Annual Review of Sociology, 27*, 307–336. ABI/INFORM Complete.

Dolan, J. E. (2016). Splicing the divide: A review of research on the evolving digital divide among K-12 students. *Journal of Research on Technology in Education, 48*(1), 16–37. https://doi.org/10.1080/15391523.2015.1103147

Drori, G. S. (2006). *Global e-litism: Digital technology, social inequality, and transnationality*. Worth Publishers.

Drori, G. S. (2010). Globalization and technology divides: Bifurcation of policy between the "digital divide" and the "innovation divide." *Sociological Inquiry, 80*(1), 63–91. https://doi.org/10.1111/j.1475-682X.2009.00316.x

Eickelmann, B. (2018). Cross-national policies on information and communication technology in primary and secondary schools: An international perspective. In J. Voogt, G. Knezek, R. Christensen, & K.-W. Lai (Eds.), *Second handbook of information technology in primary and secondary education* (pp. 1–12). Springer International Publishing. https://doi.org/10.1007/978-3-319-53803-7_84-1

Ellis, P. (2020, April 27). *Helping teachers adapt to remote teaching—3 Cambridge trainers tell their stories*. Cambridge Assessment-International Education. https://blog.cambridgeinternational.org/helping-teachers-adapt-to-remote-teaching/

Erichsen, E. A., & Salajan, F. D. (2014). A comparative analysis of e-learning policy formulation in the European Union and the United States: Discursive convergence and divergence. *Comparative Education Review, 58*(1), 135–165. https://doi.org/10.1086/674095

European Commission. (1994). *Europe and the global information society*. Office for Official Publications of the European Communities. http://ec.europa.eu/archives/ISPO/infosoc/backg/bangeman.html

European Commission. (1995). *Teaching and learning: Towards the learning society*. European Commission. http://europa.eu/documents/comm/white_papers/pdf/com95_590_en.pdf

Fairlie, R. W., Beltran, D. O., & Das, K. K. (2010). Home computers and educational outcomes: Evidence from the NLSY97 and CPS. *Economic Inquiry, 48*(3), 771–792. https://doi.org/10.1111/j.1465-7295.2009.00218.x

Fairlie, R. W., & Robinson, J. (2013). Experimental evidence on the effects of home computers on academic achievement among schoolchildren. *American Economic Journal: Applied Economics, 5*(3), 211–240. https://doi.org/10.1257/app.5.3.211

Goedhart, N. S., Broerse, J. E., Kattouw, R., & Dedding, C. (2019). 'Just having a computer doesn't make sense': The digital divide from the perspective of mothers with a low socio-economic position. *New Media & Society, 21*(11–12), 2347–2365. https://doi.org/10.1177/1461444819846059

Gonzales, A. L., Calarco, J. M., & Lynch, T. (2020). Technology problems and student achievement gaps: A validation and extension of the technology maintenance construct. *Communication Research, 47*(5), 750–770. https://doi.org/10.1177/0093650218796366

Goode, J. (2010). The digital identity divide: How technology knowledge impacts college students. *New Media & Society, 12*(3), 497–513. https://doi.org/10.1177/1461444809343560

Goolsbee, A., & Guryan, J. (2006). The impact of internet subsidies in public schools. *The Review of Economics and Statistics, 88*(2), 336–347. https://doi.org/10.1162/rest.88.2.336

Hannum, E., & Buchmann, C. (2005). Global educational expansion and socio-economic development: An assessment of findings from the social sciences. *World Development, 33*(3), 333–354. https://doi.org/10.1016/j.worlddev.2004.10.001

Hargittai, E. (2002). Second-level digital divide: Differences in people's online skills. *First Monday, 7*(4). https://doi.org/10.5210/fm.v7i4.942

Hargittai, E., & Hinnant, A. (2008). Digital inequality: Differences in young adults' use of the Internet. *Communication Research, 35*(5), 602–621.

Hassoun, D. (2015). "All over the place": A case study of classroom multitasking and attentional performance. *New Media & Society, 17*(10), 1680–1695. https://doi.org/10.1177/1461444814531756

Heyneman, S. P., & Loxley, W. A. (1983). The effect of primary-school quality on academic achievement across twenty-nine high- and low-income countries. *American Journal of Sociology, 88*(6), 1162–1194.

Hilbert, M. (2016). The bad news is that the digital access divide is here to stay: Domestically installed bandwidths among 172 countries for 1986–2014. *Telecommunications Policy, 40*(6), 567–581. https://doi.org/10.1016/j.telpol.2016.01.006

Horowitz, J. M. (2020, April 15). *Lower-income parents most concerned about their children falling behind amid COVID-19 school closures.* Pew Research Center. https://www.pewresearch.org/fact-tank/2020/04/15/lower-income-parents-most-concerned-about-their-children-falling-behind-amid-covid-19-school-closures/

Horrigan, J. B. (2015, April 20). *The numbers behind the broadband 'homework gap.'* Pew Research Center. https://www.pewresearch.org/fact-tank/2015/04/20/the-numbers-behind-the-broadband-homework-gap/

Hunley, S. A., Evans, J. H., Delgado-Hachey, M., Krise, J., Rich, T., & Schell, C. (2005). Adolescent computer use and academic achievement. *Adolescence, 40*(158), 307–318.

Iivari, N., Sharma, S., & Ventä-Olkkonen, L. (2020). Digital transformation of everyday life—How COVID-19 pandemic transformed the basic education of the young generation and why information management research should care? *International Journal of Information Management, 55*, 1–6. https://doi.org/10.1016/j.ijinfomgt.2020.102183

ITU. (2011). *Measuring the information society.* ITU. http://www.itu.int/en/ITU-D/Statistics/Pages/publications/mis2011.aspx

ITU. (2015). *Measuring the information society.* ITU.

ITU. (2018). *Measuring the information society.* ITU.

Jackson, L. A., von Eye, A., Biocca, F. A., Barbatsis, G., Zhao, Y., & Fitzgerald, H. E. (2006). Does home internet use influence the academic performance of low-income children? *Developmental Psychology, 42*(3), 429–435. https://doi.org/10.1037/0012-1649.42.3.429

Jaggars, S. S., & Xu, D. (2016). How do online course design features influence student performance? *Computers & Education, 95*, 270–284. https://doi.org/10.1016/j.compedu.2016.01.014

Kim, S. (2011). The diffusion of the Internet: Trend and causes. *Social Science Research, 40*(2), 602–613. https://doi.org/10.1016/j.ssresearch.2010.07.005

Kozma, R. B. (2008). Comparative analysis of policies for ICT in education. In J. Voogt & G. Knezek (Eds.), *International handbook of information technology in primary and secondary education* (pp. 1083–1096). Springer.

Leu, D. J., Forzani, E., Rhoads, C., Maykel, C., Kennedy, C., & Timbrell, N. (2015). The new literacies of online research and comprehension: Rethinking the reading achievement gap. *Reading Research Quarterly, 50*(1), 37–59. https://doi.org/10.1002/rrq.85

Li, C., & Lalani, F. (2020, April 29). The COVID-19 pandemic has changed education forever. This is how. *World Economic Forum*. https://www.weforum.org/agenda/2020/04/coronavirus-education-global-covid19-online-digital-learning/

Lucas, S. R. (2001). Effectively maintained inequality: Education transitions, track mobility, and social background effects. *American Journal of Sociology, 106*(6), 1642–1690. https://doi.org/10.1086/321300

Ma, J.K.-H., Vachon, T. E., & Cheng, S. (2019). National income, political freedom, and investments in R&D and education: A comparative analysis of the second digital divide among 15-year-old students. *Social Indicators Research, 144*(1), 133–166. https://doi.org/10.1007/s11205-018-2030-0

Malamud, O., & Pop-Eleches, C. (2011). Home computer use and the development of human capital. *The Quarterly Journal of Economics, 126*(2), 987–1027. https://doi.org/10.1093/qje/qjr008

Marsh, J., Plowman, L., Yamada-Rice, D., Bishop, J. C., Lahmar, J., Scott, F., Davenport, A., Davis, S., French, K., Piras, M., Thornhill, S., Robinson, P., & Winter, P. (2015). *Exploring play and creativity in pre-schoolers' use of apps: Final project report*. Technology and Play. http://www.techandplay.org

Mihelj, S. I., Leguina, A., & Downey, J. (2018). Culture is digital: Cultural participation, diversity and the digital divide. *New Media & Society, 21*(7), 1465–1485. https://journals.sagepub.com/doi/10.1177/1461444818822816

Moonen, J. (2008). Policy from a global perspective. In J. Voogt & G. Knezek (Eds.), *International handbook of information technology in primary and secondary education* (pp. 1171–1178). Springer. https://doi.org/10.1007/978-0-387-73315-9_75

Mullis, I. V. S., Martin, M. O., Foy, P., & Hooper, M. (2017). PIRLS 2016: International results in reading. In *International association for the evaluation of educational achievement*. International Association for the Evaluation of Educational Achievement (IEA). https://eric.ed.gov/?id=ED580353

National Commission on Excellence in Education. (1983). *A nation at risk: The imperative for education reform*. Government Printing Office.

Natriello, G. (2001). Bridging the second digital divide: What can sociologists of education contribute? *Sociology of Education, 74*(3), 260–265.

Norris, P. (2001). *Digital divide? Civic engagement, information poverty, and the Internet worldwide*. Cambridge University Press.

NSW. (2020a, March 31). *Laptop loans help bridge the digital divide*. NSW Government. https://education.nsw.gov.au/news/latest-news/laptop-loans-help-bridge-the-digital-divide

NSW. (2020b, October 20). *All NSW public schools to benefit from internet upgrades*. NSW Government. https://education.nsw.gov.au/news/latest-news/all-nsw-public-schools-to-benefit-from-internet-upgrades

OECD. (2011). *PISA 2009 results: Students on line: Digital technologies and performance (Volume VI)*. OECD Publishing. https://doi.org/10.1787/9789264112995-en

OECD. (2019a). *PISA 2018 results (volume II): Where all students can succeed*. PISA, OECD Publishing. https://doi.org/10.1787/b5fd1b8f-en

OECD. (2019b). *PISA 2018 results (volume III): What school life means for students' lives*. PISA, OECD Publishing. https://doi.org/10.1787/acd78851-en

OECD. (2020a). *Education responses to covid-19: Embracing digital learning and online collaboration*. OECD Publishing. https://www.oecd.org/coronavirus/policy-responses/education-responses-to-covid-19-embracing-digital-learning-and-online-collaboration-d75eb0e8/

OECD. (2020b). What is the impact of the COVID-19 pandemic on immigrants and their children? *OECD Policy Responses to Coronavirus (COVID-19)*. OECD Publishing, Paris. https://doi.org/10.1787/e7cbb7de-en

OECD Education & Skills TopClass Podcast. (2020, September 17). *Episode 25: Will the coronavirus crisis lead to a fundamental change in education?* https://www.listennotes.com/podcasts/oecd-education/episode-25-will-the-rn_0e-qcQwf/

Ottestad, G., & Gudmundsdottir, G. B. (2018). Information and communication technology policy in primary and secondary education in Europe. In J. Voogt, G. Knezek, R. Christensen, & K.-W. Lai (Eds.), *Second handbook of information technology in primary and secondary education* (pp. 1343–1362). Springer International Publishing. https://doi.org/10.1007/978-3-319-71054-9_92

Palfrey, J., & Gasser, U. (2008). *Born digital: Understanding the first generation of digital natives.* Basic Books.

Park, H., Buchmann, C., Choi, J., & Merry, J. (2016). Learning beyond the school walls: Trends and implications. *Annual Review of Sociology, 42*, 231–252. https://doi.org/10.1146/annurev-soc-081715-074341

Partnership on Measuring ICT for Development. (2011). *Measuring the WSIS targets: A statistical framework.* International Telecommunication Union (ITU). https://www.itu.int/pub/D-IND-MEAS_WSIS-2011

Plowman, L. (2015). Researching young children's everyday uses of technology in the family home. *Interacting with Computers, 27*(1), 36–46. https://doi.org/10.1093/iwc/iwu031

Powell, W. W., & Snellman, K. (2004). The knowledge economy. *Annual Review of Sociology, 30*, 199–220.

Prensky, M. (2001). Digital natives, digital immigrants Part 1. *On the Horizon, 9*(5), 1–6. https://doi.org/10.1108/10748120110424816

Puckett, C., & Rafalow, M. H. (2020). COVID-19, technology, and implications for educational equity. *American Sociological Association Footnotes, 48*(3), 34–35.

Rafalow, M. H. (2018). Disciplining play: Digital youth culture as capital at school. *American Journal of Sociology, 123*(5), 1416–1452. https://doi.org/10.1086/695766

Raftery, A. E., & Hout, M. (1993). Maximally maintained inequality: Expansion, reform, and opportunity in Irish education, 1921–75. *Sociology of Education, 66*(1), 41–62. https://doi.org/10.2307/2112784

Ragnedda, M., & Muschert, G. W. (Eds.). (2013). *The digital divide: The Internet and social inequality in international perspective.* Routledge.

Reimers, F. M., & Schleicher, A. (2020). *A framework to guide an education response to the COVID-19 pandemic of 2020.* OECD Publishing. https://learningportal.iiep.unesco.org/en/library/a-framework-to-guide-an-education-response-to-the-covid-19-pandemic-of-2020

Rideout, V. J., & Katz, V. S. (2016). *Opportunity for all? Technology and learning in lower-income families. A report of the Families and Media Project.* The Joan Ganz Cooney Center at Sesame Workshop. https://kramden.org/technology-learning-lower-income/

Robison, K. K., & Crenshaw, E. M. (2010). Reevaluating the global digital divide: Socio-demographic and conflict barriers to the Internet revolution. *Sociological Inquiry, 80*(1), 34–62. https://doi.org/10.1111/j.1475-682X.2009.00315.x

Scheerder, A. J., van Deursen, A. J., & van Dijk, J. A. (2017). Determinants of Internet skills, uses and outcomes: A systematic review of the second- and third-level digital divide. *Telematics and Informatics, 34*(8), 1607–1624. https://doi.org/10.1016/j.tele.2017.07.007

Scheerder, A. J., van Deursen, A. J., & van Dijk, J. A. (2019). Internet use in the home: Digital inequality from a domestication perspective. *New Media & Society, 21*(10), 2099–2118. https://doi.org/10.1177/1461444819844299

Sefton-Green, J., Marsh, J., Erstad, O., & Flewitt, R. (2016). *Establishing a research agenda for the digital literacy practices of young children: A white paper for COST Action IS1410.* https://doi.org/10.13140/RG.2.2.10896.30720

Selwyn, N., Gorard, S., & Williams, S. (2001). Digital divide or digital opportunity? The role of technology in overcoming social exclusion in U.S. education. *Educational Policy, 15*(2), 258–277. https://doi.org/10.1177/0895904801015002002

Selwyn, N., Potter, J., & Cranmer, S. (2009). Primary pupils' use of information and communication technologies at school and home. *British Journal of Educational Technology, 40*(5), 919–932. https://doi.org/10.1111/j.1467-8535.2008.00876.x

Starkey, L., & Finger, G. (2018). Information and communication technology in educational policies in Australia and New Zealand. In J. Voogt, G. Knezek, R. Christensen, & K.-W. Lai (Eds.), *Second handbook of information technology in primary and secondary education* (pp. 1–20). Springer International Publishing. https://doi.org/10.1007/978-3-319-53803-7_87-2

Teacher Task Force. (2020). *COVID-19 highlights the digital divide in distance learning*. International Task Force on Teachers for Education 2030. https://teachertaskforce.org/news/covid-19-highlights-digital-divide-distance-learning

UNCTAD. (2020, April 6). *Coronavirus reveals need to bridge the digital divide*. United Nations Conference on Trade and Development. https://unctad.org/news/coronavirus-reveals-need-bridge-digital-divide

UNESCO. (2000). *The Dakar framework for action: Education for all meeting our collective commitments*. United Nations Educational, Scientific and Cultural Organization. http://unesdoc.unesco.org/images/0012/001211/121147e.pdf

UNESCO. (2020a). *Adverse consequences of school closures*. United Nations Educational, Scientific and Cultural Organization. https://en.unesco.org/covid19/educationresponse/consequences

UNESCO. (2020b, August 31). *As a new academic year begins, UNESCO warns that only one third of students will return to school*. United Nations Educational, Scientific and Cultural Organization. https://en.unesco.org/news/new-academic-year-begins-unesco-warns-only-one-third-students-will-return-school

UNESCO-UIS. (2014). *Information and communication technology (ICT) in education in Asia: A comparative analysis of ICT integration and e-readiness in schools across Asia*. United Nations Educational, Scientific and Cultural Organization, Institute for Statistics. http://uis.unesco.org/sites/default/files/documents/information-communication-technologies-education-asia-ict-integration-e-readiness-schools-2014-en_0.pdf

UNESCO-UIS. (2015). *Information and communication technology (ICT) in education in sub-Saharan Africa: A comparative analysis of basic e-readiness in schools*. United Nations Educational, Scientific and Cultural Organization, Institute for Statistics. http://www.uis.unesco.org/Communication/Documents/ICT-africa.pdf

UNESCO-UIS. (2016). *Paper commissioned for the global education monitoring report 2016, education for people and planet: Creating sustainable futures for all*. http://unesdoc.unesco.org/images/0024/002455/245572e.pdf

UNESCO-UIS. (2020, April 8). *UIS COVID-19 response: Data to inform policies that mitigate setbacks in education gains*. United Nations Educational, Scientific and Cultural Organization. http://uis.unesco.org/en/news/uis-covid-19-response-data-inform-policies-mitigate-setbacks-education-gains

United Nations. (2000, September 8). *United Nations millennium declaration*. United Nations General Assembly. https://www.ohchr.org/EN/ProfessionalInterest/Pages/Millennium.aspx

U.S. Department of Education. (1996). *Getting America's students ready for the 21st century: Meeting the technology literacy challenge. A report to the nation on technology and education*. http://eric.ed.gov/?id=ED398899

van der Schuur, W. A., Baumgartner, S. E., Sumter, S. R., & Valkenburg, P. M. (2020). Exploring the long-term relationship between academic-media multitasking and adolescents' academic achievement. *New Media & Society, 22*(1), 140–158. https://doi.org/10.1177/1461444819861956

van Deursen, A. J., Helsper, E., Eynon, R., & van Dijk, J. A. (2017). The compoundness and sequentiality of digital inequality. *International Journal of Communication, 11*, 452–473.

van Deursen, A. J., & van Dijk, J. A. (2019). The first-level digital divide shifts from inequalities in physical access to inequalities in material access. *New Media & Society, 21*(2), 354–375. https://doi.org/10.1177/1461444818797082

van Dijk, J. A. G. M., & van Deursen, A. J. (2014). Solutions: Learning digital skills. In J. A. G. M. van Dijk & A. J. van Deursen (Eds.), *Digital skills: Unlocking the information society* (pp. 113–138). Palgrave Macmillan US. https://doi.org/10.1057/9781137437037_6

Vegas, E. (2020, April 14). *School closures, government responses, and learning inequality around the world during COVID-19.* The Brookings Institution. https://www.brookings.edu/research/school-closures-government-responses-and-learning-inequality-around-the-world-during-covid-19/

Vigdor, J. L., Ladd, H. F., & Martinez, E. (2014). Scaling the digital divide: Home computer technology and student achievement. *Economic Inquiry, 52*(3), 1103–1119. https://doi.org/10.1111/ecin.12089

Vogels, E. A., Perrin, A., Rainie, L., & Anderson, M. (2020, April 30). *53% of Americans say the Internet has been essential during the COVID-19 outbreak.* Pew Research Center. https://www.pewresearch.org/internet/2020/04/30/53-of-americans-say-the-internet-has-been-essential-during-the-covid-19-outbreak/

Warschauer, M. (2016). Addressing the social envelope: Education and the digital divide. In C. Greenhow, J. Sonnevend, & C. Agur (Eds.), *Education and social media: Toward a digital future* (pp. 29–48). MIT Press. https://oxfordindex.oup.com/view/10.7551/mitpress/9780262034470.003.0003?lang=en

Warschauer, M., Knobel, M., & Stone, L. (2004). Technology and equity in schooling: Deconstructing the digital divide. *Educational Policy, 18*(4), 562–588. https://doi.org/10.1177/0895904804266469

Wells, J., & Lewis, L. (2006). *Internet access in U.S. public schools and classrooms: 1994–2005 (NCES 2007–020).* U.S. Department of Education, National Center for Education Statistics.

de Werfhorst, H. G. V., & Mijs, J. J. (2010). Achievement inequality and the institutional structure of educational systems: A comparative perspective. *Annual Review of Sociology, 36*, 407–428. https://doi.org/10.1146/annurev.soc.012809.102538

Yu, J. (2020, March 20). *Covid-19 and the challenges of remote teaching in China.* Cambridge Assessment-International Education. https://blog.cambridgeinternational.org/covid-19-and-the-challenges-of-remote-teaching-in-china/

Yuen, A. H. K., & Hew, T. K. F. (2018). Information and communication technology in educational policies in the Asian region. In J. Voogt, G. Knezek, R. Christensen, & K.-W. Lai (Eds.), *Handbook of information technology in primary and secondary education* (pp. 1–20). Springer International Publishing. https://doi.org/10.1007/978-3-319-53803-7_86-1

Yuen, A. H. K., Park, J. H., Chen, L., & Cheng, M. (2018). The significance of cultural capital and parental mediation for digital inequity. *New Media & Society, 20*(2), 599–617. https://doi.org/10.1177/1461444816667084

Chapter 2
Research Literature on How Digital Inclusion Affects Adolescents' Well-Being

Abstract Despite extensive research since the 1990s, empirical studies have reported inconsistent findings in terms of the effects of ICT use on student outcomes. This chapter reviews the research literature on students' ICT use in school and at home and identifies the methodological issues that may lead to inconclusive and mixed findings. The chapter begins with a discussion of selection and omitted variable bias. This is followed by an examination of the measures of ICT access and use at home and in schools. We suggest that the considerable variation in the definitions and measures of ICT access, ICT use, and forms of educational technology used in research contributes to the inconsistent conclusions in empirical research and should receive more attention from scholars, educators, and policymakers. We also suggest that ICT use at a moderate level may have positive returns, but intensive ICT use could produce negative effects on student outcomes. Scholars should consider modeling the curvilinear relationship between ICT use and adolescent well-being in empirical analysis.

Keywords Methodological issue · Selection · Omitted variable bias · Different measurements · Educational technology · Home vs. school · Curvilinear relationship

DESPITE extensive research since the 1990s, empirical studies of effects of ICT use on student outcomes have reported inconsistent findings. These findings reflect both the mechanisms governing the relationships between ICT use and student well-being and researchers' methodological considerations. In this chapter, we focus on the methodological issues that may have led to these discrepancies. These issues include selection bias, omitted variables bias, the wide variation in the measures of ICT use, and a potentially *curvilinear* relationship between ICT use and student outcomes.

J. K.-H. Ma and S. Cheng, *Adolescent Well-being and ICT UseX*,
Human Well-Being Research and Policy Making,
https://doi.org/10.1007/978-3-031-04412-0_2

2.1 Does Digital Inclusion Promote Students' Well-Being? Incongruent Research Findings about ICT Effects

Educators often ask whether ICT use in education benefits or hinders the well-being of secondary school students, and if so, how (Aagaard, 2017). Many educators and researchers have taken the integration of ICT across a wide variety of subjects and educational fields for granted. The spike in the development of educational technology since 2000 and the COVID-19 pandemic have increased students' and teachers' reliance on ICT for schoolwork (NSW, 2020; OECD, 2020). Scholars have extensively examined the potential effect of educational technology, often with a special focus on the relationship between ICT use and academic performance. Many researchers (e.g., Attewell et al., 2003; Fairlie et al., 2010; Verbruggen et al., 2021) report positive effects of ICT on educational outcomes. Others have found evidence contradicting these findings and cast doubt on any research that seems to applaud the benefits of educational technology (e.g., Agasisti et al., 2020; Camerini et al., 2018; Vigdor et al., 2014).

What can we learn from this research literature? How do we explain these results reporting both positive and negative effects of educational technology?

2.2 Differences in the Use of Statistical Methods

In our review of the recent scholarship, we suggest that the choice and use of different statistical procedures (or research designs) determine both the magnitude and the direction of the relationship between ICT inclusion and student outcomes. This partly explains why previous empirical studies have arrived at different results. Moreover, inappropriate statistical methods may lead to biased estimates of ICT effects. We identify three sources of methodological problems and discuss each in the following subsections.

2.2.1 Selection Bias

Selection bias due to research designs and statistical methods may lead to the effects of ICT on academic achievement being overestimated or underestimated. This may partially explain the mixed research findings. ICT and online courses may be designed for and used by underperforming students for remedial purposes, or by high achievers to attain academic excellence (Barrow et al., 2009). Students who use ICT for learning also may be qualitatively different from those who exclusively use ICT for recreational purposes (Biagi & Loi, 2013). Failing to consider these issues may bias estimates of ICT effects on student outcomes.

Scholars have demonstrated the influences of selection bias in research on ICT use in education. Xu and Jaggars (2013) examine the performance of students between online course delivery and face-to-face course delivery in 34 community and technical colleges. Using the instrumental variable technique, they show that, at least in community and technical colleges, students who are more likely to take online courses are also more motivated and better prepared. As a result of this difference, analyses using only descriptive statistics or ordinary least square (OLS) cannot account for the unobserved effects of students' academic ability and motivation, and often underestimate the course grades of students in online courses. On the other hand, students in online courses are less likely to persist through the semester compared to their peers in face-to-face courses. Focusing on students who persist through online courses therefore may introduce another selection bias which, in this context, seems to underestimate the negative effects of online course delivery on course grades (Xu & Jaggars, 2013). Coates et al. (2004) suggest that "[failure] to account for the effects of selection leads to biased and inconsistent coefficient estimates in education production functions and may result in misleading inferences regarding 'no significant difference' between online and face-to-face instruction" (p. 545).

Students' sociodemographic backgrounds affect the types of information and communication technology that they use, and this technology affects their learning outcomes (Orús et al., 2016). Failure to control for the effects of sociodemographic factors therefore leads to another source of self-selection bias. Tengtrakul and Peha (2013) study the use of ICT in Thailand's schools, and find that students from high-income families and urban areas are more likely than students from low-income families and rural areas to have access to ICT. High-income and urban families are more likely than low-income and rural families to enroll their children in schools that are well equipped with ICT. Orús et al. (2016) find that participation in creating learner-generated videos on YouTube improves students' class performance. Because student participation in the online video project is voluntary, selection bias might emerge if "students participating in the activity were dedicated learners whose were highly motivated to obtain a good performance, compared to non-participant students" (Orús et al., 2016, p. 262).

Another common self-selection issue is the lack of sufficient controls for students' ICT ability, which may affect both their use of educational technology and their academic performance. Fuchs and Wößmann (2005) suggest that the decision to use computers may be a function of students' ability and is therefore not entirely random. Not controlling for student ability in the analysis of the causal relationship between computer use and academic performance therefore may lead to an "ability bias" (Fuchs & Wößmann, 2005, p. 2). Using PISA 2009 data in their cross-national study of 15-year-old students, Biagi and Loi (2013) find a positive relationship between their intensive use of computers for gaming and academic performance. To explain this counterintuitive finding, Biagi and Loi (2013) suggest that selection bias may exist if brighter students are also avid gamers.

2.2.2 Omitted Variable Bias

Scholars are also aware of *omitted variable bias*, which raises some of the same methodological concerns as selection bias. When omitted variable bias exists, it is difficult to isolate the causal effect of educational technology (often measured by access to computers or the internet) from unobserved factors such as students' characteristics and family backgrounds (Fairlie & Robinson, 2013). Vigdor et al. (2014) suggest that OLS regression analysis with unobserved omitted variable bias may overestimate the positive influence of home computer ownership "even when [the data] were drawn from a relatively rich specification" (p. 1104).

Scholars suggest that omitted measures of attitudes and motivations often confound the relationship between ICT use in education and learning outcomes. For example, students with higher cognitive ability may be more likely to purchase computers for learning. This may lead to a positive relationship between home computer ownership and academic performance (Fairlie et al., 2010; Fairlie & London, 2012). Similar spurious relationships may also occur because students with highly involved parents are more likely to own a home computer and also perform well in school. Biagi and Loi (2013) suggest that failing to control for students' attitudes toward ICT and their educational aspirations may also lead to biased estimates.

2.2.3 Other Methodological Issues

To reduce selection and omitted variable bias, scholars suggest the inclusion of both previous computer ownership at home at time 1 and *future computer ownership at home* at time 2 in statistical analysis (Fairlie et al., 2010). A positive effect of future computer ownership on academic achievement then signals concerns of computer ownership proxies for unobserved omitted individual characteristics and/or family backgrounds. In such cases, it is not computer ownership that contributes to educational performance. Instead, other omitted variables, such as household wealth and educational motivation, may shape both students' computer ownership and academic outcomes (Fairlie & London, 2012; Schmitt & Wadsworth, 2006). Vigdor et al. (2014) argue that home computer ownership may simply reflect positive income shocks or general improvements in living standards, which does not causally lead to the enhancement of school performance. With cross-sectional data, it is difficult to determine whether ICT use affects academic performance or vice versa (Jackson et al., 2006).

Scholars also suggest the use of more rigorous research designs to compensate for selection bias and omitted variable (Warschauer & Xu, 2018). Schmitt and Wadsworth (2006) recommend that random assignment of individuals into treatment and control groups (e.g., computer use vs. no computer use) is an effective way to help control for unobserved effects. Cheung and Slavin (2013) suggest that this experimental design is difficult for research on ICT use in education. Alternatively, Vigdor et al. (2014) suggest that longitudinal data allow researchers to evaluate within-student changes (before versus after gaining access to a home computer) when the sample data are not entirely random. Using panel data, Vigdor et al. (2014) find that students receive the best academic scores in years when they make moderate use of computers for homework.

Cheung and Slavin (2013) list five methodological problems in research on the education of ICT. First, some studies do not have a control group to compare students who receive the treatment to those who do not. In general, analyses with no control group tend to find a greater positive effect of ICT use in education. Second, analyses using data from short-duration observations are more likely than long-duration research to find larger effects. Third, some analyses fail to control for large pretest differences, making it difficult to determine whether the treated and control groups are comparable. Such studies are likely to overestimate the effect of educational technology. Fourth, researchers may overestimate the positive effect of ICT use when they use outcome measures that are "closely aligned with the content taught to the experimental group but not the control group" (p. 93). Fifth and finally, scholars are more likely to cite articles that support their arguments (Scheerder et al., 2017; Schulz-Hardt et al., 2000), and, occasionally, selectively report findings that are consistent with their hypotheses.

While the focus of this book is not methodological advancements in ICT research, a clear understanding of methodological issues helps us answer substantive questions: How does ICT affect students' academic and non-academic outcomes? How do researchers, educators, and policymakers interpret the modest positive effect of educational technology? What form(s) of ICT usage are more important for adolescent well-being and learning? Does educational technology unequally benefit students of different socioeconomic background and other sociodemographic characteristics?

2.3 Differences in ICT Measures

After reviewing dozens of studies, we contend that another reason for the inconclusive empirical findings in ICT research is the considerable variation in the definitions of ICT use, ICT and online activities being considered, and forms of educational technology being examined in research. For example, many studies measure digital access as a binary variable (e.g., computer ownership: 1 if yes and 0 if no; internet access: 1 if yes and 0 if no); some focus on the use of certain educational technology in school; and others focus on the level of ICT use in the household for purposes such as homework, online research, and multitasking. To our surprise, few researchers attribute inconsistent findings in ICT research to differences in ICT measures. We will discuss this issue in more detail.

2.3.1 Measures of Digital Access

Most incongruent results appear in research on the effect of digital access on academic achievement. On one hand, Attewell and Battle (1999) use data from the National Education Longitudinal Study of 1988 (NELS:88) and find students with access to computers at home have higher scores in reading, mathematics, and better school grades than those without computer access. Schmitt and Wadsworth (2006) analyze the British Household Panel Survey (BHPS) between 1991 and 2001. After controlling for unobserved household-level characteristics, they report two major findings: (1) home computer ownership at age 15 has a robust and positive effect on the grade from school examinations administered at age 16; and (2) home computer access at age 17 has a positive effect on the scores from national tests at age 18. Using both the 2000–2003 Current Population Survey (CPS) and the National Longitudinal Survey of Youth 1977 (NLSY97), Fairlie et al. (2010) report that teenagers with access to home computers are more likely to graduate from high school and have a higher GPA than those without. Wainer et al. (2015) analyze the academic achievement of Brazilian primary schoolers between 2007 and 2011 and report that computer ownership positively predicts short-term school grades. The positive effect ranges between 0.2 and 0.4 standard deviations above the mean. They find no conclusive long-term effect of computer access on educational outcomes.

On the other hand, Vigdor et al. (2014) use administrative data from the U.S. to study North Carolina public school students. Their analyses suggest that fifth- and eighth-grade students with access to a computer at home show a reduction in reading and mathematics performance. Using the PISA 2000 cross-national comparative data, Fuchs and Wößmann (2004, 2007) find a positive correlation between computer availability (both at home and at school) and academic achievement. However, after including family background and school characteristics as control variables in the analysis, the relationship turns from positive to negative. In Romania, Malamud and Pop-Eleches (2011) study 6,418 low-income families who applied for the voucher program. A random subsample of applicants received 200 Euros to purchase computers. Compared to children whose families did not receive the voucher, those whose families received a voucher scored better in computer and cognitive skills but had lower grades. Angrist and Lavy (2002) examine the influence of teachers' use of computer-aided instruction (CAI) in Israeli elementary and middle schools. Their findings suggest that the provision of computers in schools increases the likelihood of teachers' use of CAI but does not significantly improve their students' test scores.

Many studies have focused on the effects of computer access because of the persistent digital divide in computer ownership or internet access at home (Attewell & Battle, 1999; Gonzales, 2015; Gonzales et al., 2020; van Deursen & van Dijk, 2019). Scholars, educators, and policymakers wonder whether public funds should be used to provide more computers to public schools and give more free laptops to low-income students for use at home (Vigdor et al., 2014). In California, Fairlie and Robinson (2013) conducted a field experiment that gave free computers to 1,123 middle and high school students who reported not having one at home. Approximately a half of these students were randomly assigned to the treatment group and received a computer, and the other half were assigned to the control group and did not receive computers until two months later. The findings suggest that the provision of home computers had almost no effect on students' grades, test scores, and class attendance. Since 2004, a well-known initiative, the *One Laptop Per Child* (OLPC) (see James, 2010; UNESCO-UIS, 2014; Warschauer & Newhart, 2016), has offered inexpensive laptop computers or digital tablets to hundreds of millions of children in developing countries like Peru (Beuermann et al., 2013), Romania (Malamud & Pop-Eleches, 2011), and China (Mo et al., 2013). While schoolchildren who receive laptops show better basic computer skills than those without laptops, findings from several studies have suggested that the provision of laptops does not significantly improve students' academic performance (Cristia et al., 2017; James, 2010; Malamud & Pop-Eleches, 2011).

Taken together, the empirical findings from research on ICT use and educational outcomes are mixed, in large part because of inconsistent measures of digital access. To resolve this problem, researchers should more precisely measure how students use ICT, how frequently they access the internet, and what online activities and behavior they engage in. Equally important, educators and policymakers should attempt to understand why digital access may have positive or negative influences on students' learning outcomes.

2.3.2 Measures of Digital Use

Some researchers focus on the use of ICT for non-educational purposes in the course of *academic-media multitasking* (AMM) (van der Schuur et al., 2020), such as sitting in the back of classrooms and surfing websites unrelated to class material (Hassoun, 2015) and using the internet for entertainment and communication (Camerini et al., 2018). AMM leads to distraction (van der Schuur et al., 2020) and disengagement from the classroom (Hassoun, 2015). Research finds that students involved in AMM are likely to have lower academic performance.

Scholars are also interested in ICT use for educational activities (e.g., Aagaard, 2017; Cheung & Slavin, 2013; Verbruggen et al., 2021). Most researchers find a moderate positive effect of educational ICT use on academic achievement (Barrow et al., 2009; Cheung & Slavin, 2013). Some researchers suggest the effect to be negative or non-existent (Agasisti et al., 2020; Fariña et al., 2015), but report mixed findings when using different learning-related ICT measures (e.g., Hu et al., 2018).

Three groups of ICT measures are frequently used in empirical research: (1) ICT access, (2) ICT use for multitasking or non-academic activities, and (3) ICT use for other educational purposes. Obviously, different types of educational ICT activities (e.g., computer use for remedial learning, online search for academic information, and online communication with classmates about group projects) have different goals, and are likely to produce different learning results. Future studies should document these measurement differences when discussing findings from research articles and reports.

2.4 Differences in ICT Use in School

The fast growth of digital technologies has made the daily use of educational technology easier and more comprehensive. With new internet technology, people can now quickly access a massive amount of information to acquire new knowledge. As the result of the COVID-19 pandemic and school shutdowns, reliance on networked devices for online learning has increased dramatically since 2020. Online remote education is more important now than it has ever been. In this section, we discuss the prospects for ICT use in schools and examine the potential problems that are associated with the use of educational technology.

2.4.1 The Prospect of ICT in Schools

Millennials may acquire digital skills through trial and error at home, but not all of these skills can be self-taught. Without instruction and guidance from teachers, family members, or friends with ICT knowledge, millennials may become frustrated and discouraged when they encounter problems with ICT devices, and fail to find the answers that they want online.

van Dijk and van Deursen (2014) argue that it is possible for children to learn some basic operational and formal skills on their own. However, formal training is often needed if students wish to acquire more advanced content-related information, online communication, content creation, and online strategic skills. van Dijk and van Deursen (2014, pp. 121–122) suggest that:

> *[information skills] are not sufficiently learned at home, in practice or by trial and error. These skills, adapted to the context of computers and the Internet, might also be neglected at schools when teachers and school authorities equate digital skills with operational skills and only train information skills in the context of printed media and other traditional learning materials. Information skills are not automatically learned in computer and Internet operations. Many students of secondary and even tertiary education clearly lack information skills.*

Learning digital skills in formal education is even more important for students from low-income households, because these students have less digital access and adult guidance at home.

ICT use at school improves students' academic performance because, compared to the traditional "chalk and talk" method, ICT-aided instructions can increase students' motivation to attend courses or enhance their motivation to learn (Barrow et al., 2009). With a focus on the participation of Turkish college students in remote education,

Yilmaz and Keser (2016) randomly assigned students to three groups in an experimental study. Students in the first group completed a course with podcasts with the support of reflective thinking activities. Students in the second group completed the course with podcasts without those activities, and students in the last group simply watched videos. Yilmaz and Keser found that students in the first group showed greater motivation to learn than did the students in the other two groups. This suggests that online learning with well-designed reflective thinking activities can stimulate students' interest in learning.

Another study, by Orús et al. (2016), focuses on Spanish college students who participated in the creation of learner-generated videos on YouTube. Results suggest that this form of online activity is meaningful because it increases student engagement in class, enhances their interdisciplinary competence, and promotes their academic performance. Although these studies focus on college students, the results inform our study of secondary school students. In general, well-designed educational technology can help improve students' learning attitudes and their ability to stay engaged in their classwork.

Whether or not educational technology has positive effects on academic performance may depend on the type of the course and how academic performance is evaluated. Some courses require students to complete drills, practice, and memorization. The benefit of educational technology in courses like these may be limited. ICT also may not be very useful if a course requires intensive in-class discussions. In contrast, some courses are well-suited to ICT-assisted instruction. Barrow et al. (2009) studied algebra classes in several American high schools and reported that students who received computer-aided instruction (CAI) performed better in algebra tests than students who received traditional instruction. They also found that CAI is more useful in classes with a large number of students and high absentee rates. This may suggest that CAI can be an effective learning tool in mathematics courses where students feel less confident and are less engaged with the course content.

Likewise, students and teachers are likely to use e-learning strategies for different purposes, and different ICT applications may produce different learning results. A review by Cheung and Slavin (2013) highlights three forms of technology applications in schools. Supplemental CAI programs offer instruction in addition to regular courses in traditional classrooms. Computer-managed learning systems are designed to assess students' performance in courses such as mathematics and sciences, assign e-materials that fit students' ability, administer tests, and monitor progress. Finally, comprehensive models combine CAI with traditional instruction. Cheung and Slavin note that CAI has consistently moderate positive effects on students' performance in mathematics.

To summarize, the term "ICT use" may be defined and measured in several ways. Because educational technology can be applied in various forms and for different learning purposes, analysis of its effects on students should consider the ways in which ICT technology is used in school.

2.4.2 Problems Associated with ICT Use in School

At least three problems may reduce the positive effects of educational technology in school on educational outcomes. First, classroom multitasking, also known as AMM (van der Schuur et al., 2020), including texting messages, playing online games, and browsing social media sites during lecture, may impede students' academic progress and distract students from learning activities (Hassoun, 2015; Junco & Cotten, 2011). Scholars find that students who frequently use instant messaging (e.g., Facebook, Instagram, and Twitter) are more likely to have problems completing their schoolwork and have lower GPAs (Junco, 2012). van der Schuur et al. (2020) show that use of digital devices for non-academic purposes in class distracts adolescents from their educational activities. This is because using media multitasking and listening to the lecture at the same time cause information overload (Junco & Cotten, 2011, p. 370), which reduces students' capacity to concentrate on lectures and schoolwork (Mayer & Moreno, 2003). Hassoun (2015, p. 1691) notes that "students sitting in the front rows, who [were] rarely observed using media, often performed 'better' in the course and were more recognizable to [the instructor] through office hour visits."

Aagaard (2017) explains the ambivalent nature of educational technology: "when something good happens, we praise technology, but when something bad happens, we blame the students (occasionally, this blame also extends to their teachers)" (p. 1129). According to Aagaard (2017, p. 1140), "educational technologies open a gateway to the world that can be used both to bring relevant information into the space of the classroom (outside-in) and to escape educational activities in favor of off-task activity (inside-out). In both of these processes, educational technologies act neither as deciding factors nor as neutral tools." It is therefore important that researchers and educators understand how to distinguish "good ICT use" (e.g., using ICT to enhance or assist learning) from "bad ICT use" (e.g., multitasking).

Second, some courses require students to work under close supervision from instructors, considerable face-to-face interactions between students and teachers, and instant feedback from teachers. For these reasons, online teaching cannot replace traditional classroom teaching (Balkin & Sonnevend, 2016). Without a positive relationship with their instructors, students may lack confidence and feel anxious about the course (OECD, 2017). Some scholars suggest that online learning platforms should include interactive designs that enhance student–teacher relationships (Yilmaz & Keser, 2016).

Using large administrative data from 34 community and technical colleges in the U.S., Xu and Jaggars (2013) find that students who take online courses are more likely to withdraw and have lower grades than students in face-to-face courses. This is partly attributable to insufficient interpersonal interaction in online teaching environments. Jaggars and Xu (2016, p. 280) note that "[online] courses in which the instructor posted frequently, invited student questions through a variety of modalities, responded to student queries quickly, solicited and incorporated student feedback, and (perhaps most importantly) demonstrated a sense of 'caring' created an online environment that encouraged students to commit themselves to the course and perform at a stronger academic level."

Third, the extent to which teachers use classroom technology, their digital proficiency, and their experiences with or perceptions of the use of educational technology have a profound influence on students' experiences with educational technology. The attributes and attitudes of teachers play a key role in how ICT is likely to benefit students (Agasisti et al., 2020; van Dijk & van Deursen, 2014). Agasisti et al. (2020) highlight the importance of addressing "whether teachers are up to introducing ICT productively into the formal educational system" (p. 617). They suggest that educational technology can be useful to both educators and learners, but if students are not well instructed in how to use ICT in their schoolwork, they might not gain the knowledge and skills that they need. According to Agasisti et al. (2020, p. 617), remote teaching is more difficult when teachers "do not update their teaching methods to introduce more extensive use of ICT tools."

Research suggests that educational technology is most effective when students have the full support of their teachers (Verbruggen et al., 2021). This highlights the importance of proper guidance from teachers about the use of educational technology in class. For example, Kennisnet (2007) reports that in 2007, less than half of teachers in the Netherlands had enough confidence in their ICT skills, and therefore felt less capable of teaching these skills to their students. This is partly because many teachers do not often use computers in classrooms (van Dijk & van Deursen, 2014). Radovanović et al. (2015) show that in Serbia, some college professors are reluctant to adopt the new educational technology and even consider it a threat to their authority, expertise, and preferred teaching materials.

2.5 Differences in ICT Use at Home

In this section, we discuss the prospects and problems arising from the use of digital technologies at home. In our review of the literature, we highlight the importance of parents' or guardians' active participation in their children's online learning and other activities.

2.5.1 The Prospect of ICT at Home

Students can benefit from having computers, the internet, educational software, and e-tablet at home. Peck et al. (2002, pp. 475–476) suggest that "[students] became particularly tuned in academically when using computers…Technology offered these students what we called an "open door" toward improved academic work and, in some cases, fuller participation in the social side of school life." Fairlie et al. (2010) suggest that home computers may open the gate to self-learning, encourage students to stay in school, and reduce crime. Schmitt and Wadsworth (2006) argue that *[if computers] are used for information gathering and learning across a variety of subjects, or if [computers] help to increase individual experience of general computer skills, then a home computer might be reasonably considered as an input in an educational production function. This could then, theoretically, enhance children's demand for education and their future productivity. Increased familiarity with a computer, increased frequency of internet use, and computer-based learning programs could all help boost educational attainment and examination performance.* (p. 660)

In sum, just as computers have become indispensable in the workplace, computers and networked devices can be useful at home, particularly when children use them for learning and to complete school assignments. More school assignments now require extensive use of computers for word processing and other software programs in addition to online research. As a result, despite the possibility remains that ICT use may impede some students' academic progress, we cannot prevent children from accessing and using digital technologies at home. To maximize the positive effects of ICT use at home and minimize its negative effects, parents, educators, and scholars must understand the factors that may lead students to use ICT for activities that do not involve learning.

2.5.2 Problems Associated with ICT Use at Home

ICT use at home may distract students from schoolwork. Without the guidance of parents or guardians, students often struggle when using ICT at home for school tasks. Agasisti et al. (2020, p. 617) suggest that students may "over-report the amount of time they spend doing homework on their computers, providing a flawed picture of how long they really [spend] on schoolwork." The flawed picture may reflect children's immaturity or their lack of experience with educational apps, digital devices, and online learning. When using digital devices at home, children can be easily distracted by their ability to perform functions that are not related to learning, such as messaging, listening to music, and browsing other websites. As students advance, this issue becomes more critical as students stay up all night (OECD, 2019) to complete their schoolwork while engaging in other online activities.

In this connection, Vigdor et al. (2014) report that when high-speed internet connections are available in the home, students tend to spend more time on homework but less time on computers for learning. Some scholars cite the overuse of ICT for online gaming as a leading factor in the negative effects of home ICT use on educational performance (Malamud & Pop-Eleches, 2011). Without parental support and supervision, some children use digital devices only for gaming and online networking. Consequently, they struggle with "doing homework on computers without any real gain in extra skills and knowledge" (Agasisti et al., 2020, p. 617). Although policymakers and educators attempt to encourage students to integrate computers into learning activities, the effects of these efforts have been limited. This raises the concern that any potential benefits associated with educational technology may be compromised by counterproductive or inappropriate use of digital devices at home (Vigdor et al., 2014).

These issues suggest that parents and other adults at home should support, intervene in, or participate in their children's digital learning activities. Many children may find educational apps and learning websites unattractive (Attewell & Seel, 2003; Giacquinta et al., 1994), and only benefit from ICT use when their parents sit side-by-side with them to discuss what they are doing on computers (Attewell, 2001). Some researchers suggest that families should enhance the "social envelope" (Giacquinta et al., 1994) that provide both material (e.g., computers and educational software) and non-material resources (e.g., parent–child relationship, family activities, caring, and parenting) to support and scaffold children's experiences with ICT (Warschauer & Matuchniak, 2010). Without intervention or resources from their families, children may simply "turn home computers into game machines and word processors, rather than into learning resources" (Attewell, 2003, p. 27).

2.6 Effects of Digital Inclusion: Positive? Negative? Or Both?

To return to our original questions, how does digital inclusion affect adolescent students' outcomes? Why have researchers reached different conclusions regarding the relationships between ICT use and academic performance? As shown in this chapter, scholars suggest that inappropriate research designs or statistical analyses could lead to biased estimates of ICT's effects. Methodological concerns aside, it is important to understand the mechanisms that may explain the complicated relationships between ICT use and students' well-being. For instance, if researchers continue to find both positive and negative relationships between ICT use and test scores, how cautious should we be about the integration of ICT use in school settings and at home? Should teachers and parents consider restricting students' use of digital devices and online tools?

There are no simple answers to these questions. Eventually, the pressing questions that parents, teachers, and educational reformers must ask are: Why, when, and how can ICT promote or impede the well-being of young people? On one hand, inappropriate access to and use of ICT is detrimental to students' academic well-being. On the other hand, well-designed educational technology can be conducive to learning, particularly when teachers give clear instructions on how to use it for self-learning, parents can provide assistance and intervene in children's digital media activities, and students themselves know the importance of using digital devices and apps with caution. In this section, we contend that both positive and negative directions of the ICT effect coexist, leading to an inverse U-shaped relationship between ICT use and student outcomes.

2.6.1 An Inverted U-Shaped Relationship with Digital Use

This said, most empirical studies tend to conclude either positive or negative effects of ICT use. This is in part because many empirical studies model the effect of ICT use on academic outcomes as a linear relationship. Yet, a statistically insignificant linear effect does not necessarily mean that a relationship does not exist. Likewise, a negative linear association does not suggest that ICT use has no positive effect at all levels. As Thiessen and Looker (2007, p. 176) argue, "research which relies solely on direct linear measures runs the risk of underestimating the extent of the relationship, thereby ignoring important patterns which have serious practical implications." To be careful, researchers should consider examining whether or not there is a curvilinear relationship between the use of digital technologies and students' well-being.

Atteweel et al. (2003) examine the time-diary of children's daily home activities using the 1997 Panel Study of Income Dynamics data. They find that children who use computers at home for less than eight hours a week have significantly higher reading and math scores than children who do not. At the same time, home computer use for eight or more hours a week is associated with a reduction in time spent on sports or outdoor activities and an increase in body mass index. These findings suggest that *moderate* computer use at home benefits students' learning at home, but *overuse* of computers may limit the amount of time children spend on physical activities.

Using the PISA international data, other scholars have identified the curvilinear relationship between ICT use and student outcomes. For example, Fuchs and Wößmann (2004) report that compared to students who never use ICT at school, those who sometimes or occasionally use ICT perform better at school, but those who use ICT several times a week have lower school performance. They suggest that this inverse U-shaped relationship may occur because teachers might limit the use of computers in the classroom by underperforming students, or because an optimal level of ICT use (less than several times a week) might increase opportunities to learn at school. Thiessen and Looker (2007) examine Canadian students' ICT use, measured by digital access to school material, programming, and use of computers for word processing, spreadsheets, drawing, painting, and graphing, and find a curvilinear relationship between ICT use and school performance.

An official PISA report in 2009 also shows that the use of home computers, either for leisure activities or schoolwork, has an inverse U-shaped relationship (which PISA calls the mountain-shaped relationship) with students' performance in digital learning. The report suggests that moderate ICT use leads to better academic outcomes, but intensive use of ICT is likely to interfere with learning (OECD, 2011). Gubbels et al. (2020) examine the Dutch sample of the 2015 PISA data and report that students who moderately use ICT at school or at home and those with a moderate level of ICT interest have the highest performance in digitally assessed reading. In contrast, excessive access and use of ICT is associated with reductions in digital reading performance. Using propensity score matching to examine the PISA 2018 with a comparison of students across EU-15 countries, Agasisti et al. (2020) find that the intensive ICT use is negatively associated with academic performance, even when ICT is used mainly for educational purposes.

2.7 Summary and Conclusion

ICT use has altered the twenty-first-century educational landscape, a trend that has been accelerated and intensified by the COVID-19 pandemic. To date, scholars' recommendations for the optimal use of digital technologies in education, e-learning, and remote teaching are still inconclusive. In this chapter, we review the research literature to identify the methodological issues that may explain the inconsistent findings in scholarly research. The first methodological issue that may lead to under- or overestimations of ICT effects on academic achievement is selection and omitted variable bias due to research designs and choices of statistical methods. Another common methodological issue that is often overlooked by scholars is the wide variation in the measures of ICT access, ICT use, and forms of educational technology. We also suggest that the relationship between ICT use and student outcomes is likely curvilinear. Although these methodological issues may seem unintuitive and trivial for policymakers and school administrators, a careful discussion of these issues will permit a better understanding of the mechanisms that explain the relationships between ICT use and student well-being, to identify educational policies for ICT use in school, and to guide parents hoping to supervise their children's e-learning at home.

To conclude, it is important to consider if a curvilinear or inverse U-shaped relationship exists between ICT use and well-being. Our goal is to identify the patterns of ICT use, examine their effects on the lives of secondary students, and understand whether and how they affect educational outcomes. To achieve this goal, we reviewed the research literature on ICT use and education. This review provides the foundation of our empirical analysis in Chaps. 4, 5, and 6.

References

Aagaard, J. (2017). Breaking down barriers: The ambivalent nature of technologies in the classroom. *New Media & Society, 19*(7), 1127–1143. https://doi.org/10.1177/1461444816631505

Agasisti, T., Gil-Izquierdo, M., & Han, S. W. (2020). ICT use at home for school-related tasks: What is the effect on a student's achievement? Empirical evidence from OECD PISA data. *Education Economics, 28*(6), 601–620. https://doi.org/10.1080/09645292.2020.1822787

Angrist, J., & Lavy, V. (2002). New evidence on classroom computers and pupil learning. *The Economic Journal, 112*(482), 735–765.

Attewell, P. A. (2001). The first and second digital divides. *Sociology of Education, 74*(3), 252–259.

Attewell, P. A. (2003). Beyond the digital divide. In P. A. Attewell & N. M. Seel (Eds.), *Disadvantaged teens and computer technologies* (pp. 15–34). Waxmann.

Attewell, P. A., & Battle, J. (1999). Home computers and school performance. *The Information Society, 15*(1), 1–10.

Attewell, P. A., & Seel, N. M. (2003). *Disadvantaged teens and computer technologies*. Waxmann.

Attewell, P. A., Suazo-Garcia, B., & Battle, J. (2003). Computers and young children: Social benefit or social problem? *Social Forces, 82*(1), 277–296. https://doi.org/10.1353/sof.2003.0075

Balkin, J. M., & Sonnevend, J. (2016). The digital transformation of education. In C. Greenhow, J. Sonnevend, & C. Agur (Eds.), *Education and social media: Toward a digital future* (pp. 9–24). MIT Press. https://oxfordindex.oup.com/view/10.7551/mitpress/9780262034470.003.0003?lang=en, https://oxfordindex.oup.com:443/view/10.7551/mitpress/9780262034470.003.0003

Barrow, L., Markman, L., & Rouse, C. E. (2009). Technology's edge: The educational benefits of computer-aided instruction. *American Economic Journal: Economic Policy, 1*(1), 52–74. https://doi.org/10.1257/pol.1.1.52

Beuermann, D., Cristia, J., Cruz-Aguayo, Y., Cueto, S., & Malamud, O. (2013). Home computers and child outcomes: Short-term impacts from a randomized experiment in Peru. *NBER Working Paper Series, 18818*. https://doi.org/10.3386/w18818

Biagi, F., & Loi, M. (2013). Measuring ICT use and learning outcomes: Evidence from recent econometric studies. *European Journal of Education, 48*, 28–42. https://doi.org/10.2307/23357044

Camerini, A.-L., Schulz, P. J., & Jeannet, A.-M. (2018). The social inequalities of Internet access, its use, and the impact on children's academic performance: Evidence from a longitudinal study in Switzerland. *New Media & Society, 20*(7), 2489–2508. https://doi.org/10.1177/1461444817725918

Cheung, A. C. K., & Slavin, R. E. (2013). The effectiveness of educational technology applications for enhancing mathematics achievement in K-12 classrooms: A meta-analysis. *Educational Research Review, 9*, 88–113. https://doi.org/10.1016/j.edurev.2013.01.001

Coates, D., Humphreys, B. R., Kane, J., & Vachris, M. A. (2004). "No significant distance" between face-to-face and online instruction: Evidence from principles of economics. *Economics of Education Review, 23*(5), 533–546. https://doi.org/10.1016/j.econedurev.2004.02.002

Cristia, J., Ibarrarán, P., Cueto, S., Santiago, A., & Severín, E. (2017). Technology and child development: Evidence from the one laptop per child program. *American Economic Journal: Applied Economics, 9*(3), 295–320. https://doi.org/10.1257/app.20150385

Fairlie, R. W., Beltran, D. O., & Das, K. K. (2010). Home computers and educational outcomes: Evidence from the NLSY97 and CPS. *Economic Inquiry, 48*(3), 771–792. https://doi.org/10.1111/j.1465-7295.2009.00218.x

Fairlie, R. W., & London, R. A. (2012). The effects of home computers on educational outcomes: Evidence from a field experiment with community college students. *The Economic Journal, 122*(561), 727–753. https://doi.org/10.1111/j.1468-0297.2011.02484.x

Fairlie, R. W., & Robinson, J. (2013). Experimental evidence on the effects of home computers on academic achievement among schoolchildren. *American Economic Journal: Applied Economics, 5*(3), 211–240. https://doi.org/10.1257/app.5.3.211

Fariña, P., San Martín, E., Preiss, D. D., Claro, M., & Jara, I. (2015). Measuring the relation between computer use and reading literacy in the presence of endogeneity. *Computers & Education, 80*, 176–186. https://doi.org/10.1016/j.compedu.2014.08.010

Fuchs, T., & Wößmann, L. (2004). Computers and student learning: Bivariate and multivariate evidence on the availability and use of computers at home and at school. *Brussels Economic Review, 47*(3–4), 359–386.

Fuchs, T., & Wößmann, L. (2005). *Computers and student learning: Bivariate and multivariate evidence on the availability and use of computers at home and at school* (Ifo Working Paper 8). University of Munich. www.ifo.de

Fuchs, T., & Wößmann, L. (2007). What accounts for international differences in student performance? *Empirical Economics, 32*(2/3), 433–464. https://doi.org/10.1007/s00181-006-0087-0

Giacquinta, J. B., Bauer, J. A., & Levin, J. E. (1994). *Beyond technology's promise: An examination of children's educational computing at home*. Cambridge University Press.

Gonzales, A. L. (2015). The contemporary US digital divide: From initial access to technology maintenance. *Information, Communication & Society, 19*(2), 234–248. https://doi.org/10.1080/1369118X.2015.1050438

Gonzales, A. L., Calarco, J. M., & Lynch, T. (2020). Technology problems and student achievement gaps: A validation and extension of the technology maintenance construct. *Communication Research, 47*(5), 750–770. https://doi.org/10.1177/0093650218796366

Gubbels, J., Swart, N. M., & Groen, M. A. (2020). Everything in moderation: ICT and reading performance of Dutch 15-year-olds. *Large-Scale Assessments in Education, 8*(1), 17. https://doi.org/10.1186/s40536-020-0079-0

Hassoun, D. (2015). "All over the place": A case study of classroom multitasking and attentional performance. *New Media & Society, 17*(10), 1680–1695. https://doi.org/10.1177/1461444814531756

Hu, X., Gong, Y., Lai, C., & Leung, F. K. S. (2018). The relationship between ICT and student literacy in mathematics, reading, and science across 44 countries: A multilevel analysis. *Computers & Education, 125*, 1–13. https://doi.org/10.1016/j.compedu.2018.05.021

Jackson, L. A., von Eye, A., Biocca, F. A., Barbatsis, G., Zhao, Y., & Fitzgerald, H. E. (2006). Does home internet use influence the academic performance of low-income children? *Developmental Psychology, 42*(3), 429–435. https://doi.org/10.1037/0012-1649.42.3.429

Jaggars, S. S., & Xu, D. (2016). How do online course design features influence student performance? *Computers & Education, 95*, 270–284. https://doi.org/10.1016/j.compedu.2016.01.014

James, J. (2010). New technology in developing countries: A critique of the one-laptop-per-child program. *Social Science Computer Review, 28*(3), 381–390. https://doi.org/10.1177/0894439309346398

Junco, R. (2012). In-class multitasking and academic performance. *Computers in Human Behavior, 28*(6), 2236–2243. https://doi.org/10.1016/j.chb.2012.06.031

Junco, R., & Cotten, S. R. (2011). Perceived academic effects of instant messaging use. *Computers & Education, 56*(2), 370–378. https://doi.org/10.1016/j.compedu.2010.08.020

Kennisnet. (2007). *Vier in balans monitor, stand vanzaken over ict in het onderwijs*. http://web.kennisnet2.nl/portal/onderzoek/onderzoeken/monitoring/fourinbalancemonitor

Malamud, O., & Pop-Eleches, C. (2011). Home computer use and the development of human capital. *The Quarterly Journal of Economics, 126*(2), 987–1027. https://doi.org/10.1093/qje/qjr008

Mayer, R. E., & Moreno, R. (2003). Nine ways to reduce cognitive load in multimedia learning. *Educational Psychologist, 38*(1), 43–52. https://doi.org/10.1207/s15326985ep3801_6

Mo, D., Swinnen, J., Zhang, L., Yi, H., Qu, Q., Boswell, M., & Rozelle, S. (2013). Can one-to-one computing narrow the digital divide and the educational gap in China? The case of Beijing migrant schools. *World Development, 46*, 14–29.

NSW. (2020, October 20). *All NSW public schools to benefit from internet upgrades*. NSW Government. https://education.nsw.gov.au/news/latest-news/all-nsw-public-schools-to-benefit-from-internet-upgrades

OECD. (2011). *PISA 2009 results: Students on line: Digital technologies and performance* (Vol. VI). OECD. https://doi.org/10.1787/9789264112995-en

OECD. (2017). *PISA 2015 results* (Vol. III)*: Students' well-being*. OECD. https://doi.org/10.1787/9789264273856-en

OECD. (2019). *PISA 2018 results* (Vol. II)*: Where all students can succeed*. PISA, OECD. https://doi.org/10.1787/b5fd1b8f-en

OECD. (2020). *Education responses to covid-19: Embracing digital learning and online collaboration*. OECD. https://www.oecd.org/coronavirus/policy-responses/education-responses-to-covid-19-embracing-digital-learning-and-online-collaboration-d75eb0e8/

Orús, C., Barlés, M. J., Belanche, D., Casaló, L., Fraj, E., & Gurrea, R. (2016). The effects of learner-generated videos for YouTube on learning outcomes and satisfaction. *Computers & Education, 95*, 254–269. https://doi.org/10.1016/j.compedu.2016.01.007

Peck, C., Cuban, L., & Kirkpatrick, H. (2002). Techno-promoter dreams, student realities. *Phi Delta Kappan, 83*(6), 472–480. https://doi.org/10.1177/003172170208300614

Radovanović, D., Hogan, B., & Lalić, D. (2015). Overcoming digital divides in higher education: Digital literacy beyond Facebook. *New Media & Society, 17*(10), 1733–1749. https://doi.org/10.1177/1461444815588323

Scheerder, A. J., van Deursen, A. J., & van Dijk, J. A. (2017). Determinants of Internet skills, uses and outcomes: A systematic review of the second- and third-level digital divide. *Telematics and Informatics, 34*(8), 1607–1624. https://doi.org/10.1016/j.tele.2017.07.007

Schmitt, J., & Wadsworth, J. (2006). Is there an impact of household computer ownership on children's educational attainment in Britain? *Economics of Education Review, 25*(6), 659–673. https://doi.org/10.1016/j.econedurev.2005.06.001

Schulz-Hardt, S., Frey, D., Lüthgens, C., & Moscovici, S. (2000). Biased information search in group decision making. *Journal of Personality and Social Psychology, 78*(4), 655–669. https://doi.org/10.1037//0022-3514.78.4.655

Tengtrakul, P., & Peha, J. M. (2013). Does ICT in schools affect residential adoption and adult utilization outside schools? *Telecommunications Policy, 37*(6), 540–562. https://doi.org/10.1016/j.telpol.2013.01.002

Thiessen, V., & Looker, D. (2007). Digital divides and capital conversion: The optimal use of information and communication technology for youth reading achievement. *Information, Communication & Society, 10*, 159–180. https://doi.org/10.1080/13691180701307370

UNESCO-UIS. (2014). *Information and communication technology (ICT) in education in Asia: A comparative analysis of ICT integration and e-readiness in schools across Asia.* United Nations Educational, Scientific and Cultural Organization, Institute for Statistics. http://uis.unesco.org/sites/default/files/documents/information-communication-technologies-education-asia-ict-integration-e-readiness-schools-2014-en_0.pdf

van der Schuur, W. A., Baumgartner, S. E., Sumter, S. R., & Valkenburg, P. M. (2020). Exploring the long-term relationship between academic-media multitasking and adolescents' academic achievement. *New Media & Society, 22*(1), 140–158. https://doi.org/10.1177/1461444819861956

van Deursen, A. J., & van Dijk, J. A. (2019). The first-level digital divide shifts from inequalities in physical access to inequalities in material access. *New Media & Society, 21*(2), 354–375. https://doi.org/10.1177/1461444818797082

van Dijk, J. A. G. M., & van Deursen, A. J. (2014). Solutions: Learning digital skills. In J. A. G. M. van Dijk & A. J. van Deursen (Eds.), *Digital skills: Unlocking the information society* (pp. 113–138). Palgrave Macmillan US. https://doi.org/10.1057/9781137437037_6

Verbruggen, S., Depaepe, F., & Torbeyns, J. (2021). Effectiveness of educational technology in early mathematics education: A systematic literature review. *International Journal of Child-Computer Interaction, 27*. Scopus. https://doi.org/10.1016/j.ijcci.2020.100220

Vigdor, J. L., Ladd, H. F., & Martinez, E. (2014). Scaling the digital divide: Home computer technology and student achievement. *Economic Inquiry, 52*(3), 1103–1119. https://doi.org/10.1111/ecin.12089

Wainer, J., Vieira, P., & Melguizo, T. (2015). The association between having access to computers and Internet and educational achievement for primary students in Brazil. *Computers & Education, 80*, 68–76. https://doi.org/10.1016/j.compedu.2014.08.007

Warschauer, M., & Matuchniak, T. (2010). New technology and digital worlds: Analyzing evidence of equity in access, use, and outcomes. *Review of Research in Education, 34*(1), 179–225. https://doi.org/10.3102/0091732X09349791

Warschauer, M., & Newhart, V. A. (2016). Broadening our concepts of universal access. *Universal Access in the Information Society, 15*(2), 183–188. https://doi.org/10.1007/s10209-015-0417-0

Warschauer, M., & Xu, Y. (2018). Technology and equity in education. In J. Voogt, G. Knezek, R. Christensen, & K.-W. Lai (Eds.), *Second handbook of information technology in primary and secondary education* (pp. 1–17). Springer International Publishing. https://doi.org/10.1007/978-3-319-53803-7_76-1

Xu, D., & Jaggars, S. S. (2013). The impact of online learning on students' course outcomes: Evidence from a large community and technical college system. *Economics of Education Review, 37*, 46–57. https://doi.org/10.1016/j.econedurev.2013.08.001

Yilmaz, F. G. K., & Keser, H. (2016). The impact of reflective thinking activities in e-learning: A critical review of the empirical research. *Computers & Education, 95*, 163–173. https://doi.org/10.1016/j.compedu.2016.01.006

Chapter 3
Literature on the Socioeconomic Digital Learning Divide

Abstract An important goal of this study is to examine the causes of the digital learning divide and the differential effects of ICT use in education on the outcomes of students from socially advantaged and disadvantaged backgrounds. This chapter examines the research literature and discusses the theoretical foundations of the digital divide. The discussion begins with an elaboration of three types of digital divide that emerged with the rapid development of digital technology and the growing reliance on ICT in schools, followed by an analysis of digital inequalities at home and in school by students' socioeconomic status. We suggest that students from socially advantaged families are more likely to use ICT at home for educational and productive purposes, feel more comfortable to apply their digital skills in school and receive more rewards from teachers, and eventually benefit from ICT use more than students from disadvantaged families. This discussion lays the foundation for our empirical analyses in Chaps. 4 through 7.

Keywords Digital divide · Digital inequality · ICT access · Digital competence · Socioeconomic background · Parental mediation · Role of teachers · Home and school contexts

INCONSISTENT findings and policy recommendations regarding ICT use and student outcomes stem from the methodological considerations in research on ICT use in education, and from the mechanisms that underlie the causal relationships between educational use of ICT and the outcome of students from socially advantaged and disadvantaged backgrounds. In this chapter, we focus on the causes of the digital learning divide. We review the three levels of digital divide that have emerged since the 1990s and through today's COVID-19 pandemic. We examine the research literature and discuss the theoretical foundations of the digital divide. We explore the following questions: Who is excluded from ICT? In what ways? How serious is the digital learning divide as a social problem? Most importantly, how does ICT use differentially affect the learning opportunities and educational outcomes of students from different socioeconomic backgrounds?

J. K.-H. Ma and S. Cheng, *Adolescent Well-being and ICT UseX*,
Human Well-Being Research and Policy Making,
https://doi.org/10.1007/978-3-031-04412-0_3

3.1 Digital Learning Divide in the Twenty-First Century

Does the digital learning divide still exist? In the first decade of the twenty-first century, many people believed that the digital divide would no longer be a major social problem in developed societies and that digital inequality will be attenuated as time went by. As we move to the second and the third decades of the twenty-first century—even before the outbreak of COVID-19—it has become increasingly clear that the problem of the digital divide would persist. Across the globe, digital divide has evolved into several forms. The more we integrate ICT in education and the more we depend on it, the more pronounced the divide in both e-learning and ICT access, especially during the pandemic period.

In this chapter, we discuss different forms of the digital divide, elaborate upon the influence of social class, and explain how parental socioeconomic background can determine students' digital learning opportunities and their outcomes associated with ICT use. We also extend our discussion of whether ICT use reduces or widens the learning gap along socioeconomic lines and whether digital inclusion may generate new forms of educational inequality.

3.2 Theoretical Explanations on the Digital Learning Divide

This section discusses the three levels of the digital divide. The first level focuses on differences in digital access. The second level is concerned with variations in digital skills and how computers and the internet are used. In combination with the other two divides, the third level contends that there may be a growing socioeconomic disparity in the learning benefits of ICT use between socioeconomically advantaged and disadvantaged students. Figure 3.1 depicts the digital learning gap.

3.2.1 The First-Level Digital Learning Divide

Since the turn of the millennium, a burgeoning body of literature has reviewed the causes of the digital divide. Researchers have identified three types (Mihelj et al., 2018; Scheerder et al., 2017; van Deursen et al., 2017). The first level of the digital learning divide is concerned with discrepancies between those who do and do not have access to computers and the internet (DiMaggio et al., 2004; van Deursen & van Dijk, 2019). Some scholars have examined the problem of insufficient computer access in schools and the lack of ICT infrastructure (Becker, 2000; Selwyn et al., 2009; Warschauer & Newhart, 2016). Others focus on unequal access to digital technology at home (Attewell & Battle, 1999; Hilbert, 2016; Morgan & Vanlengen, 2005; Scheerder et al., 2019; Warschauer et al., 2004). To reduce this

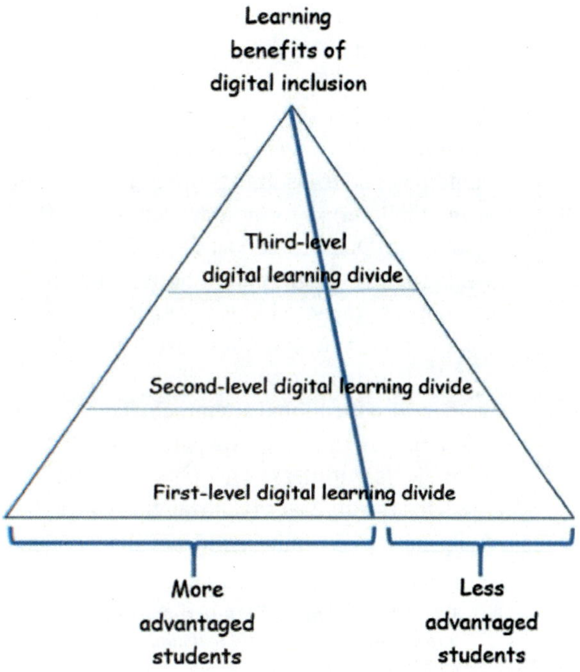

Fig. 3.1 The three levels of the digital learning divide

digital inequality, governments in developed countries have invested in educational policies, projects, and initiatives to increase computers, laptops, online interactive platforms, and internet coverage in schools (Erichsen & Salajan, 2014; Sefton-Green et al., 2016; UNESCO, 2000; Warschauer & Newhart, 2016). They have also made efforts to build an ICT infrastructure (e.g., landline, high-speed broadband services, iCloud services, and the provision of free Wi-fi in public places) in order to stimulate economic growth (Cruz-Jesus et al., 2017; Lechman, 2015; Zhang, 2013) and increase people's motivation to upgrade ICT devices in their homes (Lee et al., 2015; Ma et al., 2019).

3.2.2 The Second-Level Digital Learning Divide

Because access to digital devices and the internet does not always lead to students' use of ICT for learning at home or in school, it is important to examine variations in the types of online activities students are involved in, disparities in their digital skills, and their ICT literacy (Attewell, 2001; Dolan, 2016; Hargittai, 2002; van Deursen et al., 2014; van Deursen & van Dijk, 2014b). An underlying argument is that even if students of different sociodemographic backgrounds have equal access to computers and the internet, the socioeconomic divide in digital use and ICT skills will remain (Leu et al., 2015; Ma et al., 2019; Scheerder et al., 2019). Past empirical research has provided ample evidence that students with highly educated parents and/or from affluent families are more likely to use ICT for educational activities and for productive purposes (e.g., online information search) than are their peers from disadvantaged socioeconomic backgrounds (Attewell, 2003; Ma et al., 2019; Yuen et al., 2018).

Some students are more likely to use ICT for learning or enhancing their understanding of course subjects, whereas others are more likely to spend most of their time using the internet for non-academic activities (Attewell, 2003; Peter & Valkenburg, 2006; van Deursen & van Dijk, 2014a). On average, students from working-class backgrounds, single-parent households, and whose parents have lower educational attainment are more likely to engage in online gaming, texting, and social networking than in academic activities (Attewell, 2003; van Deursen & van Dijk, 2014a).

This socioeconomic divide is not new. In fact, scholars suggest that individuals with more educational attainment have always been more likely to acquire knowledge when they read the newspapers, watch the television, and listen to the radio than are individuals with less. This phenomenon, known as the knowledge gap thesis, long predated the digital era (DiMaggio et al., 2004; Tichenor et al., 1970). Attewell (2003, p. 28) makes a similar argument in his discussion of the "*Sesame Street* Effect":

> *This pattern of unequal outcomes is familiar to social scientists as the "Sesame Street Effect." When that children's TV program was first developed, the intention was to narrow the skills gap between poor and affluent kindergarten children, by exposing very young, disadvantaged children to numbers and letters. Unfortunately, already-advantaged children watched the TV program more often and more productively. Consequently, the skill gaps between affluent and poor children entering kindergarten increased substantially after the program became popular.*

Recent scholars have called for a closer analysis of the multidimensional construct of the digital divide. In this second-level digital learning divide, new inequalities emerge because of discrepancies in where and how people access and use ICT, what they do online, their ICT skills, and their digital literacy (van Deursen et al., 2014; van Dijk & van Deursen, 2014). Some scholars believe that, at least in developed countries, the first-level digital divide has decreased since 2000. As we discuss below, the first-level digital divide resurged along with the second in the 2010s (Calvani et al., 2012; Leu et al., 2015; Rafalow, 2018; van Deursen & van Diepen, 2013).

3.2.3 The Resurgence of the First-Level Digital Learning Divide

Since the late 2010s, the first-level digital divide has again received scholarly attention (Gonzales, 2015; Gonzales et al., 2020), partly because of the rapid development of information and communication technology, the availability of a large variety of digital devices, and "the reality that not all of the materials provide the same online opportunities" (van Deursen & van Dijk, 2019, p. 355). New laptops, tablets, smart TVs, software subscriptions, and peripherals (e.g., monitors, scanners, printers, and external hard drives) came onto the market. Most software, apps, and online cloud services are not free. Not everyone can afford the newest digital devices, unlimited high-speed internet, and the use of software. This, again, leads to the digital divide in ICT access and use of different digital devices and computer programs at home. Many studies have reported that socioeconomically disadvantaged people tend to rely on less sophisticated or poorly functioned computers for work or study (Gonzales et al., 2020; Rideout & Katz, 2016).

In response to the resurgence of the first-level digital divide, Mihelj et al. (2018, p. 1470) note that "as one divide closes, another opens up with the advent of new hardware, software, speed of connection to the Internet and so on." Van Deursen and van Dijk (2019) suggest that it is important to examine inequalities in ICT in terms of (1) differences in device opportunities, such as the availability of using other devices with different functions and capacities as replacements; (2) differences in the diversity of ICT devices and peripherals in the household; and (3) variation in the maintenance costs of devices and peripherals as well as the monthly cost of high-speed broadband. The resurgence of the first-level divide coupled with the emergence of the second-level digital divide in the 2010s has only made it more difficult for educators and educational researchers to find policy to address the digital inequality problem for the new generation.

3.2.4 The Third-Level Digital Learning Divide

Scholars have recently called for an extension to examine the third-level digital learning divide. This divide focuses on the unequal outcomes of and variations in tangible benefits derived from the use of digital technologies (Scheerder et al., 2017; Valdez & Javier, 2020; Wei et al., 2011). Scholars argue that digital inequality is present when the benefits of ICT do not accrue equally across sociodemographic groups, which may exacerbate social inequalities (Scheerder et al., 2017). This new form of digital divide suggests that it is important to assess two issues when tackling the digital inequality problem: Does the use of educational technology benefit students' learning process and their academic performance? Do the benefits accrued from educational technology differ between students of various social and economic background characteristics? Scholars generally agree that student socioeconomic background moderates the relationship between ICT use and educational outcomes (Attewell & Battle, 1999; Warschauer & Matuchniak, 2010). We now discuss how students' socioeconomic background may affect their digital learning opportunities at home and in school, which may then affect whether or not they benefit from ICT use.

3.3 Digital Learning Divide by SES in Home Environments

3.3.1 Differences in How to Use ICT

Both the first- and second-level digital divides affect families of different socioeconomic status. Home environments shape the quality and quantity of digital resources that students can use and how they use them. Early research by Attewell and Battle (1999) reports that students from high-SES families tend to receive more educational gains from home computers than did students from low-SES families. Affluent and highly educated parents are more likely to appreciate the importance of parental involvement in children's ICT activities and are more likely to provide a good learning environment at home with computers (Attewell & Battle, 1999). As Attewell (2003, p. 23) notes, "the best educational use of computers occurs when an adult sits alongside a child at the machine, discussing what the child is doing."

Studies in the United States (Leu et al., 2015; Vigdor et al., 2014), the United Kingdom (Davies, 2018; Livingstone & Helsper, 2008), the Netherlands (Peter & Valkenburg, 2006; Scheerder et al., 2019), Australia (Smith et al., 2013; Starkey & Finger, 2018), Hong Kong (Yuen et al., 2018), and South Korea (Park et al., 2016) have consistently found digital gaps among families of different socioeconomic status. In all of these countries, researchers conclude that students with highly educated or affluent parents are more likely to use ICT for learning or productive activities. In the U.S., for instance, Leu et al. (2015) report that students who grow up in high-income neighborhoods are at least one year ahead of students who grow up in middle- or low-income neighborhoods in online research skills and comprehension of online information. This digital divide extends the persistent reading achievement gap from offline to online reading. Vigdor et al. (2014, p. 1105) suggest that because parents with better parenting strategies "can serve as more effective instructors in the productive use of online resources," the introduction of home computers and broadband internet amplifies class and racial inequalities in academic achievement. Without help and supervision from their parents, students may use ICT in an unproductive way that undermines learning.

Evidence from research outside of the United States also shows that higher SES people are more likely than lower-SES people to explore the potential benefits of ICT. They are also more likely to question the validity of online information. In Britain, Davies (2018) finds that students from working-class families are more likely to use and trust whatever they find on a Google search. This is different from their high-SES peers, who are more likely to invest in the logic of practice of their e-learning field, to show their critical thinking ability, and to identify "the difference between scientific facts and pseudoscience" (p. 2773) in an online search. Researchers in South Korea have found increased demand for online private tutoring services that customize course content to help student customers prepare for and earn higher grades on the national college entrance exam (Park et al., 2016). Because only socioeconomically privileged students can afford these services, this growth in demand may widen the second digital divide (Choe, 2009).

In Switzerland, Camerini et al. (2018) find that children from low-income households are more likely to use the internet for entertainment and social networking. Because family SES mediates the types of online activities students engage in, ICT use has an indirect negative effect on the academic performance of low-income students. Leung and Lee (2012) and Yuen et al. (2018) report similar findings in Hong Kong, which suggest that students with lower-SES parents use the internet primarily for communicating with peers and gaming.

3.3.2 Differences in Computer Games and Online Gaming

Playing computer games and online gaming can stimulate cognitive development and interest in learning, and improve students' multimedia skills (Andrews, 2008; Gee, 2007; Hamari et al., 2016; Ito et al., 2013). Studies show that students from various socioeconomic backgrounds tend to play different types of games and derive different experiences from them.

Andrews (2008) examines the socioeconomic differences in students' game plays. She compares casual games (puzzles, word, and card games), computer games, fantasy games, and sports games, and concludes that socioeconomically disadvantaged students are more likely to play sports and console video games. They are less likely to play the type of games that are more sophisticated in design (e.g., MMORPGs) and require complex controls or complex simulation. In contrast, socioeconomically advantaged students may play any type of games, including games that involve strategic planning and simulation and are thought to help stimulate players' learning interest. Compared to low-SES gamers, high-SES gamers are more likely to play with other friends and read magazines or (e)articles about how to beat a game or jump levels. This is consistent with Attewell and Winston (2003), who suggest that socioeconomically advantaged students are more likely to participate in online activities that involve extensive use of search engines to learn about particular topics or intense engagement with multimedia content. In contrast, the online activities by disadvantaged students are often limited by their lack of writing and reading skills.

3.3.3 Differences in Digital Resources at Home

People in affluent societies have more access to computers and the internet at home than do people in low-income societies. However, within-society variations in the conditions and the quality of digital access are still substantial. Even in affluent societies, socioeconomically disadvantaged people are still more likely than their advantaged counterparts to use digital devices that are old, borrowed, or that have spotty internet connections. They are also more likely to share devices.

A recent study in the United States by Gonzales et al. (2020) shows that a majority of low-income and racial minority college students do their schoolwork on poorly functioning laptops. These students often experience the loss of their internet connection, slow and broken hardware, and data limits. Gonzales et al. (2020) also find that students tend to have lower GPAs when they have cell phone plans with limited internet access, have others who pay for their data overage, or have poorly functioning laptops.

Using the term "technology maintenance," Gonzales (2014) explains that "participants described a variety of [ICT] access barriers that demonstrate the constant effort to ensure stable access, even after initial access, defined as in-home or public access, was acquired" (p. 241). Technology maintenance consists of (1) coping with disruptions in access, (2) sustaining access, and (3) achieving access. Socioeconomically and racially disadvantaged students tend to be stuck in the first stage, and often struggle to gain digital equality (Gonzales et al., 2020). This form of the digital access divide is problematic. When students use computers that are too slow or outdated for school-related tasks, those students are less likely to benefit from their use of digital technology (Agasisti et al., 2020).

3.4 Digital Learning Divide by SES in School Context

ICT resources are more equally distributed across schools in affluent societies than in poor and developing societies (ITU, 2018; Ma et al., 2019; UNESCO-UIS, 2014). However, a clear second-level digital learning divide in school remains. This form of persistent digital inequality is often closely related to differences in teachers' ICT knowledge and computer experience (Graves, 2019; Hughes et al., 2015; Warschauer, 2016), the educational expectations teachers have of their students (Rafalow, 2014, 2018), whether teachers treat ICT as a source of skills or distractions (Davies, 2018; Rafalow, 2018), and the institutional settings and cultural features of schools (Agirdag et al., 2012; Jack, 2016).

3.4.1 Differences in Digital Resources in School

Scholars have offered at least two explanations for the digital divide in schools. The first explanation highlights the importance of school resources and suggests that variations in school-level resources—both in the forms of material (e.g., classroom equipment, the provision of ICT devices and applications, and financial support) and non-material resources (e.g., teacher quality, teachers' expertise on educational technology, and students' prior knowledge on ICT and other course subjects)—determine e-learning opportunities in the classroom. For example, Warschauer et al. (2004) suggest that high-SES schools are more likely than low-SES schools to hire full-time ICT staff and develop digital support networks among teachers and other personnel in order to use educational technology. In contrast, the teachers' digital competence and experiences in ICT instruction in low-SES schools are low (Warschauer, 2016). Perhaps teachers in lower-SES schools are less confident in their ICT use and are more reluctant to integrate advanced e-materials into their class instructions. In this connection, Robinson (2014) suggests that disadvantaged students are more likely to attend schools that do not offer enough ICT training or provide advanced-level computer courses.

When most students in a school come from a disadvantaged socioeconomic background, teachers often feel unsure whether their students have digital access at home and know how to use a computer and digital technology (Hughes et al., 2015). Consequently, teachers focus on teaching basic digital literacy such as basic computer and software use. In high-SES schools, in contrast, teachers tend to assume that students have already learned these skills at home and therefore spend more class time on how to use ICT for research and analytics, how to master software programs (e.g., PowerPoint), and how to make better presentations using multimedia (Warschauer et al., 2004). Becker (2000) suggests that teachers in high-SES schools are more likely to teach students how to make presentations, how to analyze online information, and how to participate in complex simulations on computers. This is a stark difference from teachers in low-SES schools, who seem to adopt less constructive and more traditional teaching strategies in classrooms and devote much of their attention to the use of computers for remedial activities (e.g., drills and practice exercises).

Resource-poor and low-SES schools are likely to encounter barriers to the integration of ICT. These barriers include the lack of qualified or certified teachers, staff shortages, and dilapidated classrooms. Additionally, a significant number of students in resource-poor and low-SES schools not only are economically or socially underprivileged but also have lower academic performance in core subjects such as reading and math. Consequently, even when low-SES or academically underperforming schools invest in ICT devices and infrastructure (e.g., desktops, tablets, and head projectors), the improvement of students' learning of ICT skills and other subjects is limited. Often, other expenditures that are vital to run these resource-poor schools drain the investment on educational technology, and school administrations struggle with the allocation or misallocation of educational resources for different needs (Natriello, 2001).

3.4.2 Differences in the Culture and Institutional Contexts of School

The second explanation of the digital divide in school focuses on the influence of schools' cultural contexts and their institutional arrangements (Agirdag et al., 2012; Bowles & Gintis, 2002, 2011; Goode, 2010; Ma, 2021; Rafalow, 2020). Even among schools with similar levels of digital access and e-learning resources, teachers may evaluate students' educational performance, attitudes, and digital competencies very differently because of the institutional settings of schools, their cultures, and their students' socioeconomic characteristics (Rafalow, 2018). Cultural differences in social class exist not only in school, but also in the family and community. According to Bowles and Gintis' (2002, 2011) correspondence principle, schools socialize middle-class students to learn advanced skills and develop critical thinking and creativity competencies, which prepare these students for managerial or professional positions. In contrast, teachers tend to guide working-class students to accept authority and obey rules, which, then, leads to working-class jobs. In schools with mostly low-income and disadvantaged students, teachers are more likely to undervalue students' cognitive development and underestimate their learning potential as well as their chances to succeed. In schools with mostly upper- and middle-class students, teachers are more likely to encourage students to engage in interactive, creative, and self-learning activities. Overall, schools with resources have more positive teacher–student interaction than resource-poor schools (Jack, 2016).

The cultural distinction within and between schools determines how students experience e-learning, the kinds of online learning activities they participate in, and how they perceive the potential benefits of educational technology (Goode, 2010; Graves, 2019; Rafalow, 2014; Warschauer, 2016). Rafalow (2018) proposes the notion of "digital play" to describe the idea that young people develop digital skills through online play with their peers. With government-led educational reforms and emphasis on the importance of digital skills for learning in the twenty-first century, these skills could help students' learning in school.

In his field study of American high schools, Rafalow (2018) illustrates how the social class composition of a school interacts with the way teachers discipline students' digital play, regardless of the students' ICT competence and their teachers' technical expertise. Students develop digital skills and online experiences at home and bring these experiences and online communication and production skills to school. When they enter schools, however, they discover that teachers take very different disciplinary approaches to their digital play and ICT skills. In high-SES schools, teachers tell students that their ICT skills are valuable and essential for learning; in low-SES schools, teachers perceive students' ICT skills as a threat to classroom discipline or as irrelevant to their education. Rafalow (2018, p. 1446) writes:

> *…only Heathcliff students, [which were predominantly wealthy and white], reported an overlap between digital play and schooling that led them to pursue their interest-driven digital play during class. A key effect wat that these privileged students came to see schooling itself as a malleable setting where they could tinker with institutional norms and shape educational ideals. Social reproduction of inequality still occurred, however, because it is only privileged students—not minority and working-class youth—who were given the pedestal needed to go "under the hood" and ramp schooling up for the digital age. Disciplining play is thus how schools shape students' consciousness by differently cultivating digital laborers, rule followers, and 21st-century tinkerers.*

Paino and Renzulli (2013) use the concept of digital cultural capital to expand the span of cultural capital. They suggest that teachers give higher evaluations to students when they see or believe that those students have good computer proficiency.

This suggests that ICT experiences and digital skills may become another indicator that teachers use for evaluating, judging, rewarding, or disciplining students. There is no doubt that as "institutional gatekeepers" (Rafalow, 2018, p. 1446), teachers' evaluations of students' performance online or offline are affected by students' family backgrounds, the socioeconomic and demographic composition of the student body in school, and features of students and the school (Graves, 2019; Rafalow, 2018; Warschauer, 2016).

3.5 Differential Benefits of ICT Use by SES

We have explained how socioeconomic background affects students' digital access (the first-level digital learning divide) and the ways they use ICT (the second-level digital learning divide) at home and in school. In this section, we elaborate on the third-level digital learning divide and examine whether students' socioeconomic background moderates the outcomes/benefits derived from ICT use.

Empirical studies have begun to examine how ICT use may differentially benefit students of different socioeconomic groups. Scholars contend that the effects of computer use and internet access are less positive and sometimes negative on the test score of low-SES and racial minority students and positive on those of high-SES and white students (Warschauer & Matuchniak, 2010). At least three related mechanisms may explain this third-level digital divide. First, computer use for remedial, drill, and practice purposes, such as the improvement of grammar and punctuations, in the school environment is less effective (Natriello, 2001; Warschauer & Xu, 2018), and thus has limited effects on the improvement of educational outcomes. Socioeconomically disadvantaged students are more likely to engage in this form of e-learning activities at school. In contrast, socioeconomically privileged students are more likely to use ICT for constructive or integrative activities (e.g., games, word processing, simulations, and data analysis). As a result, ICT use more positively affects the educational achievement of advantaged students than those of disadvantaged students (Wenglinsky, 2005).

Second, students who "have more connection point through which to access the internet" and "[more] freedom to use the technology when and where one wants without constraint from others" have more "autonomy of use" and better experience with the internet (Hargittai & Hinnant, 2008, p. 607). Consequently, these students tend to benefit the most from ICT use (Mascheroni & Ólafsson, 2016). As noted earlier, socioeconomically underprivileged people are more likely to use poorly functioning computers for work and study, and have limited or intermittent internet connections (Gonzales, 2015; Gonzales et al., 2020). Disadvantaged students are also more likely to rely on mobile phones instead of desktops or laptops to access the internet (Donner et al., 2011; Gonzales et al., 2020; Marler, 2018). This may generate digital inequality, because some websites, online services, and computer software (e.g., job application websites and Microsoft Office) are not designed and thus not suitable for mobile phone users. Therefore, those who mainly use mobile phones to access the internet are often stymied when they attempt to search for advanced information, work on programming, present multimedia content, and process Word or Excel documents (Napoli & Obar, 2014; Tsetsi & Rains, 2017).

Third, earlier research by Attewell and Battle (1999) suggests that in the U.S., students with high-SES backgrounds gain more educational benefits from the use of home computers than students with low-SES backgrounds. More recent research on Brazilian students finds that home internet access is positively associated with test scores for higher SES students but not for lower-SES students (Wainer et al., 2015). Whereas parents with lower educational attainment tend to apply restrictive mediation practices to regulate children's internet access and computer use, parents with higher educational attainment tend to use an active and instructive style of parental mediation to help enhance their children's digital skills (Cabello-Hutt et al., 2018). Taken together, ICT use is potentially counterproductive for some groups of students than others, and is particularly detrimental to students living in households without effective parental monitoring strategies (Vigdor et al., 2014).

Recent research by Scheerder et al. (2019) may generate additional insights into the mechanisms underlying the third-level digital divide by SES. In their qualitative fieldwork, Scheerder et al. (2019) observe that students of higher-SES families learn how to use digital devices and build a strong interest in learning ICT at a very young age. These students enroll in computer clubs or ICT camps for children. After school, they observe and learn how their parents use different digital devices to work at home. Often, parents and children in high-SES families help each other to solve problems they encounter with digital technology. In contrast, parents from lower-SES families feel less empowered and therefore are less likely to help their children solve problems they encounter with digital technology. When buying new digital devices, higher-SES families tend to focus on the functionalities of the device, such as processor speed and computer memory. Their goals are to integrate different digital devices and peripherals to increase their productivity and make their life more convenient. In contrast, lower-SES families tend to focus on the price of new ICT devices. Whereas higher-SES families tend to incorporate ICT into their professional and educational activities, lower-SES households tend to use ICT exclusively for entertainment and maintaining social contacts.

3.6 Summary and Conclusion

Since the 1990s, research on ICT use in education has undergone several important changes in research focus, from inequalities in ICT access, digital skills, and literacy, to the resurgent digital inequality in access to new technologies, devices, and, most recently, the differential effects of ICT use on the outcomes of students of different backgrounds. In this chapter, we review the research literature on the three levels of the digital learning divide and discuss the differential effects of ICT use in education on the outcomes of students from advantaged and disadvantaged socioeconomic backgrounds. This research review informs our empirical analyses in Chaps. 4–7. In these chapters, we present the research findings from our analyses of data from the 2018 Programme for International Student Assessment (PISA) survey regarding the three levels of digital inequality and their effects on secondary school students.

References

Agasisti, T., Gil-Izquierdo, M., & Han, S. W. (2020). ICT Use at home for school-related tasks: What is the effect on a student's achievement? Empirical evidence from OECD PISA data. *Education Economics, 28*(6), 601–620. https://doi.org/10.1080/09645292.2020.1822787

Agirdag, O., Van Houtte, M., & Van Avermaet, P. (2012). Why does the ethnic and socio-economic composition of schools influence math achievement? The role of sense of futility and futility culture. *European Sociological Review, 28*(3), 366–378. https://doi.org/10.1093/esr/jcq070

Andrews, G. 'Gus.' (2008). Gameplay, gender, and socioeconomic status in two American high schools. *E-Learning and Digital Media, 5*(2), 199–213. https://doi.org/10.2304/elea.2008.5.2.199

Attewell, P. A. (2001). The first and second digital divides. *Sociology of Education, 74*(3), 252–259.

Attewell, P. A. (2003). Beyond the digital divide. In P. A. Attewell & N. M. Seel (Eds.), *Disadvantaged teens and computer technologies* (pp. 15–34). Waxmann.

Attewell, P. A., & Battle, J. (1999). Home computers and school performance. *The Information Society, 15*(1), 1–10.

Attewell, P. A., & Winston, H. (2003). Children of the digital divide. In P. A. Attewell & N. M. Seel (Eds.), *Disadvantaged teens and computer technologies* (pp. 117–136). Waxmann.

Becker, H. J. (2000). Who's wired and who's not: Children's access to and use of computer technology. *The Future of Children, 10*(2), 44–75.

Bowles, S., & Gintis, H. (2002). Schooling in capitalist America revisited. *Sociology of Education, 75*(1), 1–18.

Bowles, S., & Gintis, H. (2011). *Schooling in capitalist America: Educational reform and the contradictions of economic life* (Reprint edition). Haymarket Books.

Cabello-Hutt, T., Cabello, P., & Claro, M. (2018). Online opportunities and risks for children and adolescents: The role of digital skills, age, gender and parental mediation in Brazil. *New Media & Society, 20*(7), 2411–2431. https://doi.org/10.1177/1461444817724168

Calvani, A., Fini, A., Ranieri, M., & Picci, P. (2012). Are young generations in secondary school digitally competent? A study on Italian teenagers. *Computers & Education, 58*(2), 797–807. https://doi.org/10.1016/j.compedu.2011.10.004

Camerini, A.-L., Schulz, P. J., & Jeannet, A.-M. (2018). The social inequalities of Internet access, its use, and the impact on children's academic performance: Evidence from a longitudinal study in Switzerland. *New Media & Society, 20*(7), 2489–2508. https://doi.org/10.1177/1461444817725918

Choe, S.-H. (2009, June 1). Tech company helps South Korean students ace entrance tests. *The New York Times*. https://www.nytimes.com/2009/06/02/business/global/02cram.html?_r=0

Cruz-Jesus, F., Oliveira, T., Bacao, F., & Irani, Z. (2017). Assessing the pattern between economic and digital development of countries. *Information Systems Frontiers, 19*(4), 835–854. https://doi.org/10.1007/s10796-016-9634-1

Davies, H. C. (2018). Learning to Google: Understanding classed and gendered practices when young people use the Internet for research. *New Media & Society, 20*(8), 2764–2780. https://doi.org/10.1177/1461444817732326

DiMaggio, P., Hargittai, E., Celeste, C., & Shafer, S. (2004). Digital inequality: From unequal access to differentiated use. In K. Neckerman (Ed.), *Social inequality* (pp. 355–400). Russell Sage Foundation.

Dolan, J. E. (2016). Splicing the divide: A review of research on the evolving digital divide among K-12 students. *Journal of Research on Technology in Education, 48*(1), 16–37. https://doi.org/10.1080/15391523.2015.1103147

Donner, J., Gitau, S., & Marsden, G. (2011). Exploring mobile-only Internet use: Results of a training study in urban South Africa. *International Journal of Communication, 5*, 574–597.

Erichsen, E. A., & Salajan, F. D. (2014). A comparative analysis of e-learning policy formulation in the European Union and the United States: Discursive convergence and divergence. *Comparative Education Review, 58*(1), 135–165. https://doi.org/10.1086/674095

Gee, J. P. (2007). *What video games have to teach us about learning and literacy* (2nd ed.). St. Martin's Griffin.

Gonzales, A. L. (2014). Health benefits and barriers to cell phone use in low-income urban U.S. neighborhoods: Indications of technology maintenance. *Mobile Media & Communication, 2*(3), 233–248. https://doi.org/10.1177/2050157914530297

Gonzales, A. L. (2015). The contemporary US digital divide: From initial access to technology maintenance. *Information, Communication & Society, 19*(2), 234–248. https://doi.org/10.1080/1369118X.2015.1050438

Gonzales, A. L., Calarco, J. M., & Lynch, T. (2020). Technology problems and student achievement gaps: A validation and extension of the technology maintenance construct. *Communication Research, 47*(5), 750–770. https://doi.org/10.1177/0093650218796366

Goode, J. (2010). The digital identity divide: How technology knowledge impacts college students. *New Media & Society, 12*(3), 497–513. https://doi.org/10.1177/1461444809343560

Graves, K. E. (2019). *Disrupting the digital norm in the new digital divide: Toward a conceptual and empirical framework of technology leadership for social justice through multilevel latent class analysis.* Doctoral dissertation, Columbia University.

Hamari, J., Shernoff, D. J., Rowe, E., Coller, B., Asbell-Clarke, J., & Edwards, T. (2016). Challenging games help students learn: An empirical study on engagement, flow and immersion in game-based learning. *Computers in Human Behavior, 54*, 170–179. https://doi.org/10.1016/j.chb.2015.07.045

Hargittai, E. (2002). Second-level digital divide: Differences in people's online skills. *First Monday, 7*(4). https://doi.org/10.5210/fm.v7i4.942

Hargittai, E., & Hinnant, A. (2008). Digital inequality: Differences in young adults' use of the Internet. *Communication Research, 35*(5), 602–621.

Hilbert, M. (2016). The bad news is that the digital access divide is here to stay: Domestically installed bandwidths among 172 countries for 1986–2014. *Telecommunications Policy, 40*(6), 567–581. https://doi.org/10.1016/j.telpol.2016.01.006

Hughes, J. E., Read, M. F., Jones, S., & Mahometa, M. (2015). Predicting middle school students' use of web 2.0 technologies out of school using home and school technological variables. *Journal of Research on Technology in Education, 47*(4), 211–228. https://doi.org/10.1080/15391523.2015.1065156

Ito, M., Horst, H. A., Baumer, S., Bittanti, M., boyd, danah, Cody, R., Stephenson, B. H., Lange, P. G., Mahendran, D., Martínez, K. Z., Pascoe, C. J., Perkel, D., Robinson, L., Sims, C., Tripp, L., Antin, J., Finn, M., Law, A., Manion, A., … Yardi, S. (2013). *Hanging out, messing around, and geeking out: Kids living and learning with new media.* The MIT Press.

ITU. (2018). *Measuring the information society.* ITU.

Jack, A. A. (2016). (No) harm in asking class, acquired cultural capital, and academic engagement at an elite university. *Sociology of Education, 89*(1), 1–19. https://doi.org/10.1177/0038040715614913

Lechman, E. (2015). *ICT diffusion in developing countries: Towards a new concept of technological takeoff*. Springer International.

Lee, H., Park, N., & Hwang, Y. (2015). A new dimension of the digital divide: Exploring the relationship between broadband connection, smartphone use and communication competence. *Telematics and Informatics, 32*(1), 45–56. https://doi.org/10.1016/j.tele.2014.02.001

Leu, D. J., Forzani, E., Rhoads, C., Maykel, C., Kennedy, C., & Timbrell, N. (2015). The new literacies of online research and comprehension: Rethinking the reading achievement gap. *Reading Research Quarterly, 50*(1), 37–59. https://doi.org/10.1002/rrq.85

Leung, L., & Lee, P. S. N. (2012). Impact of Internet literacy, Internet addiction symptoms, and Internet activities on academic performance. *Social Science Computer Review, 30*(4), 403–418. https://doi.org/10.1177/0894439311435217

Livingstone, S., & Helsper, E. J. (2008). Parental mediation and children's Internet use. *Journal of Broadcasting & Electronic Media, 52*(4), 581–599. https://doi.org/10.1080/08838150802437396

Ma, J.K.-H. (2021). The digital divide at school and at home: A comparison between schools by socioeconomic level across 47 countries. *International Journal of Comparative Sociology, 62*(2), 115–140. https://doi.org/10.1177/00207152211023540

Ma, J.K.-H., Vachon, T. E., & Cheng, S. (2019). National income, political freedom, and investments in R&D and education: A comparative analysis of the second digital divide among 15-year-old students. *Social Indicators Research, 144*(1), 133–166. https://doi.org/10.1007/s11205-018-2030-0

Marler, W. (2018). Mobile phones and inequality: Findings, trends, and future directions: *New Media & Society*. https://doi.org/10.1177/1461444818765154

Mascheroni, G., & Ólafsson, K. (2016). The mobile Internet: Access, use, opportunities and divides among European children. *New Media & Society, 18*(8), 1657–1679. https://doi.org/10.1177/1461444814567986

Mihelj, S. I., Leguina, A., & Downey, J. (2018). Culture is digital: Cultural participation, diversity and the digital divide. *New Media & Society, 21*(7), 1465–1485. https://journals.sagepub.com/doi/10.1177/1461444818822816

Morgan, J. N., & Vanlengen, C. A. (2005). The digital divide and K-12 student computer use. *Issues in Informing Science and Information Technology, 2*, 705–722.

Napoli, P. M., & Obar, J. A. (2014). The emerging mobile internet underclass: A critique of mobile internet access. *The Information Society, 30*(5), 323–334. https://doi.org/10.1080/01972243.2014.944726

Natriello, G. (2001). Bridging the second digital divide: What can sociologists of education contribute? *Sociology of Education, 74*(3), 260–265.

Paino, M., & Renzulli, L. A. (2013). Digital dimension of cultural capital: The (in)visible advantages for students who exhibit computer skills. *Sociology of Education, 86*(2), 124–138. https://doi.org/10.1177/0038040712456556

Park, H., Buchmann, C., Choi, J., & Merry, J. (2016). Learning beyond the school walls: Trends and implications. *Annual Review of Sociology, 42*, 231–252. https://doi.org/10.1146/annurev-soc-081715-074341

Peter, J., & Valkenburg, P. M. (2006). Adolescents' Internet use: Testing the "disappearing digital divide" versus the "emerging digital differentiation" approach. *Poetics, 34*(4–5), 293–305. https://doi.org/10.1016/j.poetic.2006.05.005

Rafalow, M. H. (2014). The digital divide in classroom technology use: A comparison of three schools. *International Journal of Sociology of Education, 3*(1), 67–100. https://doi.org/10.4471/rise.2014.04

Rafalow, M. H. (2018). Disciplining play: Digital youth culture as capital at school. *American Journal of Sociology, 123*(5), 1416–1452. https://doi.org/10.1086/695766

Rafalow, M. H. (2020). *Digital divisions: How schools create inequality in the tech era* (1st ed.). University of Chicago Press.

Rideout, V. J., & Katz, V. S. (2016). *Opportunity for all? Technology and learning in lower-income families. A report of the Families and Media Project*. The Joan Ganz Cooney Center at Sesame Workshop. https://kramden.org/technology-learning-lower-income/

Robinson, L. (2014). Freeways, detours, and dead ends: Search journeys among disadvantaged youth. *New Media & Society, 16*(2), 234–251. https://doi.org/10.1177/1461444813481197

Scheerder, A. J., van Deursen, A. J., & van Dijk, J. A. (2017). Determinants of Internet skills, uses and outcomes: A systematic review of the second- and third-level digital divide. *Telematics and Informatics, 34*(8), 1607–1624. https://doi.org/10.1016/j.tele.2017.07.007

Scheerder, A. J., van Deursen, A. J., & van Dijk, J. A. (2019). Internet use in the home: Digital inequality from a domestication perspective. *New Media & Society, 21*(10), 2099–2118. https://doi.org/10.1177/1461444819844299

Sefton-Green, J., Marsh, J., Erstad, O., & Flewitt, R. (2016). *Establishing a research agenda for the digital literacy practices of young children: A white paper for COST Action IS1410*. https://doi.org/10.13140/RG.2.2.10896.30720

Selwyn, N., Potter, J., & Cranmer, S. (2009). Primary pupils' use of information and communication technologies at school and home. *British Journal of Educational Technology, 40*(5), 919–932. https://doi.org/10.1111/j.1467-8535.2008.00876.x

Smith, J., Skrbis, Z., & Western, M. (2013). Beneath the 'digital native' myth: Understanding young Australians' online time use. *Journal of Sociology, 49*(1), 97–118. https://doi.org/10.1177/1440783311434856

Starkey, L., & Finger, G. (2018). Information and communication technology in educational policies in Australia and New Zealand. In J. Voogt, G. Knezek, R. Christensen, & K.-W. Lai (Eds.), *Second handbook of information technology in primary and secondary education* (pp. 1–20). Springer International Publishing. https://doi.org/10.1007/978-3-319-53803-7_87-2

Tichenor, P. J., Donohue, G. A., & Olien, C. N. (1970). Mass media flow and differential growth in knowledge. *Public Opinion Quarterly, 34*(2), 159–170. https://doi.org/10.1086/267786

Tsetsi, E., & Rains, S. A. (2017). Smartphone Internet access and use: Extending the digital divide and usage gap. *Mobile Media & Communication, 5*(3), 239–255. https://doi.org/10.1177/2050157917708329

UNESCO. (2000). *The Dakar framework for action: Education for all meeting our collective commitments*. United Nations Educational, Scientific and Cultural Organization. http://unesdoc.unesco.org/images/0012/001211/121147e.pdf

UNESCO-UIS. (2014). *Information and communication technology (ICT) in education in Asia: A comparative analysis of ICT integration and e-readiness in schools across Asia*. United Nations Educational, Scientific and Cultural Organization, Institute for Statistics. http://uis.unesco.org/sites/default/files/documents/information-communication-technologies-education-asia-ict-integration-e-readiness-schools-2014-en_0.pdf

Valdez, V. B., & Javier, S. P. (2020). Digital divide: From a peripheral to a core issue for all SDGs. In W. Leal Filho, A. M. Azul, L. Brandli, A. Lange Salvia, P. G. Özuyar, & T. Wall (Eds.), *Reduced inequalities, encyclopedia of the UN sustainable development goals* (pp. 1–14). Springer International Publishing. https://doi.org/10.1007/978-3-319-71060-0_107-1

van Deursen, A. J., Helsper, E. J., & Eynon, R. (2014). *Measuring digital skills: From digital skills to tangible outcomes project report*. www.oii.ox.ac.uk/research/projects/?id=112

van Deursen, A. J., Helsper, E. J., Eynon, R., & van Dijk, J. A. (2017). The compoundness and sequentiality of digital inequality. *International Journal of Communication, 11*, 452–473.

van Deursen, A. J., & van Diepen, S. (2013). Information and strategic Internet skills of secondary students: A performance test. *Computers & Education, 63*, 218–226. https://doi.org/10.1016/j.compedu.2012.12.007

van Deursen, A. J., & van Dijk, J. A. (2014a). The digital divide shifts to differences in usage. *New Media & Society, 16*(3), 507–526. https://doi.org/10.1177/1461444813487959

van Deursen, A. J., & van Dijk, J. A. (2014b). *Digital skills: Unlocking the information society*. Palgrave Macmillan.

van Deursen, A. J., & van Dijk, J. A. (2019). The first-level digital divide shifts from inequalities in physical access to inequalities in material access. *New Media & Society, 21*(2), 354–375. https://doi.org/10.1177/1461444818797082

van Dijk, J. A. G. M., & van Deursen, A. J. (2014). Solutions: Learning digital skills. In J. A. G. M. van Dijk & A. J. van Deursen (Eds.), *Digital skills: Unlocking the information society* (pp. 113–138). Palgrave Macmillan US. https://doi.org/10.1057/9781137437037_6

Vigdor, J. L., Ladd, H. F., & Martinez, E. (2014). Scaling the digital divide: Home computer technology and student achievement. *Economic Inquiry, 52*(3), 1103–1119. https://doi.org/10.1111/ecin.12089

Wainer, J., Vieira, P., & Melguizo, T. (2015). The association between having access to computers and Internet and educational achievement for primary students in Brazil. *Computers & Education, 80*, 68–76. https://doi.org/10.1016/j.compedu.2014.08.007

Warschauer, M. (2016). Addressing the social envelope: Education and the digital divide. In C. Greenhow, J. Sonnevend, & C. Agur (Eds.), *Education and social media: Toward a digital future* (pp. 29–48). MIT Press. https://oxfordindex.oup.com/view/10.7551/mitpress/9780262034470.003.0003?lang=en, https://oxfordindex.oup.com:443/view/10.7551/mitpress/9780262034470.003.0003

Warschauer, M., Knobel, M., & Stone, L. (2004). Technology and equity in schooling: Deconstructing the digital divide. *Educational Policy, 18*(4), 562–588. https://doi.org/10.1177/0895904804266469

Warschauer, M., & Matuchniak, T. (2010). New technology and digital worlds: Analyzing evidence of equity in access, use, and outcomes. *Review of Research in Education, 34*(1), 179–225. https://doi.org/10.3102/0091732X09349791

Warschauer, M., & Newhart, V. A. (2016). Broadening our concepts of universal access. *Universal Access in the Information Society, 15*(2), 183–188. https://doi.org/10.1007/s10209-015-0417-0

Warschauer, M., & Xu, Y. (2018). Technology and equity in education. In J. Voogt, G. Knezek, R. Christensen, & K.-W. Lai (Eds.), *Second handbook of information technology in primary and secondary education* (pp. 1–17). Springer International Publishing. https://doi.org/10.1007/978-3-319-53803-7_76-1

Wei, K.-K., Teo, H.-H., Chan, H. C., & Tan, B. C. Y. (2011). Conceptualizing and testing a social cognitive model of the digital divide. *Information Systems Research, 22*(1), 170–187. https://doi.org/10.1287/isre.1090.0273

Wenglinsky, H. (2005). *Using technology wisely: The keys to success in schools.* Teachers College Press.

Yuen, A. H. K., Park, J. H., Chen, L., & Cheng, M. (2018). The significance of cultural capital and parental mediation for digital inequity. *New Media & Society, 20*(2), 599–617. https://doi.org/10.1177/1461444816667084

Zhang, X. (2013). Income disparity and digital divide: The internet consumption model and cross-country empirical research. *Telecommunications Policy, 37*(6), 515–529. https://doi.org/10.1016/j.telpol.2012.12.011

Chapter 4
Digital Inclusion and Academic Performance

Abstract As ICT continues to change the educational landscape in ways beyond many of our imaginations, how digital inclusion affects adolescent students' learning and their academic achievement have also become an important topic for scholars. Using 2018 PISA data, this chapter examines the effects of ICT use at home and in school on adolescents' reading performance, with a focus on 21 developed countries and societies. Results from multilevel regression analyses suggest that: (1) ICT use in school has no positive effects on students' reading achievement in most developed countries. In a small number of countries (e.g., Australia, New Zealand, the United States, and Scandinavian nations), a moderate level of school ICT use has positive effects on reading, but the effects become negative when students use ICT in school at a high level. When school ICT use shows positive effects, the effects on low-SES students are often greater than the effects on high-SES students, especially when they are using ICT for core subjects in school. (2) Inverted U-shaped curvilinear relationships between ICT use at home and reading performance are apparent in most countries. These curvilinear effects suggest that a moderate level of home ICT use would help improve adolescents' reading performance. As ICT use at home increases, however, its positive effect diminishes, and may have negative impacts on academic achievement if students use ICT at home at a high level. Taken together, these findings suggest that the relationships between adolescents' ICT use and academic achievement vary both across countries and by students' socioeconomic background within countries.

Keywords Digital inclusion · Academic performance · Reading scores · Home vs. school · Curvilinear relationship

DIGITAL learning inequality has become a new component of educational inequality. It will remain unavoidable if Information and Communication Technology (ICT) continues to change the educational landscape in ways far beyond our imagination. This newly emergent e-learning gap will become an ever more important topic for educational researchers and social scientists across the globe.

J. K.-H. Ma and S. Cheng, *Adolescent Well-being and ICT UseX*,
Human Well-Being Research and Policy Making,
https://doi.org/10.1007/978-3-031-04412-0_4

Beginning from this chapter, we report empirical findings concerning the effect of digital inclusion on adolescents' well-being, including their academic performance, learning attitudes, psychological well-being, and digital competence. Specifically, this chapter uses data from the 2018 Programme for International Student Assessment (PISA) survey to examine the relationships between digital inclusion and academic achievement among secondary school students. Following the discussions in the previous chapters, our analyses include ICT use for general schoolwork and for core subjects both within and outside of schools. We are concerned with how the relationship between ICT use and well-being is contingent on *where* students use digital technology—at home vs. at school. Taking a comparative approach, our analyses span 21 affluent countries and societies, which allows us to grasp the general patterns of the digital learning divide in this part of the world. Since our analyses are conducted separately in each of the analyzed countries/societies, we will also be able to identify specific patterns in each of them.

4.1 Methodology

Our goals are to assess the differences in the effects of digital inclusion at home *versus* the effects at school on academic achievement and examine whether the magnitudes and directions of these effects vary by students' socioeconomic background and differ cross-nationally. Digital inclusion—broadly defined as the use of digital technologies for learning-related activities or school-related work—is measured by students' ICT use for general schoolwork and for core subjects. Academic achievement is measured by students' performance in reading, mathematics, and science.

4.1.1 Outcome Variables

During the study period, students were asked to take a set of internationally comparable assessments for different academic subjects, including reading, mathematics, and science. To account for the influence of the assessment/research design that may affect test reliability and cause measurement error, PISA reports a set of 10 plausible values (PV) for each subject based on weighted likelihood estimates (WLE) rather than definitive performance scores. For our analyses, we average the 10 plausible values to measure each individual student's average performance scores in reading, mathematics, and science. The scores range from 0 to 1,000, with an OECD mean of 500 and an OECD standard deviation of 100. Higher scores indicate higher levels of academic performance. Full descriptions of how these indices are created, calculated, and assessed are available from the OECD's official reports (OECD, 2021).

4.1.2 Explanatory Variables

We use four explanatory variables to measure ICT use for learning- or school-related activities (OECD, 2021). The first explanatory variable, *home ICT use for general schoolwork*, is a PISA-created IRT index (*HOMESCH*) that is standardized with an OECD mean of 0 and an OECD standard deviation of 1. In the survey, student respondents were asked "How often do you use digital devices for the following activities outside of school?" The response categories from lower to higher values include: "Never or hardly ever," "Once or twice a month," "Once or twice a week," "Almost every day," and "Every day." This index is based on the following 11 activities.

- Browsing the internet for schoolwork (e.g., for preparing an essay or presentation).
- Browsing the internet to follow up on lessons, e.g., for finding explanations.
- Using email for communication with other students about schoolwork.
- Using email for communication with teachers and submission of homework or other schoolwork.
- Using social networks for communication with teachers (e.g., Facebook and MySpace).
- Downloading, uploading, or browsing material from my school's website (e.g., timetable or course materials).
- Checking the school's website for announcements (e.g., absence of teachers).
- Doing homework on a computer.
- Doing homework on a mobile device.
- Using learning apps or learning websites on a computer.
- Using learning apps or learning websites on a mobile device.

The second explanatory variable, *home ICT use for core subjects*, is also a PISA-created IRT index (*ICTOUTSIDE*) that is standardized with an OECD mean of 0 and an OECD standard deviation of 1. In the survey, student respondents were asked "In a typical school week, how much time do you spend using digital devices outside of classroom lessons (regardless of whether at home or in school) for the following subjects?" The response categories from lower to higher values include: "I do not study this subject," "No time," "1–30 min a week," "31–60 min a week," and "More than 60 min a week." This index is calculated from student responses in the following five subjects.

- Test language lessons.
- Mathematics.
- Science.
- Foreign language.
- Social sciences.

The third explanatory variable is *school ICT use for general schoolwork*, again a PISA-created IRT index (*USESCH*) that is standardized with an OECD mean of 0 and an OECD standard deviation of 1. In the survey, student respondents were asked "How often do you use digital devices for the following activities at school?"

The response categories from lower to higher values include: "Never or hardly ever," "Once or twice a month," "Once or twice a week," "Almost every day," and "Every day." The index is based on the following 10 activities.

- Chatting online at school.
- Using email at school.
- Browsing the internet for schoolwork.
- Downloading, uploading, or browsing material from the school's website (e.g., intranet).
- Posting my work on the school's website.
- Playing simulations at school.
- Practicing and drilling, such as for foreign language learning or mathematics.
- Doing homework on a school computer.
- Using school computers for group work and communication with other students.
- Using learning apps or learning websites.

The fourth explanatory variable is *school ICT use for core subjects*, a PISA-created IRT index (*ICTCLASS*) that is standardized with an OECD mean of 0 and an OECD standard deviation of 1. In the survey, student respondents were asked "In a typical school week, how much time do you spend using digital devices during classroom lessons?" The response categories from lower to higher values include: "I do not study this subject," "No time," "1–30 min a week," "31–60 min a week," and "More than 60 min a week." This index is calculated from student responses to the following five subjects.

- Test language lessons.
- Mathematics.
- Science.
- Foreign language.
- Social sciences.

4.1.3 Family SES and Other Control Variables

We use *family SES* to measure students' social class backgrounds, a composite measure of parental educational level, parental occupational status, and household possessions. The variable is derived from the index of economic, social, and cultural status (*ESCS*) constructed by the PISA research team (OECD, 2021). It is standardized with an OECD mean of 0 and an OECD standard deviation of 1.

Our analyses include a range of individual- and school-level variables to control for students' personal and family background characteristics and schools' quality. These variables are likely associated with both our key independent variables and the outcome measures. The control variables at the individual-student-level include *country-specific program, school grade, student age, gender, immigration status, foreign language use at home, available ICT resources at home*, and *perceived digital competence*. When we analyze the effect of *home* ICT use on academic performance, we control for *school ICT use for general schoolwork*. Likewise, we control *home ICT use for general schoolwork* in the analyses that examine the effect of *school* ICT use on academic performance. At the school-level, we control for *school average SES*, *school type* (public versus private), urbanity (*rural, town, or urban school*), *shortage of educational staff*, and *shortage of educational material*. We assume that these control factors are associated with both our key explanatory variable of interest (family SES) and outcome variables (e.g., reading achievement).

4.1.4 Analytical Strategies and Methods

To examine the relationships between digital inclusion and academic achievement, we run separate multilevel models for each of the 21 countries and societies included in our analysis. Each multilevel model includes explanatory variables at both the student-level (*Level 1*) and the school-level (*Level 2*). Compared to analyses that aggregate all countries in a single multilevel model, an advantage of using separate multilevel models for each country is that it allows us to see the different effect patterns more clearly across countries.

Our presentation of the empirical patterns focuses on four points. First, we examine whether there are cross-national variations in the relationships between ICT use and students' academic achievement. Second, we examine whether the effect of ICT use for schoolwork at home differs from the effect of ICT use for schoolwork at school after controlling for individual-level and school-level factors. Third, we examine whether the relationships between ICT use and student well-being vary by family SES within countries. Fourth, we examine whether the relationship between ICT use and academic achievement is linear. More specifically, we want to see whether there is an inverted U-shaped relationship between ICT use and academic outcomes. For each student *i* at a school *s*, the multilevel model we use in the analysis can be written as,

$$Y_{is} = \beta_{0s} + \beta_{1s}(\text{SES})_{is} + \beta_{2s}(\text{ICT use})_{is} + \beta_{3s}(\text{ICT use})^2_{is} + \beta_{4s}(\text{SES} \times \text{ICT use})_{is} + \beta_{5s}\left[\text{SES} \times (\text{ICT use}^2)\right]_{is} + \sum_{6}^{k} \beta_{ks} x_{is} + e_{is} \quad (4.1)$$

At the student-level (Eq. 4.1), Y_{is} is the dependent variable. β_{0s} is the intercept, which is adjusted for other student-level explanatory variables (i.e., SES, ICT use, ICT use^2, SES $\times$ ICT use, SES $\times$ ICT use^2, and control variables x_{6s} to x_{ks}) as well as school-level controls Z_1 to Z_k, as shown in Eq. 4.2 below. The intercept is assumed to vary randomly across schools.

$$\beta_{0s} = \gamma_{00} + \sum_{1}^{k} \gamma_{0k} Z_{ks} + \mu_{0s} \tag{4.2}$$

To ease the presentation of the results, we use graphs to visualize the predicted values for the curvilinear effects of ICT use conditional on students' family SES for each country. The predicted values are calculated from the multilevel models after controlling for all student-level and school-level characteristics. After each set of analyses, we summarize the major findings in a table.

4.2 Home ICT Use for General Schoolwork, Reading Performance, and Family SES

4.2.1 Overall Results

Figure 4.1 presents the plots from multilevel regression analyses to illustrate the curvilinear relationship between home ICT use for general schoolwork (*x*-axis) and predicted reading performance (*y*-axis) for each country and society after controlling for individual-level and school-level characteristics. In each plot, we show the relationships for high-SES students, middle-SES students, and low-SES students. Table 4.1 summarizes the major findings from these plots. In the Appendix, we further report predicted plots that illustrate the curvilinear effect of home ICT use for schoolwork on students' achievement in mathematics (Fig. A.1) and science (Fig. A.5).

In Fig. 4.1, we observe clear inverted U-shaped curves in 14 of the 21 developed countries and societies in the analyses, including: Australia, Finland, Hong Kong, Iceland, Ireland, Japan, South Korea, Macao, New Zealand, Singapore, Sweden, Taiwan, the United Kingdom, and the United States. These inverted U-shaped curves suggest that a moderate level of ICT use at home for school-related activities is associated with an improvement in reading performance. As ICT use at home increases, its positive effect on reading diminishes and begins to reduce students' reading performance after reaching the inflection point of the curve at high levels of ICT use. Compared to students who use ICT at home for schoolwork at a moderate level, those who use ICT at home at a very high level have substantially lower reading performance.

In some countries, such as Austria, Belgium, and Switzerland, we observe clear and consistently negative effects of home ICT use for school-related tasks or activities on reading performance. As summarized in Table 4.1, with the exception of the United Kingdom, home use of ICT for schoolwork generally does not improve the academic performance of students in Western and Southern Europe, at least for the countries in our analyses. Together, these patterns suggest that the relationships between home ICT use for school-related work and reading performance vary across countries; within countries, they also differ substantially by students' socioeconomic background.

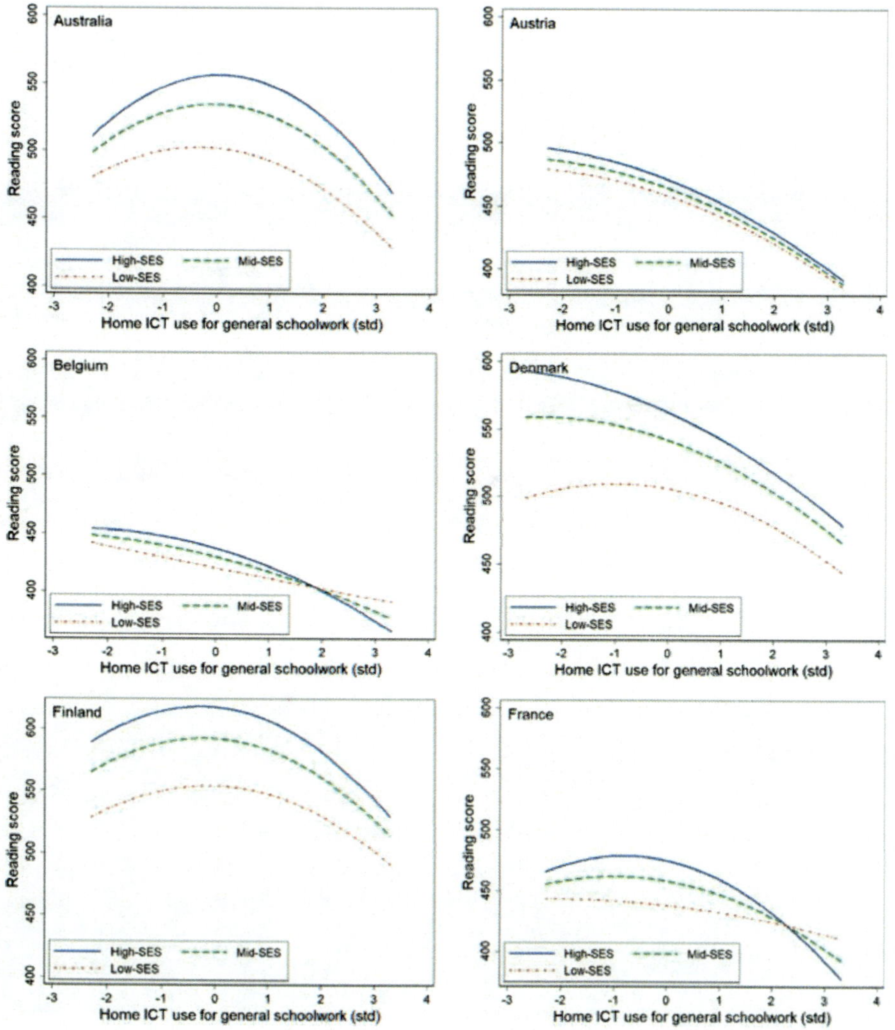

Fig. 4.1 Curvilinear effects of home ICT use for general schoolwork on reading performance by family SES (*Data source* The 2018 Programme for International Student Assessment [PISA] survey. *Note* Countries/societies are listed alphabetically. High-SES refers to students who are at the 90th percentile in family SES. Mid-SES and Low-SES refer to those at the 50th and 10th percentiles in family SES, respectively. Predicted values are calculated based on two-level multilevel models for each country, where student-level variables are used in the Level-1 equation and schools' characteristics are used in the Level-2 equation. All multilevel models include country-specific educational program, school grade, student age, gender, immigration status, foreign language use at home, ICT resources at home, school ICT use for general schoolwork, and perceived digital competence as Level-1 controls. School average SES, public/private school, rural/town/urban school, shortage of educational staff, and shortage of educational material are Level-2 control variables. All Level-1 equations include the interaction effects between family SES and home ICT use for general schoolwork and between family SES and the squared term of home ICT use for general schoolwork. The following countries are not included in these analyses because key independent or dependent variables are unavailable from the country's PISA data: Canada, Germany, the Netherlands, Portugal, Spain, Norway, and China)

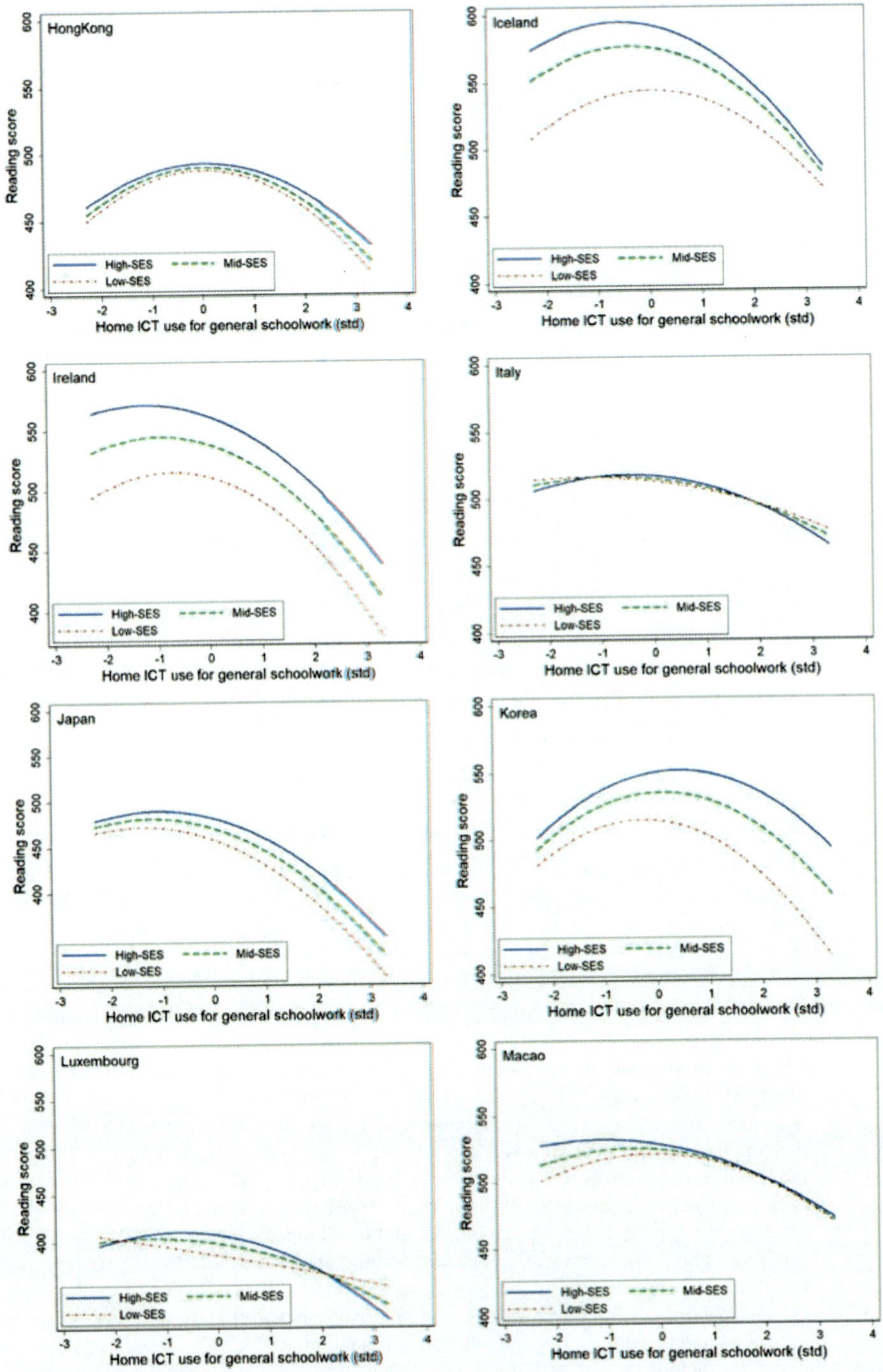

Fig. 4.1 (continued)

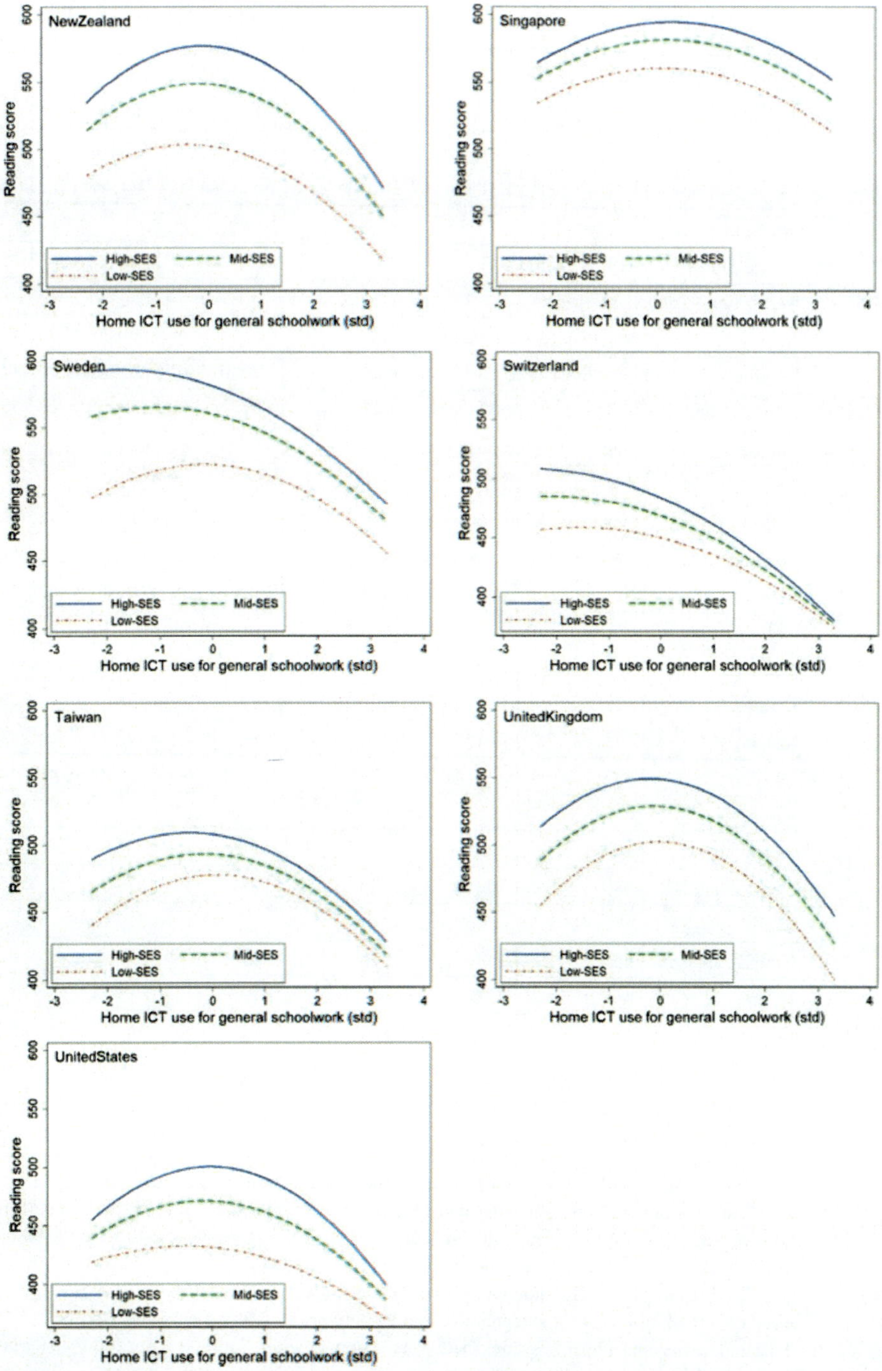

Fig. 4.1 (continued)

Table 4.1 Differences in predicted reading scores between students who do not use ICT for schoolwork at home and students who moderately use ICT for schoolwork at home: Summary of 21 countries/societies in Fig. 4.1

	Low-SES student			High-SES student		
	No ICT use (1)[a]	Moderate ICT use (2)[b]	Difference (2)–(1)[c]	No ICT use (1)[a]	Moderate ICT use (2)[b]	Difference (2)–(1)[c]
North America						
United States	419	433	14	455	500	**46**
Western and Southern Europe						
Austria	Negative (or no positive) effect[d]			Negative (or no positive) effect[d]		
Belgium	Negative (or no positive) effect[d]			Negative (or no positive) effect[d]		
United Kingdom	455	502	**47**	513	549	**35**
France	Negative (or no positive) effect[d]			466	479	13
Ireland	494	515	21	564	571	7
Italy	Negative (or no positive) effect[d]			506	518	12
Luxembourg	Negative (or no positive) effect[d]			395	409	14
Switzerland	Negative (or no positive) effect[d]			Negative (or no positive) effect[d]		
Scandinavia						
Denmark	499	509	10	Negative (or no positive) effect[d]		
Finland	528	554	25	589	618	29
Iceland	508	544	**36**	574	595	21
Sweden	497	522	25	Negative (or no positive) effect[d]		
Pacific						
Australia	480	502	22	511	556	**45**
New Zealand	480	503	23	534	577	**42**
Asia						
Hong Kong	450	488	**38**	461	493	**32**
Japan	465	472	6	479	489	11
Korea	481	514	**34**	501	551	**50**
Macao	501	521	20	Negative (or no positive) effect[d]		
Singapore	534	560	26	564	594	**30**
Taiwan	440	478	**37**	489	509	20

Data source The 2018 Programme for International Student Assessment (PISA) survey
Note Countries/societies in each geographical region are listed alphabetically. Low-SES students refer to those who are at the 10th percentile in family SES. High-SES students refer to those at the 90th percentile in family SES
[a]Predicted reading scores for students who do not use ICT for schoolwork at home
[b]Predicted reading scores for students who moderately use ICT for schoolwork at home
[c]Differences in gains of reading scores between Columns 1 and 2. Scores that are above 30 (approximately 1/3 of a standard deviation in reading performance) are highlighted in bold
[d]ICT use at home has no positive effect on reading performance

4.2.2 The United Kingdom, Scandinavia, and Asia

How does digital inclusion at home influence the academic performance among socioeconomically disadvantaged students? As shown in Table 4.1, in the United Kingdom and several Scandinavian and Asian countries/societies, the role of home ICT use is at least equally or more important for low-SES than for high-SES students. For instance, in the United Kingdom, low-SES students who moderately use ICT at home for schoolwork are 47 points higher in reading scores than other low-SES students who do not use ICT at home for schoolwork. This improvement in reading performance is greater than those of high-SES students, who average 513 points if they do not use ICT for schoolwork at home and 549 points if they moderately use ICT for schoolwork at home.

Except for Finland, the effects of moderate use of ICT at home versus no use of ICT at home are generally more positive for low-SES than for high-SES students in Scandinavian countries. In Iceland, the improvements are 36 and 21 points respectively for low- and high-SES students. In Sweden, the use of ICT at home has no positive effects on high-SES students but improves the reading scores of low-SES students by 25 points.

In Asia, with South Korea as an exception (which we return to shortly), moderate ICT use compared to no ICT use at home either favors low-SES students or has similar positive effects for low- and high-SES students. In Japan and Singapore, for example, the positive effects are similar (6 and 11 points respectively for low- and high-SES students in Japan; 26 and 30 points respectively for low- and high-SES students in Singapore). In Macao, moderate use of ICT at home has no positive effect on high-SES students but improves the reading scores of low-SES students by 20 points. In Taiwan, the improvements are 37 points and 20 points respectively for low- and high-SES students. In Hong Kong, the improvements are 38 points and 32 points respectively for low- and high-SES students.

4.2.3 South Korea, the United States, Australia, and New Zealand

As noted, South Korea is an exception among the Asian countries and societies in our analysis. In South Korea, the academic benefits of ICT use at home are visibly greater for socioeconomically privileged students than for socioeconomically disadvantaged peers (50 versus 34 points). This pattern of the *third*-level digital divide similarly appears in the United States, Australia, and New Zealand. In the United States, the use of ICT at home for schoolwork, on average, increases high-SES students' reading performance by 46 points but increases low-SES students' reading performance only by 14 points. In both Australia and New Zealand, the positive effects are also greater for high-SES students than for low-SES students (45 vs. 22 in Australia; 42 vs. 23 in New Zealand).

4.3 Home ICT Use for Core Subjects, Reading Performance, and Family SES

4.3.1 Overall Results

Figure 4.2 presents plots of multilevel regression analyses to illustrate the curvilinear relationship between home ICT use for core subjects (x-axis) and predicted reading performance (y-axis) for each country and society after controlling for individual- and school-level characteristics. In each plot, we show the relationships for high-SES students, middle-SES students, and low-SES students. Table 4.2 summarizes the major findings from these plots. In the Appendix, we report predicted plots that illustrate the curvilinear effect of home ICT use for core subjects on students' achievement in mathematics (Fig. A.2) and science (Fig. A.6).

Overall, the results suggest that the relationships between home ICT use for core subjects and reading performance vary substantially across countries and differ by students' socioeconomic background within countries. In Fig. 4.2, we observe that home ICT use for core subjects has either negative or no effects on reading performance in countries such as Belgium, Italy, and Denmark. At the same time, we also observe clear inverted U-shaped curves in 15 of the 21 countries and societies, including: Australia, Finland, France, Germany, Ireland, Japan, South Korea, Luxembourg, Macao, New Zealand, Singapore, Sweden, Switzerland, the United Kingdom, and the United States. These inverted U-shaped curves suggest that a moderate level of ICT use at home for core subjects (e.g., reading and mathematics) is associated with a moderate improvement in reading performance. Again, as ICT use at home increases, its positive effect on reading diminishes and begins to reduce students' reading performance after reaching the inflection point of the curve at high levels of ICT use. Compared to students who use ICT at home at a moderate level, those who use ICT at home at a very high level have lower reading performance.

4.3.2 The United Kingdom, New Zealand, Ireland, and Sweden

In the United Kingdom and New Zealand, Table 4.2 further suggests that the effects of home ICT use for core subjects are large on the reading performance among both low- and high-SES students (45 points vs. 59 points for United Kingdom; 43 points vs. 50 points for New Zealand). Similarly, home ICT use also produces similar positive effects among low- and high-SES students in Ireland (25 points vs. 23 points) and Sweden (28 points vs. 24 points), but the effect size in these two countries is relatively smaller than the effect size in the United Kingdom and New Zealand.

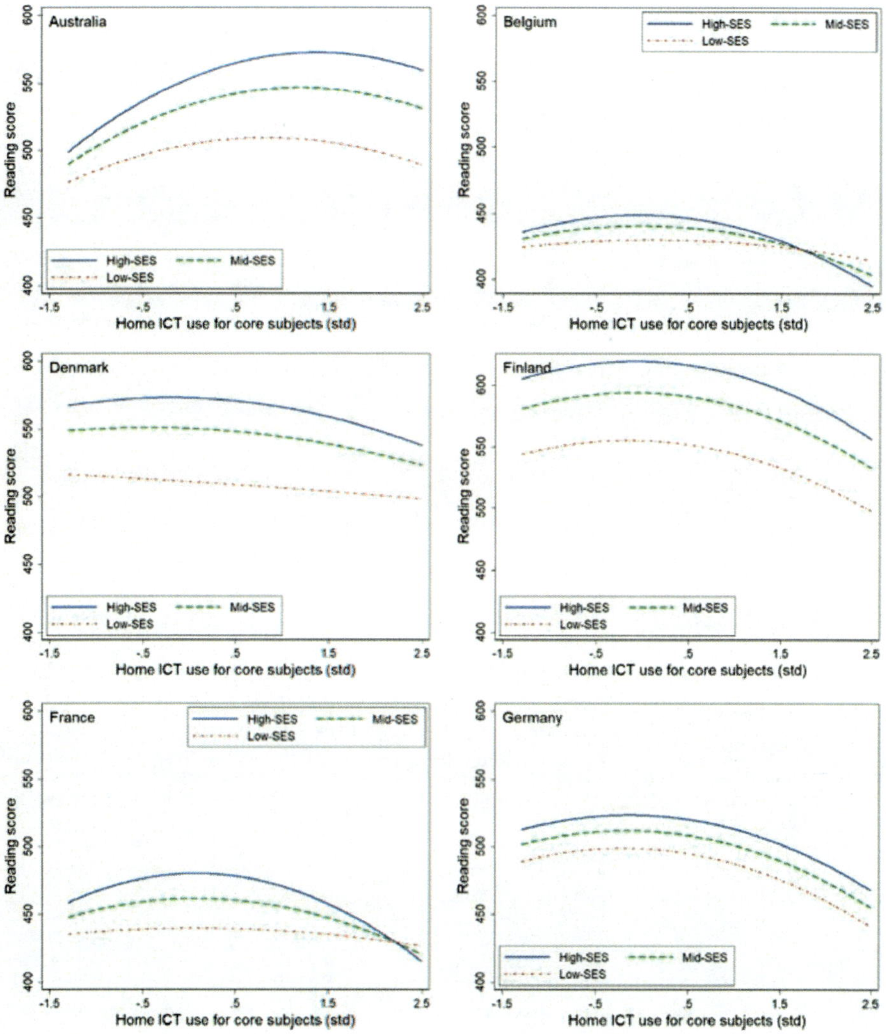

Fig. 4.2 Curvilinear effects of home ICT use for core subjects on reading performance by family SES (*Data source* The 2018 Programme for International Student Assessment [PISA] survey. *Note*: Countries/societies are listed alphabetically. High-SES refers to students who are at the 90th percentile in family SES. Mid-SES and Low-SES refer to those at the 50th and 10th percentiles in family SES, respectively. Predicted values are calculated based on two-level multilevel models for each country, where student-level variables are used in the Level-1 equation and schools' characteristics are used in the Level-2 equation. All multilevel models include country-specific educational program, school grade, student age, gender, immigration status, foreign language use at home, ICT resources at home, school ICT use for general schoolwork, and perceived digital competence as Level-1 controls. School average SES, public/private school, rural/town/urban school, shortage of educational staff, and shortage of educational material are Level-2 control variables. All Level-1 equations include the interaction effects between family SES and home ICT use for core subjects, and between family SES and the squared term of home ICT use for core subjects. The following countries are not included in these analyses because key independent or dependent variables are unavailable from the country's PISA data: Canada, Austria, the Netherlands, Portugal, Spain, Norway, and China)

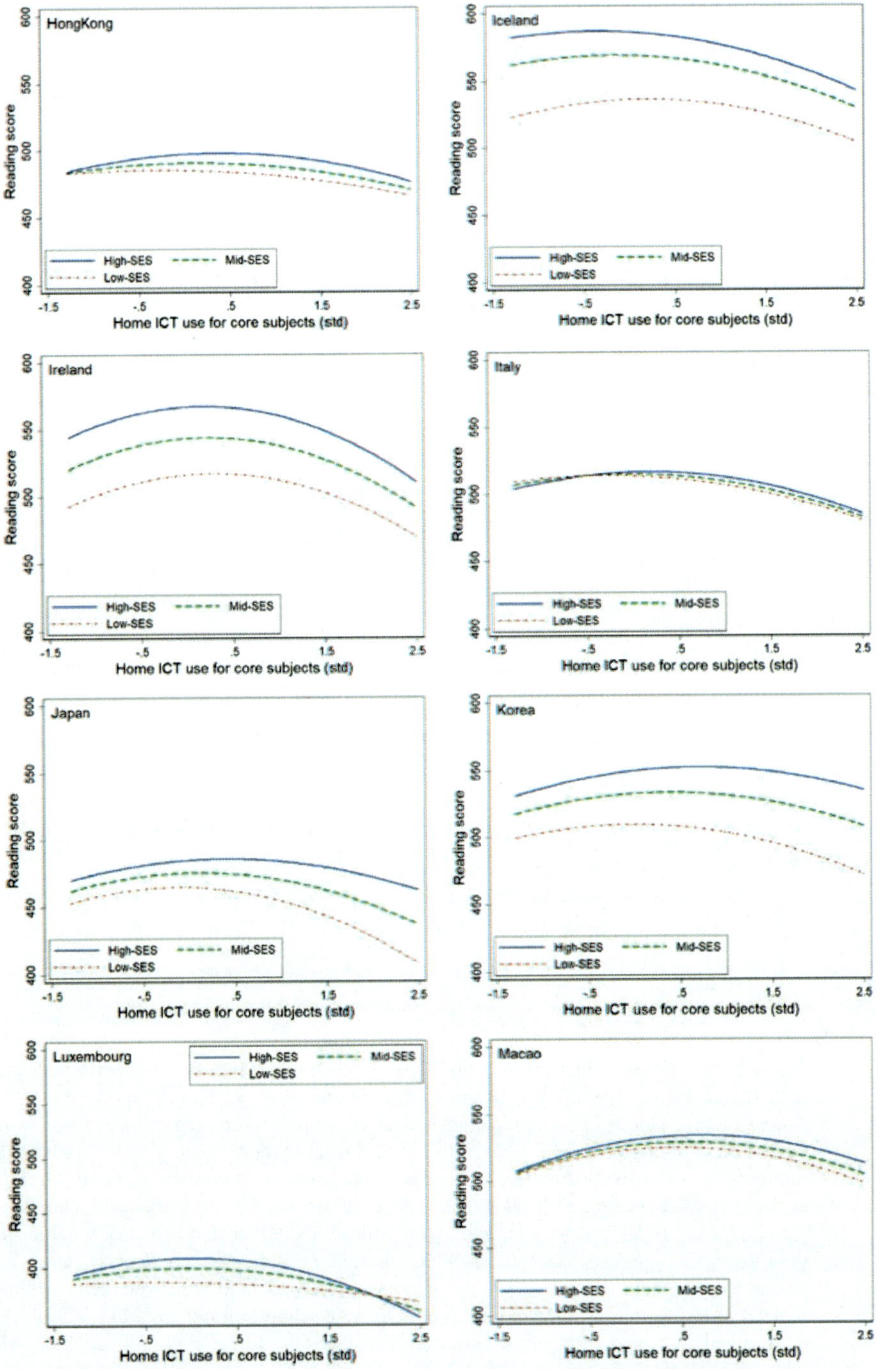

Fig. 4.2 (continued)

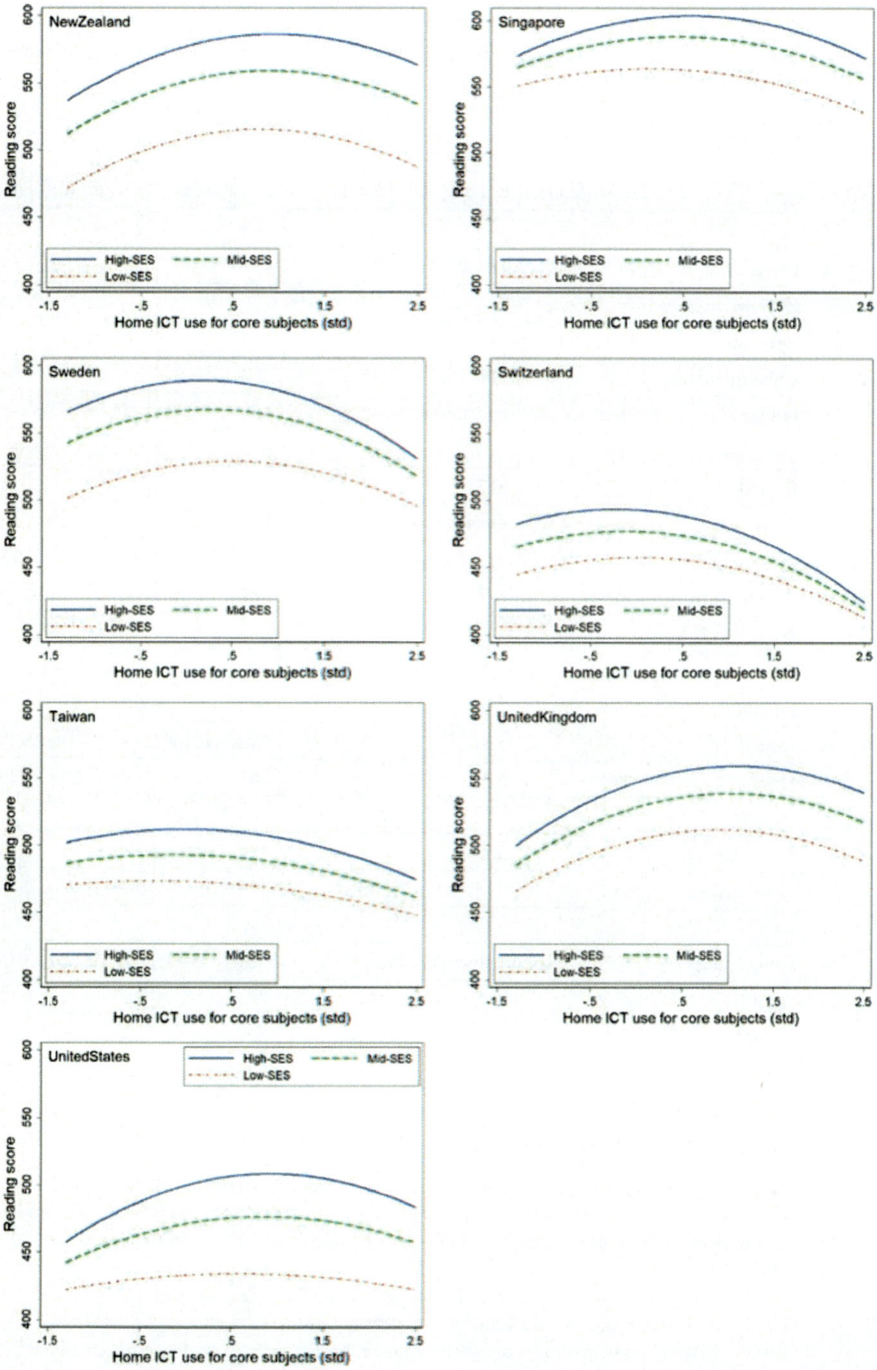

Fig. 4.2 (continued)

Table 4.2 Differences in predicted reading scores between students who do not use ICT for core subjects at home and students who moderately use ICT for core subjects at home: Summary of 21 countries/societies in Fig. 4.2

	Low-SES student			High-SES student		
	No ICT use (1)[a]	Moderate ICT use (2)[b]	Difference (2)–(1)[c]	No ICT use (1)[a]	Moderate ICT use (2)[b]	Difference (2)–(1)[c]
North America						
United States	422	434	12	457	508	**51**
Western and Southern Europe						
Belgium	Negative (or no positive) effect[d]			436	449	13
United Kingdom	466	511	**45**	500	559	**59**
France	Negative (or no positive) effect[d]			459	480	21
Germany	489	499	10	513	523	11
Ireland	492	517	25	544	567	23
Italy	Negative (or no positive) effect[d]			504	516	13
Luxembourg	Negative (or no positive) effect[d]			393	408	15
Switzerland	445	457	13	482	493	11
Scandinavia						
Denmark	Negative (or no positive) effect[d]			Negative (or no positive) effect[d]		
Finland	544	555	11	605	619	14
Iceland	523	536	13	Negative (or no positive) effect[d]		
Sweden	502	529	28	565	589	24
Pacific						
Australia	476	509	**33**	499	572	**74**
New Zealand	472	515	**43**	537	586	**50**
Asia						
Hong Kong	Negative (or no positive) effect[d]			484	498	13
Japan	453	465	12	470	486	15
Korea	500	509	10	531	552	21
Macao	505	525	19	508	534	26
Singapore	551	564	13	574	604	**30**
Taiwan	Negative (or no positive) effect[d]			502	512	10

Data source The 2018 Programme for International Student Assessment (PISA) survey
Note Countries/societies in each geographical region are listed alphabetically. Low-SES students refer to those who are at the 10th percentile in family SES. High-SES students refer to those at the 90th percentile in family SES
[a]Predicted reading scores for students who do not use ICT for core subjects at home
[b]Predicted reading scores for students who moderately use ICT for core subjects at home
[c]Differences in gains of reading scores between Columns 1 and 2. Scores that are above 30 (approximately 1/3 of a standard deviation in reading performance) are highlighted in bold
[d]ICT use at home has no positive effect on reading performance

4.3.3 The United States, France, Australia, South Korea, and Singapore

We have found a clear third-level digital divide in the United States, France, Australia, South Korea, and Singapore. As shown in Table 4.2, the academic benefits of ICT use at home are visibly greater for socioeconomically privileged students than for their socioeconomically disadvantaged peers. In the United States, the use of ICT at home for core subjects, on average, increases high-SES students' reading performance by 51 points, which is about four times larger than the effect on low-SES students (12 points). In France, the use of ICT at home moderately increases the reading performance for high-SES students (21 points), but it does not improve low-SES students' reading performance. In Australia, the use of ICT at home for core subjects increases high-SES students' reading performance by 74 points, more than two times greater than the effect on low-SES students (33 points). Similarly, the effects of home ICT use are substantially greater for high-SES students than for low-SES students in South Korea (21 points vs. 10 points) and Singapore (30 points vs. 13 points).

4.4 School ICT Use for General Schoolwork, Reading Performance, and Family SES

4.4.1 Overall Results

Figure 4.3 presents the plots from multilevel regression analyses to illustrate the curvilinear relationship between school ICT use for general schoolwork (*x*-axis) and predicted reading performance (*y*-axis) for each country and society after controlling for individual-level and school-level characteristics. In each plot, we show the relationships for high-SES students, middle-SES students, and low-SES students. Table 4.3 summarizes the major findings from these plots. In the appendix, we further report predicted plots that illustrate the curvilinear effect of school ICT use for general schoolwork on students' achievement in mathematics (Fig. A.3) and science (Fig. A.7).

In general, our analyses in Fig. 4.3 show either negative or no relationships between the use of ICT at school for general schoolwork and students' reading. This suggests that classroom ICT use for general activities does not improve students' academic performance in many developed countries. As shown in Table 4.3, this pattern applies to most of the countries and societies in Western Europe, Southern Europe, and Asia. The exceptions to this general pattern include Australia, Denmark, New Zealand, Sweden, the United Kingdom, and the United States. In these countries, we still observe inverted U-shaped curves, which suggests a moderate level of ICT use for school-related tasks in class enhances students' academic performance. However, students with a high-level use of ICT in schools tend to have lower academic achievement than those who have a moderate level of ICT use in school.

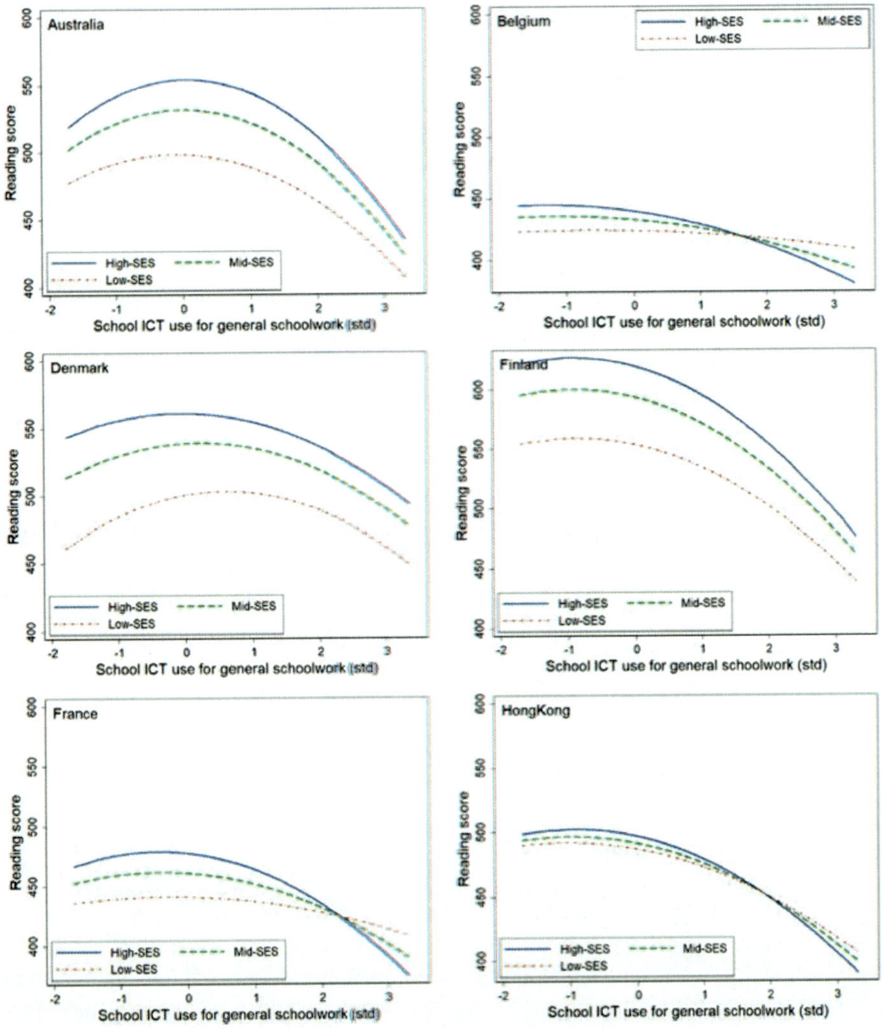

Fig. 4.3 Curvilinear effects of school ICT use for general schoolwork on reading performance by family SES (*Data source* The 2018 Programme for International Student Assessment [PISA] survey. *Note*: Countries/societies are listed alphabetically. High-SES refers to students who are at the 90th percentile in family SES. Mid-SES and Low-SES refer to those at the 50th and 10th percentiles in family SES, respectively. Predicted values are calculated based on two-level multilevel models for each country, where student-level variables are used in the Level-1 equation and schools' characteristics are used in the Level-2 equation. All multilevel models include country-specific educational program, school grade, student age, gender, immigration status, foreign language use at home, ICT resources at home, home ICT use for general schoolwork, and perceived digital competence as Level-1 controls. School average SES, public/private school, rural/town/urban school, shortage of educational staff, and shortage of educational material are Level-2 control variables. All Level-1 equations include the interaction effects between family SES and school ICT use for general schoolwork, and between family SES and the squared term of school ICT use for general schoolwork. The following countries are not included in these analyses because key independent or dependent variables are unavailable from the country's PISA data: Canada, Austria, Germany, the Netherlands, Portugal, Spain, Norway, and China)

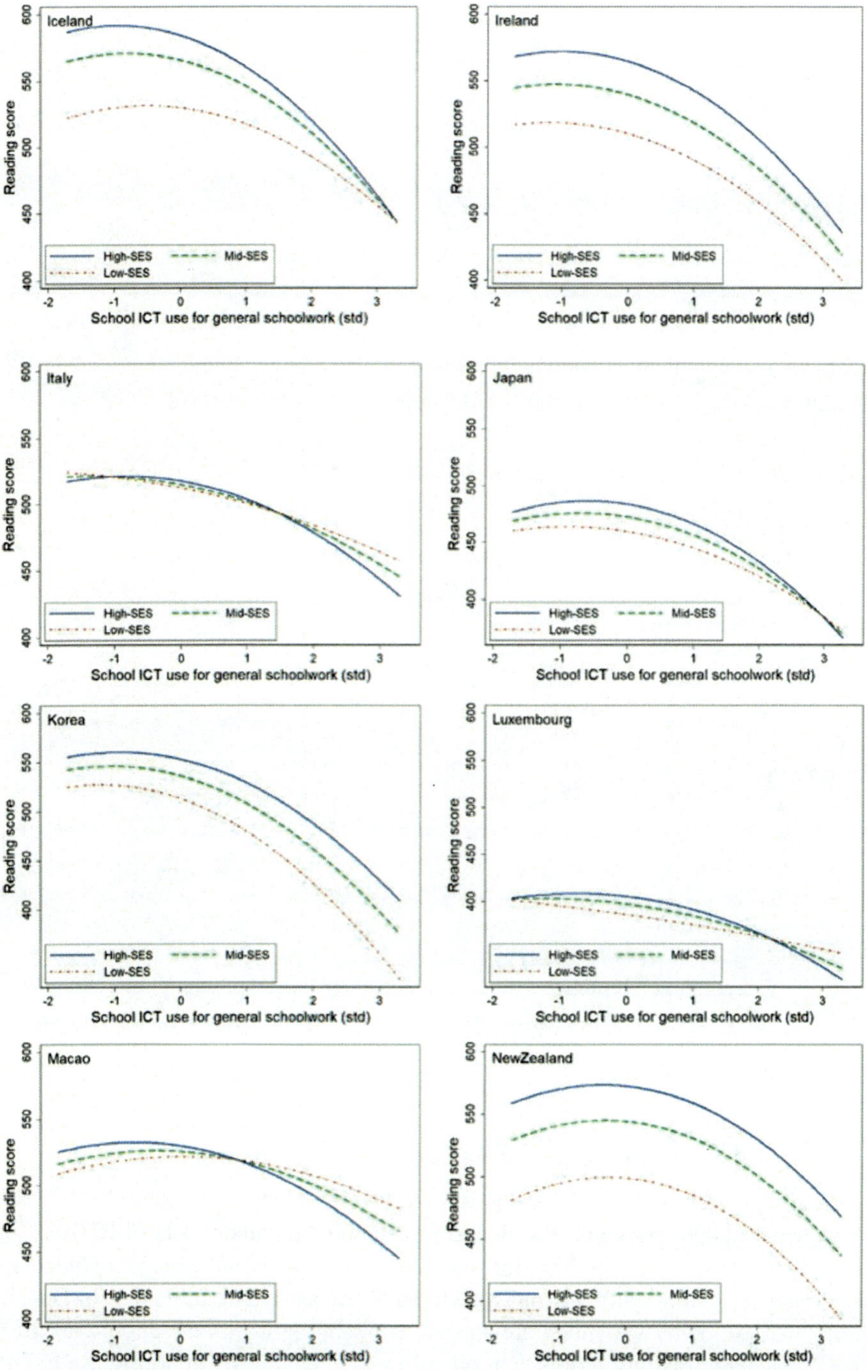

Fig. 4.3 (continued)

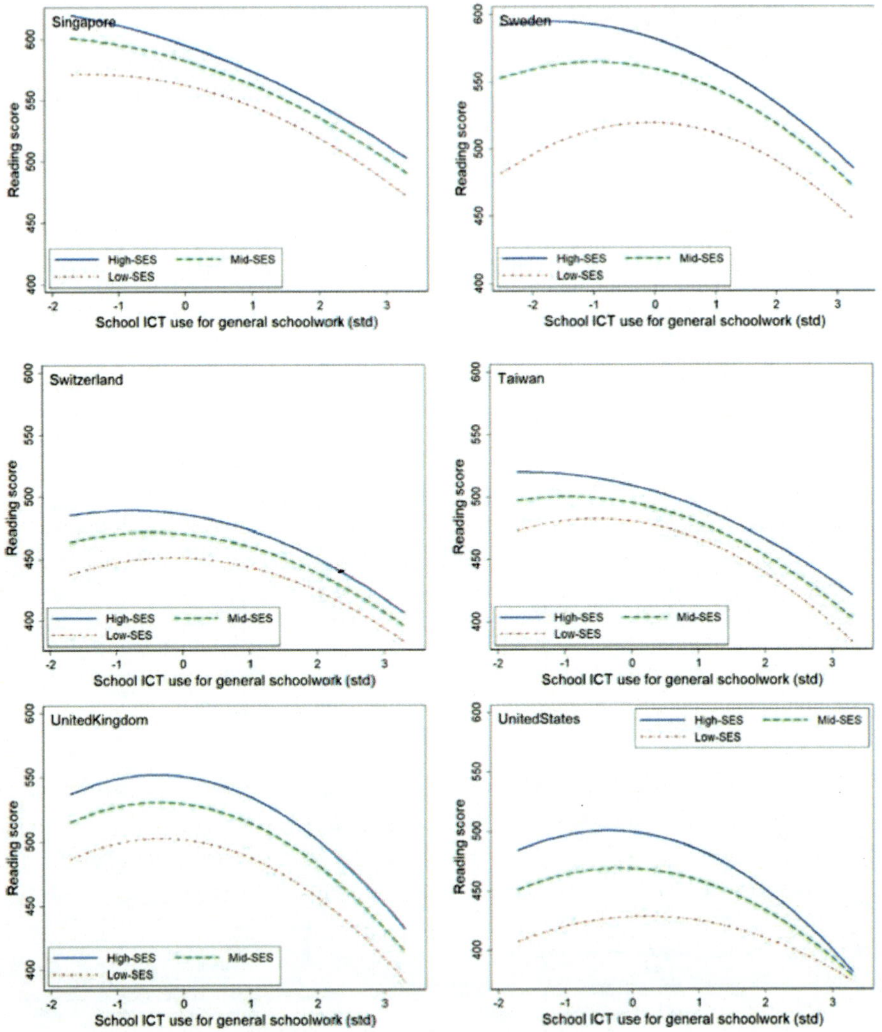

Fig. 4.3 (continued)

4.4.2 Denmark and Sweden

In both Denmark and Sweden, the academic benefits of school ICT use for general schoolwork are greater for socioeconomically disadvantaged students than for socioeconomically advantaged students. As shown in Table 4.3, in Denmark, low-SES students who moderately use ICT in school for general schoolwork are 42 points higher in reading scores than other low-SES students who rarely use ICT in school. This improvement in reading performance is greater than those of high-SES students,

Table 4.3 Differences in predicted reading scores between students who do not use ICT for schoolwork at school and students who moderately use ICT for schoolwork at school: Summary of 20 countries/societies in Fig. 4.3

	Low-SES student			High-SES student		
	No ICT use (1)[a]	Moderate ICT use (2)[b]	Difference (2)–(1)[c]	No ICT use (1)[a]	Moderate ICT use (2)[b]	Difference (2)–(1)[c]
North America						
United States	407	428	21	484	500	17
Western and Southern Europe						
Belgium	Negative (or no positive) effect[d]			Negative (or no positive) effect[d]		
United Kingdom	486	502	16	537	552	15
France	Negative (or no positive) effect[d]			466	478	12
Ireland	Negative (or no positive) effect[d]			Negative (or no positive) effect[d]		
Italy	Negative (or no positive) effect[d]			Negative (or no positive) effect[d]		
Luxembourg	Negative (or no positive) effect[d]			Negative (or no positive) effect[d]		
Switzerland	437	451	14	Negative (or no positive) effect[d]		
Scandinavia						
Denmark	461	503	**42**	543	561	17
Finland	Negative (or no positive) effect[d]			Negative (or no positive) effect[d]		
Iceland	522	531	9	Negative (or no positive) effect[d]		
Sweden	482	519	**37**	Negative (or no positive) effect[d]		
Pacific						
Australia	478	498	21	519	554	**35**
New Zealand	481	499	19	559	573	15
Asia						
Hong Kong	Negative (or no positive) effect[d]			Negative (or no positive) effect[d]		
Japan	Negative (or no positive) effect[d]			476	486	10
Korea	Negative (or no positive) effect[d]			Negative (or no positive) effect[d]		
Macao	509	522	13	525	532	7
Singapore	Negative (or no positive) effect[d]			Negative (or no positive) effect[d]		
Taiwan	473	482	9	Negative (or no positive) effect[d]		

Data source The 2018 Programme for International Student Assessment (PISA) survey

Note Countries/societies in each geographical region are listed alphabetically. Low-SES students refer to those who are at the 10th percentile in family SES. High-SES students refer to those at the 90th percentile in family SES

[a]Predicted reading scores for students who do not use ICT for schoolwork at school

[b]Predicted reading scores for students who moderately use ICT for schoolwork at school

[c]Differences in gains of reading scores between Columns 1 and 2. Scores that are above 30 (approximately 1/3 of a standard deviation in reading performance) are highlighted in bold

[d]ICT use at school has no positive effect on reading performance

who average 543 points if they do not use ICT for general schoolwork in school and 561 points if they moderately use ICT for general schoolwork in school. Similarly, in Sweden, ICT use in school improves low-SES students' reading by 37 points but has no positive effects on the reading performance of high-SES students.

4.4.3 Australia

Australia appears to be one of the few countries in this set of analyses that shows inverted U-shaped curves for low-, mid-, and high-SES students. The inverted U-shaped curves suggest that a moderate level of digital use in classrooms is associated with an improvement in reading performance. A high level of digital use in classrooms, however, may have negative influence on student learning. We also observe class inequalities in the effects of school ICT use on student outcomes in Australia—a phenomenon also known as the *third*-level digital divide. For high-SES students, the improvement of reading scores from school ICT use for general schoolwork is 35 points. For low-SES students, the improvement is 21 points.

4.5 School ICT Use for Core Subjects, Reading Performance, and Family SES

4.5.1 Overall Results

Figure 4.4 presents the plots from multilevel regression analyses to illustrate the curvilinear relationship between school ICT use for core subjects (x-axis) and predicted reading performance (y-axis) for each country and society after controlling for individual-level and school-level characteristics. In each plot, we show the relationships for high-SES students, middle-SES students, and low-SES students. Table 4.4 summarizes the major findings from these plots. In the appendix, we further report predicted plots that illustrate the curvilinear effect of school ICT use on students' achievement in mathematics (Fig. A.4) and science (Fig. A.8).

In Fig. 4.4, we observe a notable difference between two groups of countries and societies. In the first group, we observe clear inverted U-shaped curvilinear relationships between the use of digital technologies for core subjects and reading performance, including Australia, South Korea, New Zealand, the United States, and most of the Scandinavian countries (except for Finland). This suggests that a moderate level of ICT use in classrooms for core subjects is associated with an improvement in reading performance. As ICT use in classrooms increases, its moderate positive effect diminishes and begins to negatively impact students' reading performance after reaching the inflection point of the curves at high levels of ICT use. Compared

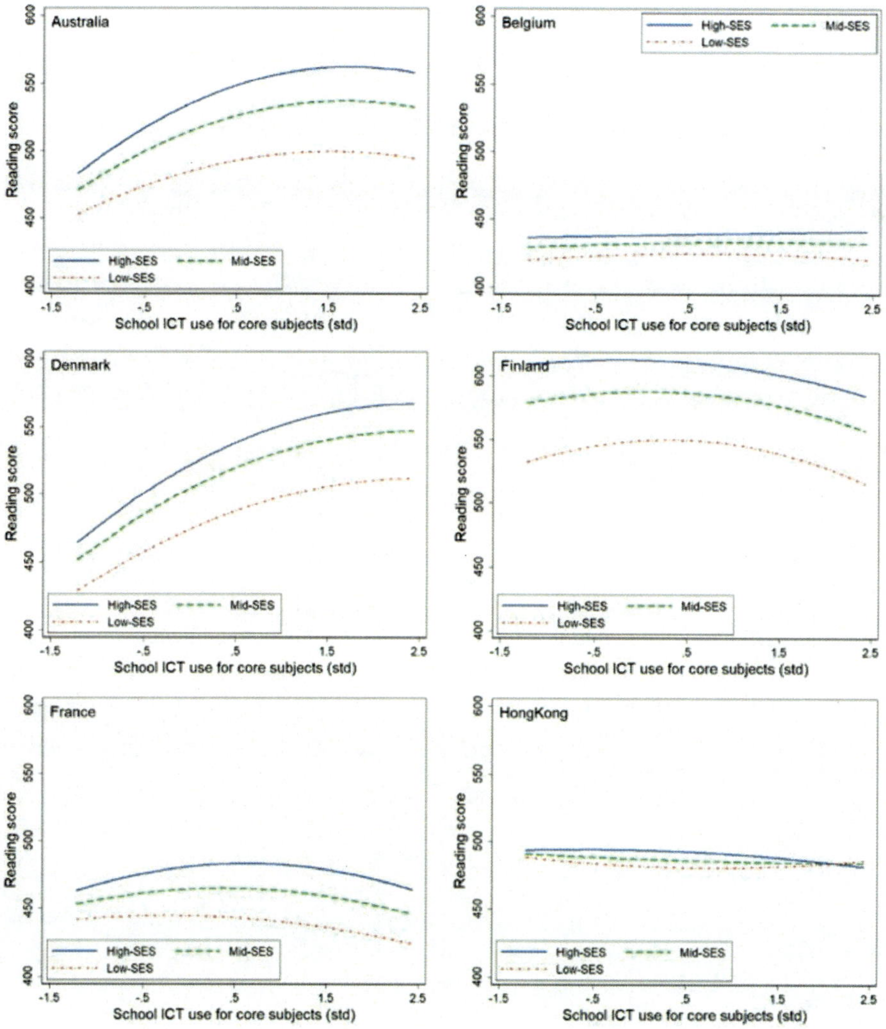

Fig. 4.4 Curvilinear effects of school ICT use for core subjects on reading performance by family SES (*Data source* The 2018 Programme for International Student Assessment [PISA] survey. *Note*: Countries/societies are listed alphabetically. High-SES refers to students who are at the 90th percentile in family SES. Mid-SES and Low-SES refer to those at the 50th and 10th percentiles in family SES, respectively. Predicted values are calculated based on two-level multilevel models for each country, where student-level variables are used in the Level-1 equation and schools' characteristics are used in the Level-2 equation. All multilevel models include country-specific educational program, school grade, student age, gender, immigration status, foreign language use at home, ICT resources at home, home ICT use for general schoolwork, and perceived digital competence as Level-1 controls. School average SES, public/private school, rural/town/urban school, shortage of educational staff, and shortage of educational material are Level-2 control variables. All Level-1 equations include the interaction effects between family SES and school ICT use for core subjects, and between family SES and the squared term of school ICT use for core subjects. The following countries are not included in these analyses because key independent or dependent variables are unavailable from the country's PISA data: Canada, Austria, Germany, the Netherlands, Portugal, Spain, Norway, and China)

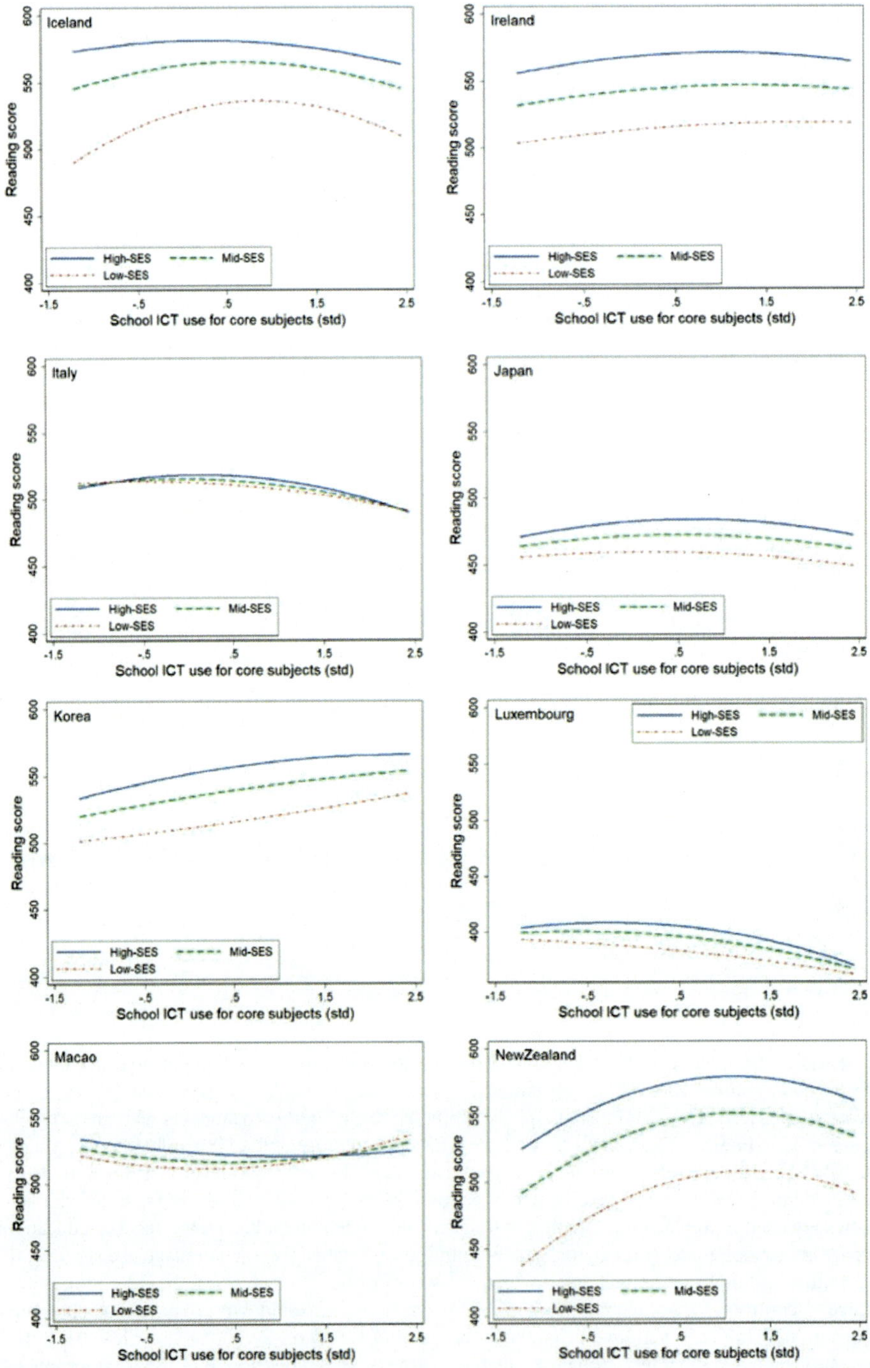

Fig. 4.4 (continued)

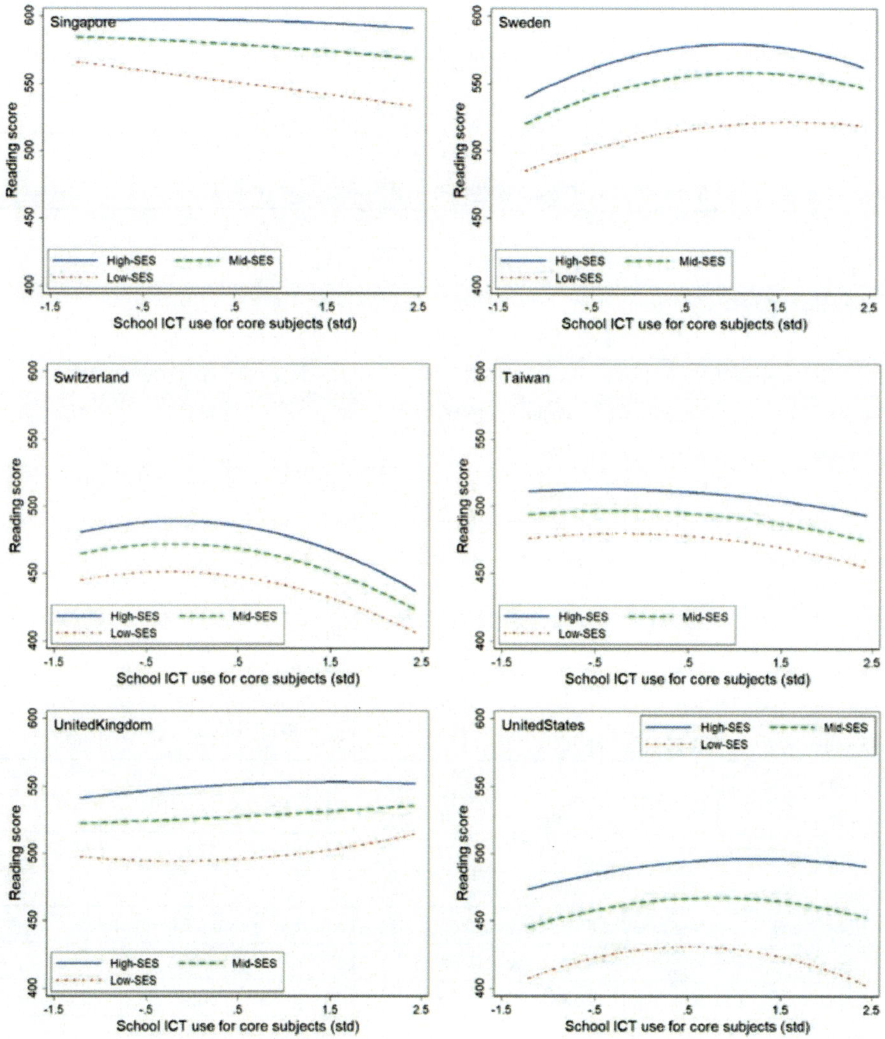

Fig. 4.4 (continued)

to students who use ICT in classrooms at moderate levels, those who use ICT in classrooms at high levels may have lower reading performance.

In the second group of countries, the use of ICT directly for core subjects in classrooms has either negative or zero effects on reading performance. This group includes Belgium, Luxembourg, Switzerland, the United Kingdom, and most Asian countries and societies (except for South Korea). Together, these patterns suggest that the relationships between school ICT use for core subjects and reading performance both vary across countries/societies and differ by students' socioeconomic background within countries/societies.

Table 4.4 Differences in predicted reading scores between students who do not use ICT for core subjects at school and students who moderately use ICT for core subjects at school: Summary of 20 countries/societies in Fig. 4.4

	Low-SES student			High-SES student		
	No ICT use (1)[a]	Moderate ICT use (2)[b]	Difference (2)–(1)[c]	No ICT use (1)[a]	Moderate ICT use (2)[b]	Difference (2)–(1)[c]
North America						
United States	408	431	23	474	496	23
Western and Southern Europe						
Belgium	Negative (or no positive) effect[d]			Negative (or no positive) effect[d]		
United Kingdom	Negative (or no positive) effect[d]			Negative (or no positive) effect[d]		
France	Negative (or no positive) effect[d]			463	483	20
Ireland	503	519	15	556	571	15
Italy	Negative (or no positive) effect[d]			509	518	10
Luxembourg	Negative (or no positive) effect[d]			Negative (or no positive) effect[d]		
Switzerland	Negative (or no positive) effect[d]			481	489	8
Scandinavia						
Denmark	429	512	**83**	464	567	**102**
Finland	533	550	17	Negative (or no positive) effect[d]		
Iceland	490	536	**46**	573	581	8
Sweden	485	521	**36**	539	579	**40**
Pacific						
Australia	453	500	**46**	483	562	**79**
New Zealand	438	508	**71**	525	579	**54**
Asia						
Hong Kong	Negative (or no positive) effect[d]			Negative (or no positive) effect[d]		
Japan	Negative (or no positive) effect[d]			471	484	13
Korea	501	537	**35**	533	566	**32**
Macao	521	536	15	Negative (or no positive) effect[d]		
Singapore	Negative (or no positive) effect[d]			Negative (or no positive) effect[d]		
Taiwan	Negative (or no positive) effect[d]			Negative (or no positive) effect[d]		

Data source The 2018 Programme for International Student Assessment (PISA) survey
Note Countries/societies in each geographical region are listed alphabetically. Low-SES students refer to those who are at the 10th percentile in family SES. High-SES students refer to those at the 90th percentile in family SES
[a]Predicted reading scores for students who do not use ICT for core subjects at school
[b]Predicted reading scores for students who moderately use ICT for core subjects at school
[c]Differences in gains of reading scores between Columns 1 and 2. Scores that are above 30 (approximately 1/3 of a standard deviation in reading performance) are highlighted in bold
[d]ICT use at school has no positive effect on reading performance

4.5.2 *Scandinavia, the United States, Ireland, New Zealand, South Korea, and Macao*

As shown in Table 4.4, the effects of school ICT use for core subjects are equally or more important for low-SES students than for high-SES students among a number of countries/societies, including most Scandinavian countries (except for Denmark), the United States, Ireland, New Zealand, South Korea, and Macao. For instance, in Iceland, low-SES students gain 46 points in reading scores with moderate ICT use in school, compared to a gain of 8 points for high-SES students. In New Zealand, the gains from low- and high-SES students are respectively 71 and 54 points. In Finland and Macao, the effects of school ICT use are positive for low-SES students but negative or zero for high-SES students. In the United States, Ireland, Sweden, and South Korea, the gains for low- and high-SES students are almost the same.

4.5.3 *France, Denmark, Australia, and Japan*

Again, several countries appear to have a third-level digital divide in the effects of school ICT for core subjects on reading performance. In Denmark, for example, we observe an improvement of 102 points in reading scores for high-SES students versus 83 points for low-SES students. In Australia, the gain for high-SES students is 79 points, compared to a gain of 46 points for low-SES students. In France and Japan, the effects of moderate ICT use in school on high-SES students are positive, but zero or negative on low-SES students.

4.6 Summary and Conclusion

Nearly 40 years after the world's first ICT learning policy initiative, *A Nation at Risk*, from the United States in 1983, the question "Does ICT use save the world's formal education from a system at risk?" is more pressing than ever. In the midst of the pandemic, the answer to this question is a quick yes. Indeed, without the advancement of digital and communication technologies over the past few decades, it is difficult to imagine how our education systems would have adjusted to the crisis of school shutdowns across the globe. At the same time, however, it is now also clear to educators and policymakers that new forms of educational inequalities have emerged because of pervasive ICT use.

In this chapter, we examine the effects of ICT use at home and in school on adolescents' reading performance, using 2018 PISA data. Overall, our multilevel analyses show that the relationships between adolescents' ICT use and academic achievement vary across countries and differ by students' socioeconomic background within countries. In most countries, ICT use in school has no visibly positive effects on students' reading achievement. When school ICT use does show positive effects, however, the effects on low-SES students are often greater than the effects on high-SES students, especially when students use ICT for core subjects in classrooms. Because children in developed countries have more opportunities to use ICT applications and are more likely to grow up as "digital natives" than children from less developed countries, these findings lend support to the argument by scholars that public education serves the role of teaching basic digital skills and knowledge to students and reducing the achievement gap by social class.

Still, our analyses show an inverted U-shaped curvilinear relationship between school ICT use and reading achievement in a small number of countries, including Australia, South Korea, New Zealand, the United Kingdom, the United States, and most Scandinavian countries. This may suggest that policymakers and educators can still design effective curricula to further improve the application of digital technologies in school.

In contrast, inverted U-shaped curvilinear relationships between ICT use at home and reading performance are apparent in most countries and societies in our analysis—14 out of 21 countries/societies for home ICT use for general schoolwork, and 15 of 21 for home ICT use for core subjects. These curvilinear effects suggest that a moderate level of home ICT use helps improve adolescents' reading performance. As ICT use at home increases, however, its positive effect diminishes, and may cause negative impacts on academic achievement if students use ICT at home at a high level. Taken together, the results in this chapter suggest that as digital technologies continue to develop, home environments may play a more important role than schools in shaping adolescents' e-learning experiences and digital competencies, and thus determines whether ICT use may reduce or widen educational inequalities in the twenty-first century.

Reference

OECD. (2021). *PISA 2018 technical report*. PISA, OECD Publishing. https://www.oecd.org/pisa/data/pisa2018technicalreport/

Chapter 5
Digital Inclusion and Learning Attitudes

Abstract To further answer the question, "How does digital technology use influence adolescents' well-being in developed countries?," this chapter examines the effects of ICT use at home and in school on adolescent students' learning attitudes and enjoyment of reading, using 2018 PISA data. Results of multilevel analyses suggest that although adolescents may engage in digital activities in school and at home, home environments are more important in shaping adolescents' learning attitudes and reading enjoyment. However, intensive ICT use at home may yield diminishing returns or even have negative effects on students' learning attitudes and enjoyment of reading. As in Chapter 4, our analyses suggest that the effect of ICT use depends on students' socioeconomic background and differs across countries. In the United Kingdom and Scandinavian countries, ICT use tends to reduce the gaps in learning attitudes between low- and high-SES students. In contrast, in most Western and Asian developed countries, the unequal returns of ICT use widen the disparities between socially advantaged and disadvantaged students.

Keywords Digital inclusion · Learning attitudes · Reading enjoyment · Home vs. school · Curvilinear relationship

THE extent to which digital technologies affect students' academic achievement and well-being is unclear, in part because of the limited measures of ICT use and student outcomes included in empirical analyses. One of the understudied outcome factors is learning attitudes. As a student outcome itself that may be affected by adolescents' digital experience at home and in school, learning attitudes are associated with students' interest in and attention to different academic subjects. Therefore, learning attitudes are determinants of students' academic performance. As an extension, enjoyment of reading is an important component of learning attitudes which are associated with students' cognitive development. Reading enjoyment is also an indicator of learning interest and reading involvement, and a component of intrinsic motivation that can affect students' academic achievement. In this chapter, we analyze

J. K.-H. Ma and S. Cheng, *Adolescent Well-being and ICT UseX*,
Human Well-Being Research and Policy Making,
https://doi.org/10.1007/978-3-031-04412-0_5

the relationship between ICT use and reading enjoyment and the motivation of trying hard at school to answer the question, "How does ICT use influence adolescents' well-being?".

5.1 Methodology

Using data from the 2018 Programme for International Student Assessment (PISA) survey, this chapter has three goals: (1) To assess the differences in the effects of digital inclusion at home versus the effects of digital inclusion in school on learning attitudes, (2) to address cross-national variations in the effects of educational technology, and (3) to examine whether both the magnitude and the direction of these effects vary by students' socioeconomic background.

5.1.1 Outcome Variables

In this chapter, the outcome variables are adolescent students' (1) attitudes toward reading and their (2) attitudes toward learning, such as whether they perceive working hard at school to be important. The first outcome variable, *enjoyment of reading*, is a PISA-created IRT index (*JOYREAD*) based on students' responses to five statements, with an OECD standardized mean of 0 and an OECD standard deviation of 1. In the questionnaire, student respondents were asked "How much do you agree or disagree with these statements about reading?" The response categories from lower to higher values are "Strongly disagree," "Disagree," "Agree," and "Strongly agree." The five statements are:

- I read only if I have to (reverse coding).
- Reading is one of my favorite hobbies.
- I like talking about books with other people.
- For me, reading is a waste of time (reverse coding).
- I read only to get information that I need (reverse coding).

The second outcome variable, *attitudes towards learning at school*, is also a PISA-created IRT index (*ATTLNACT*), based on students' responses to three statements, with an OECD standardized mean of 0 and an OECD standard deviation of 1. In the questionnaire, student respondents were asked "Thinking about your school: to what extent do you agree with the following statements?" The response categories from lower to higher values are "Strongly disagree," "Disagree," "Agree," and "Strongly agree." The three statements are:

- Trying hard at school will help me get a good job.
- Trying hard at school will help me get into a good <college>.
- Trying hard at school is important.

5.1.2 Explanatory Variables

We use two explanatory variables to measure the extent to which students use ICT for school activities at *home* and in *school* (OECD, 2021). The first explanatory variable, *home ICT use for general schoolwork*, is a PISA-created IRT index (*HOMESCH*) based on students' responses to 11 activities and is standardized with an OECD mean of 0 and an OECD standard deviation of 1. In the questionnaire, student respondents were asked "How often do you use digital devices for the following activities outside of school?" The response categories from lower to higher values include "Never or hardly ever," "Once or twice a month," "Once or twice a week," "Almost every day," and "Every day." The 11 activities are:

- Browsing the internet for schoolwork (e.g., for preparing an essay or presentation).
- Browsing the internet to follow up on lessons, e.g., for finding explanations.
- Using email for communication with other students about schoolwork.
- Using email for communication with teachers and submission of homework or other schoolwork.
- Using social networks for communication with teachers (e.g., Facebook and MySpace).
- Downloading, uploading, or browsing material from my school's website (e.g., timetable or course materials).
- Checking the school's website for announcements, e.g., absence of teachers.
- Doing homework on a computer.
- Doing homework on a mobile device.
- Using learning apps or learning websites on a computer.
- Using learning apps or learning websites on a mobile device.

The second explanatory variable is *school ICT use for general schoolwork*. It is also a PISA-created IRT index (*USESCH*), based on students' answers to 10 activities, and is standardized with an OECD mean of 0 and an OECD standard deviation of 1. In the questionnaire, student respondents were asked "How often do you use digital devices for the following activities at school?" The response categories from lower to higher values are "Never or hardly ever," "Once or twice a month," "Once or twice a week," "Almost every day," and "Every day." The 10 activities are:

- Chatting online at school.
- Using email at school.
- Browsing the internet for schoolwork.
- Downloading, uploading, or browsing material from the school's website (e.g., intranet).
- Posting my work on the school's website.
- Playing simulations at school.
- Practicing and drilling, such as for foreign language learning or mathematics.
- Doing homework on a school computer.
- Using school computers for group work and communication with other students.
- Using learning apps or learning websites.

5.1.3 Family SES and Other Control Variables

We use *family SES* to measure students' social class backgrounds. This variable is derived from the index of economic, social, and cultural status (*ESCS*) by PISA (OECD, 2021) as a composite of parental educational level, parental occupational status, and a set of household possessions. It is also standardized with an OECD mean of 0 and an OECD standard deviation of 1. Our analyses include the following control variables at the student-level, including *country-specific program, school grade, student age, gender, immigration status, foreign language use at home, available ICT resources at home*, and *perceived digital competence.* When analyzing the effect of *home* ICT use on academic performance, we control for *school ICT use for general schoolwork.* Likewise, our analyses of the effect of *school* ICT use on academic performance include *home ICT use for general schoolwork* as a control. We also include the following control variables at the school-level: *school average SES*; *public or private school*; *rural, town, or urban school*; *shortage of educational staff*; and *shortage of educational material.* Full descriptions of how OECD constructs the composite variables are available in the OECD's official reports (OECD, 2021).

5.1.4 Analytical Strategies and Methods

To account for cross-national variations, we use the same analytical strategies as in Chapter 4 by running separate multilevel models for *each* country using the OECD PISA 2018 datasets. Each multilevel model includes explanatory variables at both the student-level and the school-level. Our empirical analyses focus on four general areas: First, there may be cross-national variations in the relationship between ICT use and learning attitudes among secondary school students. Second, after controlling for individual- and school-level factors, the influence of ICT use for schoolwork at *home* is likely to differ from that of ICT use for schoolwork in *school.* Third, within countries, the relationship between ICT use and well-being may substantially differ by family SES. Fourth, we examine whether ICT use and learning attitudes have a linear or an inverted U-shaped relationship. The general form of the model for a student i at school s can be written as,

$$\begin{aligned} Y_{is} = &\beta_{0s} + \beta_{1s}(\text{SES})_{is} + \beta_{2s}(\text{ICT use})_{is} + \beta_{3s}(\text{ICT use})^2_{is} \\ &+ \beta_{4s}(\text{SES} \times \text{ICT use})_{is} + \beta_{5s}\left[\text{SES} \times (\text{ICT use}^2)\right]_{is} + \sum_{6}^{k} \beta_{ks} x_{is} + e_{is} \end{aligned} \tag{5.1}$$

At the student-level (Eq. 5.1), Y is the dependent variable. β_{0s} represents the intercept, which is adjusted for other student-level explanatory variables (i.e., SES, ICT use, ICT use^2, SES $\times$ ICT use, SES $\times$ ICT use^2, and β_{6s} to β_{ks}) as well as several school-level control variables (Z_1 to Z_k), as shown in Eq. 5.2 below. The intercept is assumed to vary randomly across schools (μ_{0s}).

$$\beta_{0s} = \gamma_{00} + \sum_{1}^{k} \gamma_{0k} Z_{ks} + \mu_{0s} \tag{5.2}$$

To ease interpretation of the results, we use graphs to visualize the predicted values for the curvilinear effect of digital inclusion (i.e., the use of ICT for school-related work at home or at school) for each country conditioned on student SES. The predicted values reflect the results of multilevel modeling after controlling for all individual-level and school-level characteristics.

5.2 Home ICT Use for General Schoolwork, Enjoyment of Reading, and Family SES

5.2.1 Overall Results

Figure 5.1 presents plots of the predicted values from multilevel regression analyses to illustrate the curvilinear relationship between home ICT use for general schoolwork (x-axis) and enjoyment of reading (y-axis) for each country conditioned on family SES and controlling for individual-level and school-level characteristics. Table 5.1 summarizes and compares the effect size of home ICT use between low- and high-SES students.

Overall, Fig. 5.1 shows clear inverted U-shaped relationships in all of the countries and societies in the analyses. The curvilinear and inverted U-shaped effects suggest that, on one hand, a moderate level of ICT use for schoolwork at home is associated with an increase in students' enjoyment in reading. With the exception of Austria and Japan, the size of this positive effect is substantial for almost all countries. On the other hand, a high level of ICT use at home does not further increase, but instead decreases students' reading enjoyment. Students who use ICT at home at a high level have similar or lower levels of reading enjoyment than their peers who use ICT at a moderate level. The curvilinear relationships between home ICT use for school-related work and reading enjoyment not only vary substantially across countries but also differ by students' socioeconomic background.

Next, we discuss whether digital inclusion at home can enhance low-SES students' reading enjoyment and whether high-SES students receive more learning benefits from e-learning than their low-SES peers.

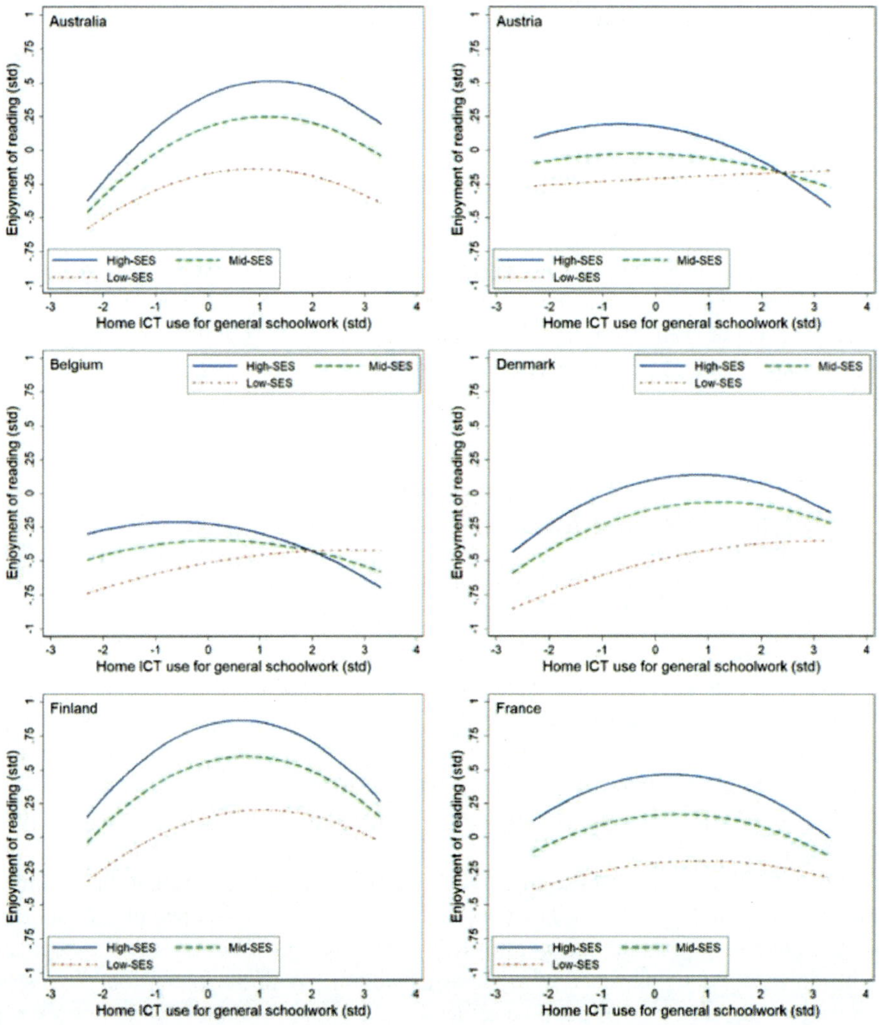

Fig. 5.1 Curvilinear effects of home ICT use for general schoolwork on reading enjoyment by family SES (*Data source* The 2018 Programme for International Student Assessment [PISA] survey. *Note* Countries/societies are listed alphabetically. High-SES refers to students who are at the 90th percentile in family SES. Mid-SES and Low-SES refer to those at the 50th and 10th percentiles in family SES, respectively. Predicted values are calculated based on two-level multilevel models for each country, where student-level variables are used in the Level-1 equation and schools' characteristics are used in the Level-2 equation. All multilevel models include country-specific educational program, school grade, student age, gender, immigration status, foreign language use at home, ICT resources at home, school ICT use for general schoolwork, and perceived digital competence as Level-1 controls. School average SES, public/private school, rural/town/urban school, shortage of educational staff, and shortage of educational material are Level-2 control variables. All Level-1 equations include the interaction effects between family SES and home ICT use for general schoolwork, and between family SES and the squared term of home ICT use for general schoolwork. The following countries are not included in these analyses because key independent or dependent variables are unavailable from the country's PISA data: Canada, Germany, the Netherlands, Portugal, Norway, and China)

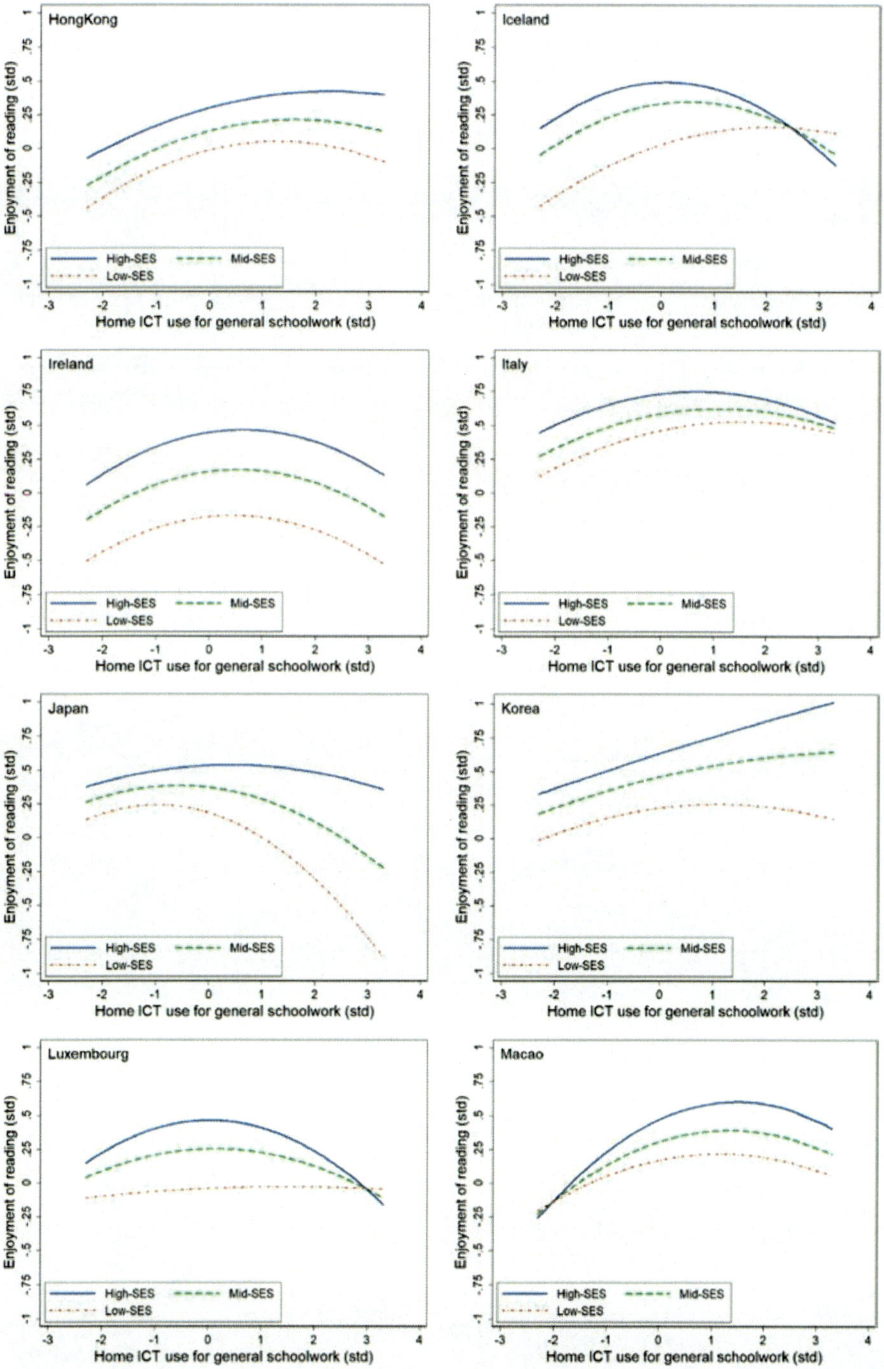

Fig. 5.1 (continued)

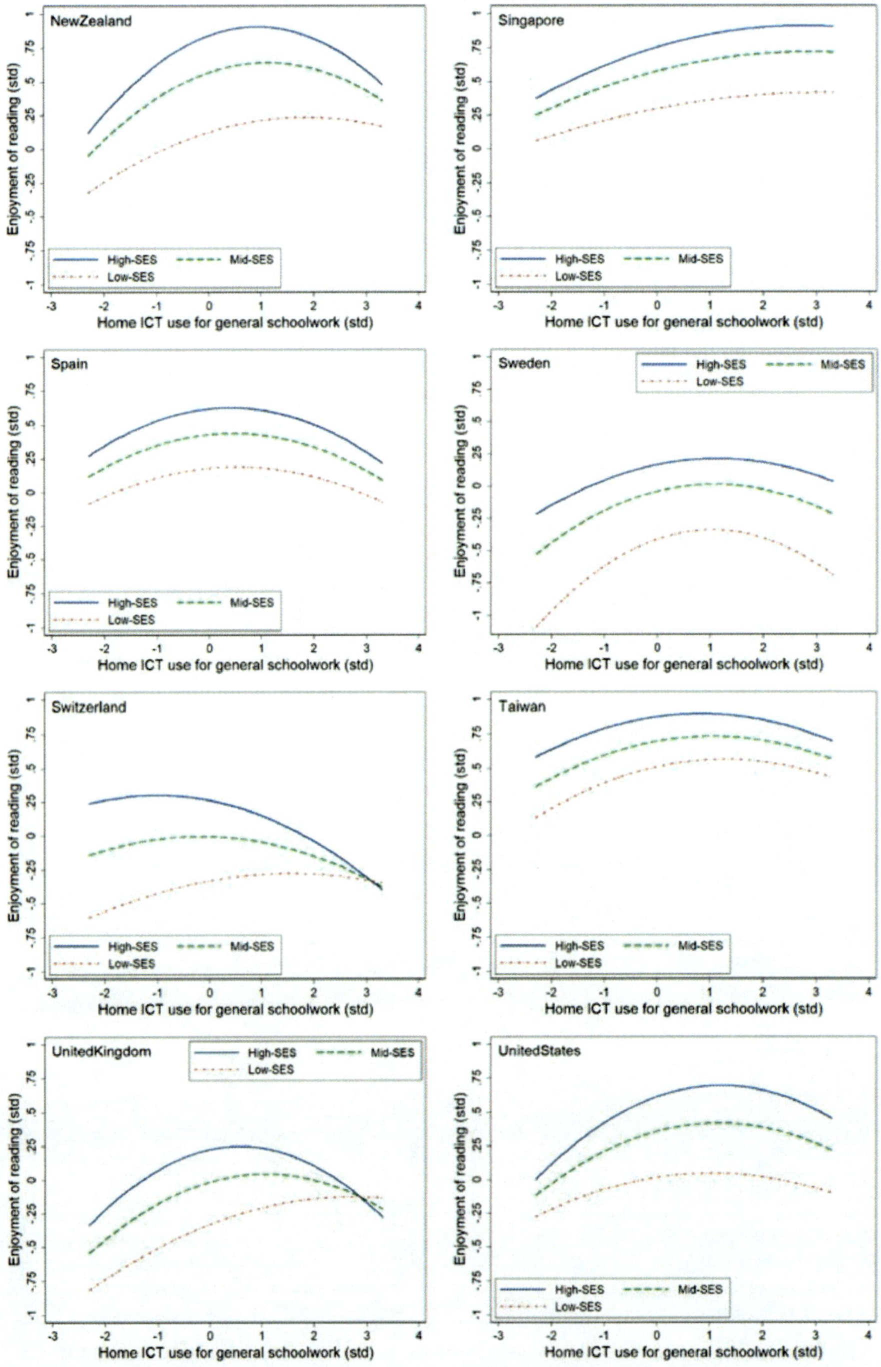

Fig. 5.1 (continued)

Table 5.1 Differences in predicted reading enjoyment between students who do not use ICT for schoolwork at home and students who moderately use ICT for schoolwork at home: Summary of 22 countries/societies in Fig. 5.1

	Low-SES student			High-SES student		
	No ICT use (1)[a]	Moderate ICT use (2)[b]	Difference (2)–(1)[c]	No ICT use (1)[a]	Moderate ICT use (2)[b]	Difference (2)–(1)[c]
North America						
United States	−0.28	0.05	**0.32**	0.00	0.69	**0.69**
Western & Southern Europe						
Austria	−0.26	−0.15	0.11	0.09	0.19	0.10
Belgium	−0.74	−0.42	**0.32**	−0.30	−0.21	0.09
United Kingdom	−0.82	−0.13	**0.69**	−0.34	0.25	**0.58**
France	−0.39	−0.18	0.21	0.12	0.46	**0.34**
Ireland	−0.50	−0.17	**0.33**	0.06	0.46	**0.40**
Italy	0.12	0.53	**0.40**	0.45	0.75	**0.30**
Luxembourg	Negative (or no positive) effect[d]			0.15	0.46	**0.31**
Spain	−0.08	0.19	0.27	0.27	0.62	**0.35**
Switzerland	−0.61	−0.28	**0.33**	Negative (or no positive) effect[d]		
Scandinavia						
Denmark	−0.85	−0.35	**0.50**	−0.44	0.14	**0.57**
Finland	−0.33	0.20	**0.52**	0.15	0.86	**0.71**
Iceland	−0.42	0.16	**0.58**	0.15	0.49	**0.34**
Sweden	−1.09	−0.34	**0.75**	−0.22	0.21	**0.43**
Pacific						
Australia	−0.58	−0.14	**0.44**	−0.38	0.51	**0.89**
New Zealand	−0.32	0.24	**0.55**	0.12	0.91	**0.79**
Asia						
Hong Kong	−0.44	0.05	**0.49**	−0.07	0.42	**0.49**
Japan	0.13	0.24	0.11	0.37	0.53	0.16
Korea	−0.01	0.25	0.27	0.33	1.02	**0.69**
Macao	−0.21	0.22	**0.42**	−0.26	0.60	**0.86**
Singapore	0.06	0.42	**0.36**	0.37	0.91	**0.54**
Taiwan	0.13	0.56	**0.43**	0.58	0.90	**0.32**

Data source The 2018 Programme for International Student Assessment (PISA) survey
Note Countries/societies in each geographical region are listed alphabetically. Low-SES students refer to those who are at the 10th percentile in family SES. High-SES students refer to those at the 90th percentile in family SES
[a]Predicted reading enjoyment for students who do not use ICT for schoolwork at home
[b]Predicted reading enjoyment for students who moderately use ICT for schoolwork at home
[c]Differences in gains of reading enjoyment between Columns 1 and 2. Scores that are above 30 (approximately 1/3 of a standard deviation in reading enjoyment) are highlighted in bold
[d]ICT use at home has no positive effect on reading enjoyment

5.2.2 *Scandinavia*

Table 5.1 shows that in Denmark, Iceland, and Sweden, the role of home ICT use is equally or more important for low-SES students than for high-SES students. In Denmark, for example, moderate home ICT use for schoolwork increases low-SES students' reading enjoyment by 0.50 standard deviations, similar to the increase of 0.57 standard deviations for high-SES students. In Iceland, moderate home ICT use for schoolwork increases low-SES students' reading enjoyment by 0.58 standard deviations, compared to an increase of 0.34 standard deviations for high-SES students. In Sweden, the effects for low- and high-SES students are, respectively, 0.75 and 0.43 standard deviations.

Besides, there is also an inverted U-shaped curvilinear relationship between home ICT use and reading enjoyment in Finland. Unlike the other three Scandinavian countries, however, the positive effect is greater for high-SES students than for low-SES students (0.71 and 0.52 standard deviations, respectively). This greater positive return for high-SES students suggests the problem of the third-level digital divide that exists in Finland.

5.2.3 *Western and Southern Europe*

The results for the Western and Southern European countries are mixed. First, in Austria, although the predicted values of reading enjoyment for moderate ICT use at home are higher than those for no ICT use, the positive effects are small. Second, in Belgium, the United Kingdom, Italy, and Switzerland, the positive relationship between ICT use at home and reading enjoyment is greater for low-SES students than that for high-SES students. In Belgium and Switzerland, for example, although home ICT use only moderately increases low-SES students' reading enjoyment by 0.32 and 0.33 standard deviations, these effects are close to zero among high-SES students. In the case of United Kingdom, home ICT use substantially increases the reading enjoyment of students from both low- and high-SES backgrounds (0.69 and 0.58 standard deviations, respectively).

Third, we also see a third-level digital divide in France and Luxembourg. In these two countries, the effect of home ICT use on reading enjoyment is greater for socioeconomically privileged students than for students of disadvantaged social backgrounds. In Luxembourg, in particular, the regression line predicting low-SES students' reading enjoyment is flat; this suggests that the home ICT use does not increase their reading enjoyment.

5.2.4 *The United States, Australia, and New Zealand*

Home ICT use is important in shaping the reading attitudes of students in the United States, Australia, and New Zealand, but we also see a problem of the third-level digital divide in these countries. In the United States and Australia, home ICT use increases high-SES students' reading enjoyment, respectively, by 0.69 and 0.89 standard deviations, approximately twice as big as the effects for low-SES students (0.32 and 0.44 standard deviations). In New Zealand, the effect is 0.79 standard deviations for high-SES students and 0.55 standard deviations for low-SES students.

5.2.5 *Asia*

Likewise, we observe the third-level digital divide among several Asian countries and societies, such as South Korea, Macao, and Singapore. Taking South Korea and Macao as an example, home ICT use increases high-SES students' reading enjoyment by 0.69 and 0.86 standard deviations, approximately twice as big as the effects for low-SES students (0.27 and 0.42 standard deviations). In contrast, in Hong Kong and Taiwan, the effects of home ICT use at home on reading enjoyment are similar between high- and low-SES students.

5.3 Home ICT Use for General Schoolwork, Learning Attitudes in School, and Family SES

5.3.1 *Overall Results*

Figure 5.2 presents plots of the predicted values from multilevel regression analyses to illustrate the curvilinear relationship between adolescent students' home ICT use for schoolwork (x-axis) and their learning attitudes at school (y-axis) for each country by family SES, after controlling for individual- and school-level characteristics. Table 5.2 summarizes and compares the effect size of home ICT use between low- and high-SES students.

We observe clear inverted U-shaped relationships across all countries and societies that are in the multilevel analyses. Again, these curvilinear and inverted U-shaped effects suggest that, on one hand, a moderate level of home ICT use for schoolwork is associated with an increase in students' positive learning attitudes in school. These positive effects are substantial in magnitudes across all countries. On the other hand, a high level of ICT use at home does not further improve students' learning attitudes in schools. Students who heavily use ICT at home have similar or more negative

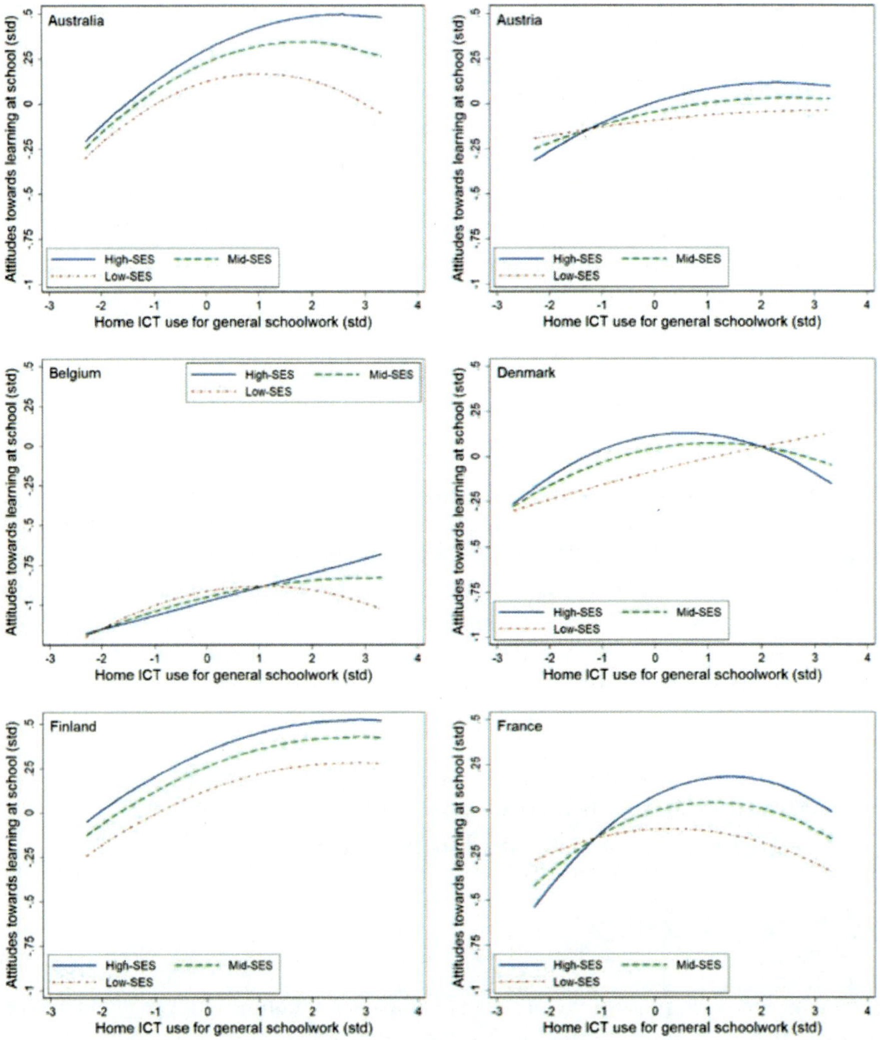

Fig. 5.2 Curvilinear effects of home ICT use for general schoolwork on learning attitudes in school by family SES (*Data source* The 2018 Programme for International Student Assessment [PISA] survey. *Note* Countries/societies are listed alphabetically. High-SES refers to students who are at the 90th percentile in family SES. Mid-SES and Low-SES refer to those at the 50th and 10th percentiles in family SES, respectively. Predicted values are calculated based on two-level multilevel models for each country, where student-level variables are used in the Level-1 equation and schools' characteristics are used in the Level-2 equation. All multilevel models include country-specific educational program, school grade, student age, gender, immigration status, foreign language use at home, ICT resources at home, school ICT use for general schoolwork, and perceived digital competence as Level-1 controls. School average SES, public/private school, rural/town/urban school, shortage of educational staff, and shortage of educational material are Level-2 control variables. All Level-1 equations include the interaction effects between family SES and home ICT use for general schoolwork, and between family SES and the squared term of home ICT use for general schoolwork. The following countries are not included in these analyses because key independent or dependent variables are unavailable from the country's PISA data: Canada, Germany, the Netherlands, Portugal, Norway, and China)

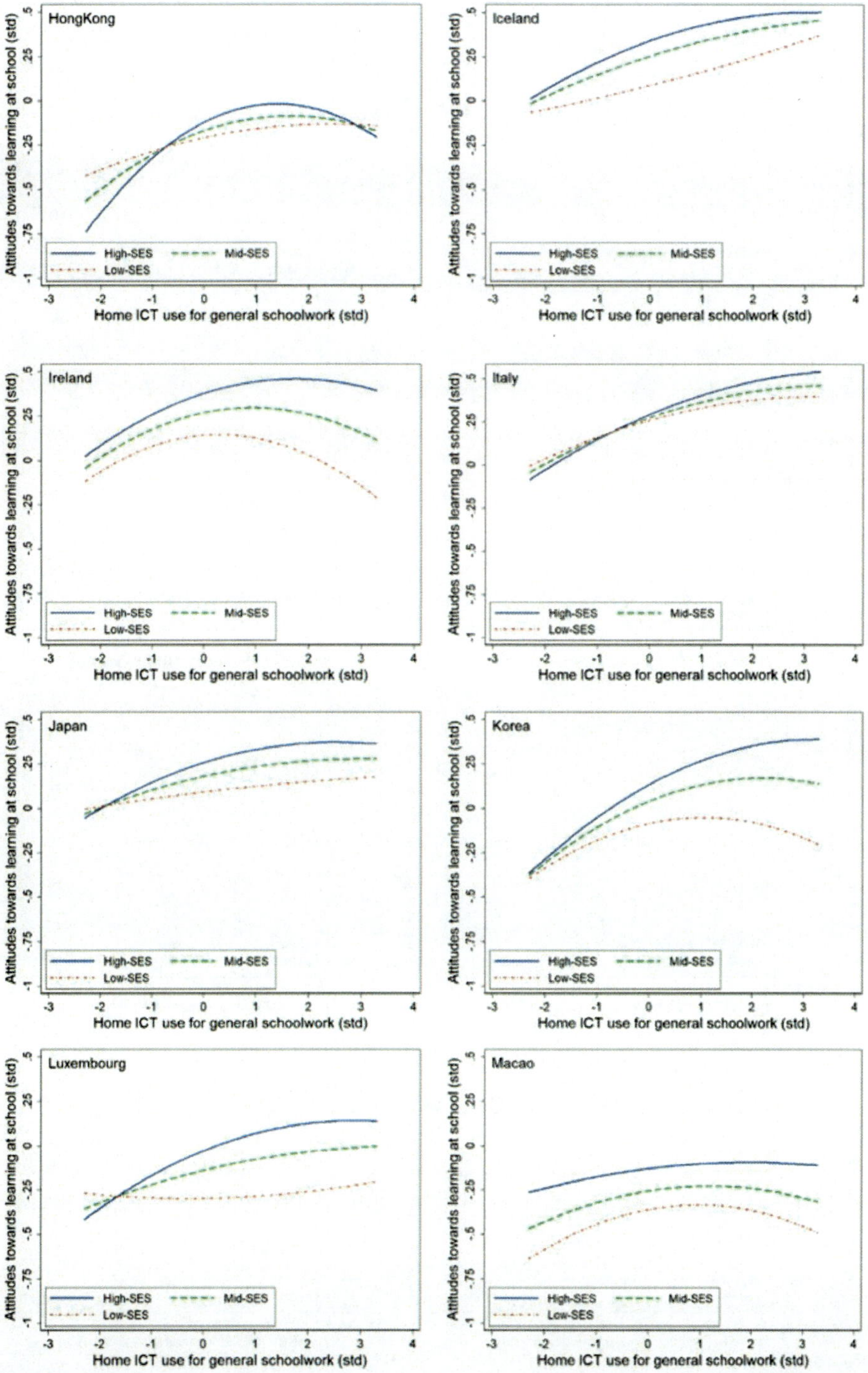

Fig. 5.2 (continued)

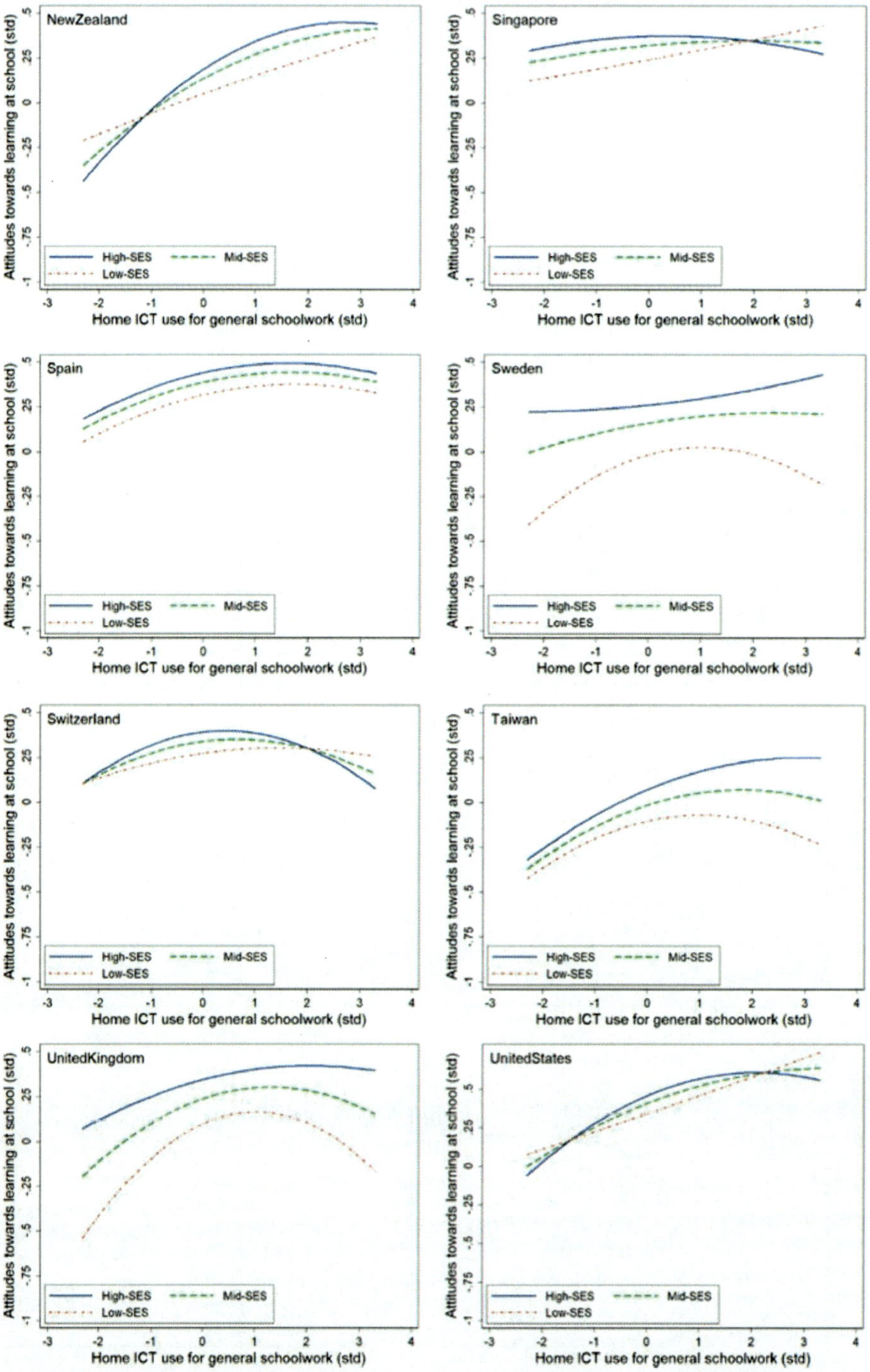

Fig. 5.2 (continued)

Table 5.2 Differences in predicted learning attitudes between students who do not use ICT for schoolwork at home and students who moderately use ICT for schoolwork at home: Summary of 22 countries/societies in Fig. 5.2

	Low-SES student			High-SES student		
	No ICT use (1)[a]	Moderate ICT use (2)[b]	Difference (2)–(1)[c]	No ICT use (1)[a]	Moderate ICT use (2)[b]	Difference (2)–(1)[c]
North America						
United States	0.08	0.74	**0.66**	−0.06	0.61	**0.67**
Western and Southern Europe						
Austria	−0.19	−0.04	0.16	−0.32	0.11	**0.43**
Belgium	−1.20	−0.88	**0.32**	−1.18	−0.68	**0.50**
United Kingdom	−0.54	0.16	**0.70**	0.07	0.42	**0.35**
France	−0.28	−0.11	0.17	−0.54	0.18	**0.72**
Ireland	−0.12	0.14	0.26	0.02	0.46	**0.43**
Italy	−0.01	0.39	**0.40**	−0.08	0.54	**0.62**
Luxembourg	Negative (or no positive) effect[d]			−0.42	0.14	**0.56**
Spain	0.06	0.38	**0.32**	0.18	0.49	**0.31**
Switzerland	0.10	0.30	0.20	0.11	0.40	0.29
Scandinavia						
Denmark	−0.30	0.13	**0.43**	−0.26	0.13	**0.39**
Finland	−0.24	0.28	**0.52**	−0.05	0.52	**0.58**
Iceland	−0.06	0.38	**0.44**	0.01	0.50	**0.49**
Sweden	−0.41	0.02	**0.43**	0.22	0.43	0.21
Pacific						
Australia	−0.30	0.17	**0.47**	−0.21	0.50	**0.70**
New Zealand	−0.21	0.37	**0.58**	−0.44	0.45	**0.89**
Asia						
Hong Kong	−0.42	−0.13	0.29	−0.74	−0.02	**0.72**
Japan	−0.01	0.18	0.18	−0.05	0.37	**0.43**
Korea	−0.39	−0.05	**0.34**	−0.37	0.39	**0.76**
Macao	−0.64	−0.34	**0.30**	−0.27	−0.09	0.17
Singapore	0.12	0.43	**0.31**	0.29	0.37	0.08
Taiwan	−0.42	−0.07	**0.35**	−0.32	0.25	**0.57**

Data source The 2018 Programme for International Student Assessment (PISA) survey
Note Countries/societies in each geographical region are listed alphabetically. Low-SES students refer to those who are at the 10th percentile in family SES. High-SES students refer to those at the 90th percentile in family SES
[a]Predicted learning attitudes for students who do not use ICT for schoolwork at home
[b]Predicted learning attitudes for students who moderately use ICT for schoolwork at home
[c]Differences in improvement of learning attitudes between Columns 1 and 2. Scores that are above 30 (approximately 1/3 of a standard deviation in learning attitudes) are highlighted in bold
[d]ICT use at home has no positive effect on learning attitudes

learning attitudes in school than their peers who moderately use ICT at home. The curvilinear relationships between home ICT use for schoolwork and learning attitudes not only vary substantially across countries but also differ by students' socioeconomic background.

5.3.2 *Scandinavia*

Table 5.2 shows that home ICT use is equally or more important for low-SES students' learning attitudes than for high-SES students among all Scandinavian countries. In Denmark and Finland, moderate home ICT use increases low-SES students' positive learning attitudes, respectively, by 0.43 and 0.52 standard deviations; these effects are approximately the same as for high-SES students (0.39 and 0.58 standard deviations, respectively). In Sweden, the positive effects of moderate home ICT use on learning attitudes are greater for low-SES students (0.43 standard deviations) than for high-SES students (0.21 standard deviations).

5.3.3 *Western and Southern Europe*

We find the problem of the third-level digital divide in six of nine Western or Southern European countries, including Austria, Belgium, France, Ireland, Italy, and Luxembourg. In these countries, the positive effects of home ICT use for schoolwork on learning attitudes are greater among high-SES students compared to their low-SES peers. These unequal returns of ICT use further increase the disparities between socially advantaged and disadvantaged students.

In contrast, in Spain and Switzerland, the positive effects of home ICT use on learning attitudes are similar for low-SES (0.32 and 0.20 standard deviations, respectively) and high-SES students (0.31 and 0.29 standard deviations, respectively). In Britain, moderate home ICT use increases low-SES students' positive learning attitudes by 0.70 standard deviations, approximately twice as big as the positive effect on high-SES students (0.35 standard deviations).

5.3.4 *The United States, Australia, and New Zealand*

In the United States, the positive effects of home ICT use on learning attitudes are approximately equal for low- and high-SES students (0.66 and 0.67 standard deviations). In contrast, the third-level digital divide is also present in Australia and New Zealand, where using ICT at home can improve high-SES students' learning attitudes by 0.70 and 0.89 standard deviations, respectively, which are greater than the improvement gained by low-SES students (0.47 and 0.58 standard deviations).

5.3.5 Asia

We also observe the problem of the third-level digital divide in most of the Asian countries and societies, including Hong Kong, Japan, South Korea, and Taiwan. Taking Hong Kong and Japan as an example, the sizes of the positive effect of ICT use at home on learning attitudes are 0.72 and 0.43 standard deviations, respectively, for high-SES students. But these positive effects for low-SES students are much smaller (0.29 and 0.18 standard deviations, respectively). In Macao and Singapore, on the contrary, the positive effects of home ICT use seem greater for low-SES students (0.30 and 0.31 standard deviations) than for high-SES students (0.17 and 0.08 standard deviations).

5.4 School ICT Use for General Schoolwork, Enjoyment of Reading, and Family SES

5.4.1 Overall Results

In this section, we examine the effects of ICT use in school. Figure 5.3 presents plots of the predicted values from multilevel regression analyses to illustrate the curvilinear relationship between students' ICT use in school (x-axis) and their enjoyment of reading (y-axis) for each country conditioned on family SES and controlling for individual- and school-level characteristics. Table 5.3 summarizes and compares the effect size of school ICT use between low- and high-SES students.

Overall, school ICT use seems less important than home ICT use in terms of their influences on students' reading enjoyment. Figure 5.3 shows inverted U-shaped relationships between ICT use and reading enjoyment in 11 of the 21 countries and societies included the analyses. These include Australia, Belgium, Denmark, France, Iceland, Japan, Macao, New Zealand, Sweden, the United Kingdom, and the United States. For students in these countries, a moderate level of ICT use at school is associated with an increase in students' reading enjoyment, but the size of the effect is modest. In other countries, such as Italy, Spain, and Switzerland, ICT use in school has a consistently negative effect on reading enjoyment. Table 5.3 further highlights this pattern: In most of the Western European, Southern European, and Asian developed countries, the relationship between ICT use in school and the level of students' reading enjoyment is negative.

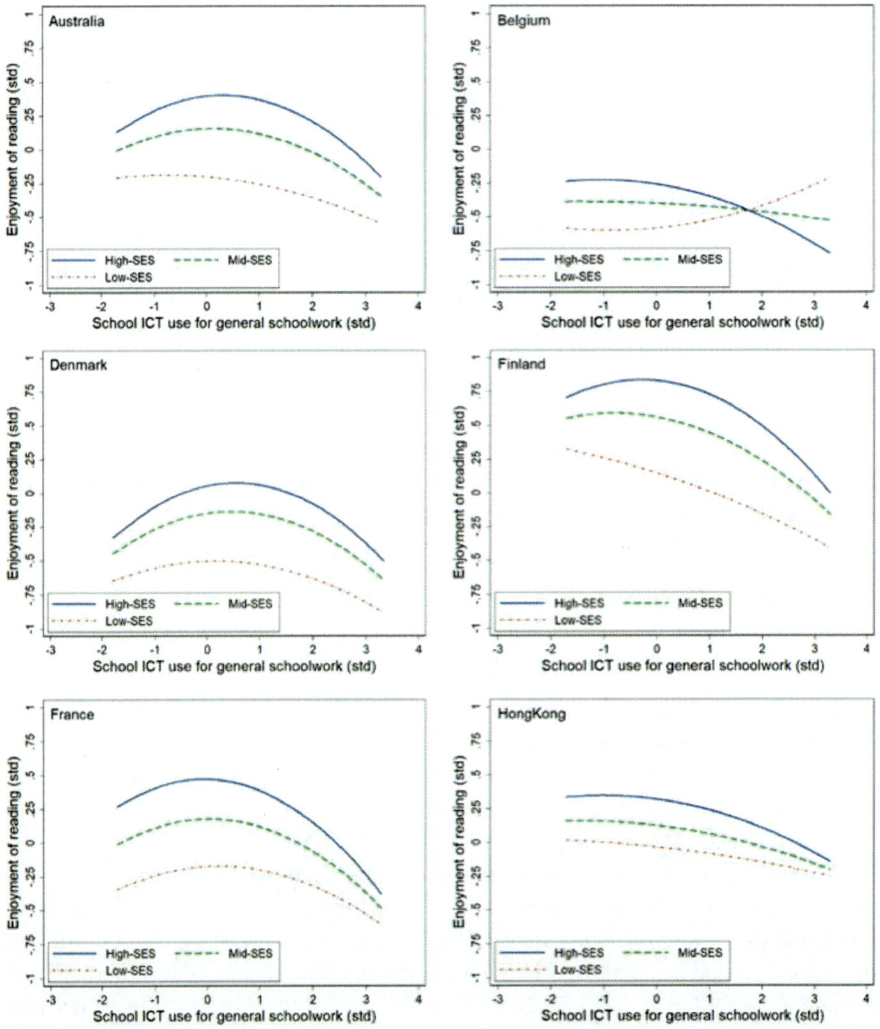

Fig. 5.3 Curvilinear effects of school ICT use for general schoolwork on reading enjoyment by family SES (*Data source* The 2018 Programme for International Student Assessment [PISA] survey. *Note* Countries/societies are listed alphabetically. High-SES refers to students who are at the 90th percentile in family SES. Mid-SES and Low-SES refer to those at the 50th and 10th percentiles in family SES, respectively. Predicted values are calculated based on two-level multilevel models for each country, where student-level variables are used in the Level-1 equation and schools' characteristics are used in the Level-2 equation. All multilevel models include country-specific educational program, school grade, student age, gender, immigration status, foreign language use at home, ICT resources at home, home ICT use for general schoolwork, and perceived digital competence as Level-1 controls. School average SES, public/private school, rural/town/urban school, shortage of educational staff, and shortage of educational material are Level-2 control variables. All Level-1 equations include the interaction effects between family SES and school ICT use for general schoolwork, and between family SES and the squared term of school ICT use for general schoolwork. The following countries are not included in these analyses because key independent or dependent variables are unavailable from the country's PISA data: Canada, Austria, Germany, the Netherlands, Portugal, Norway, and China)

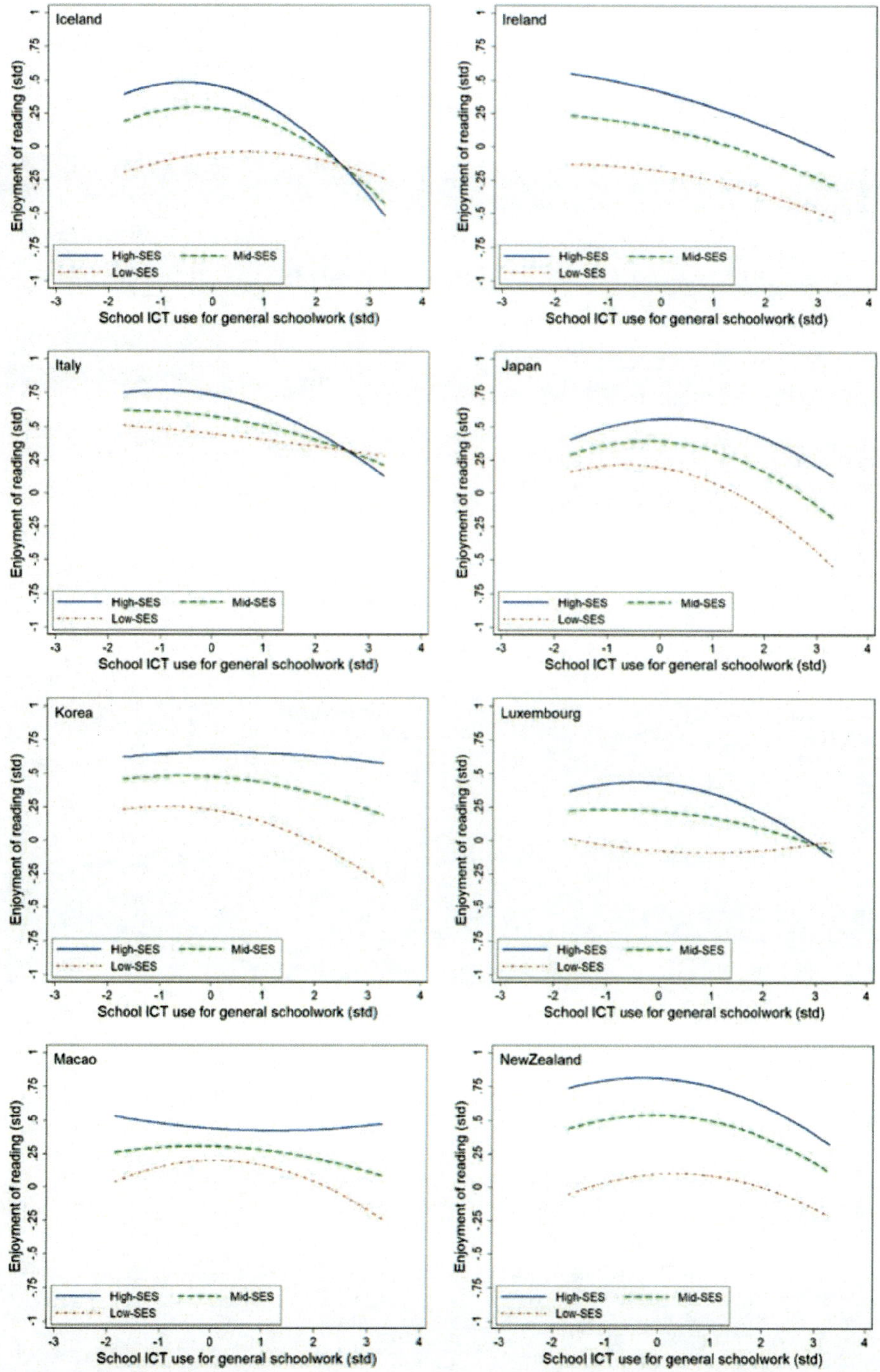

Fig. 5.3 (continued)

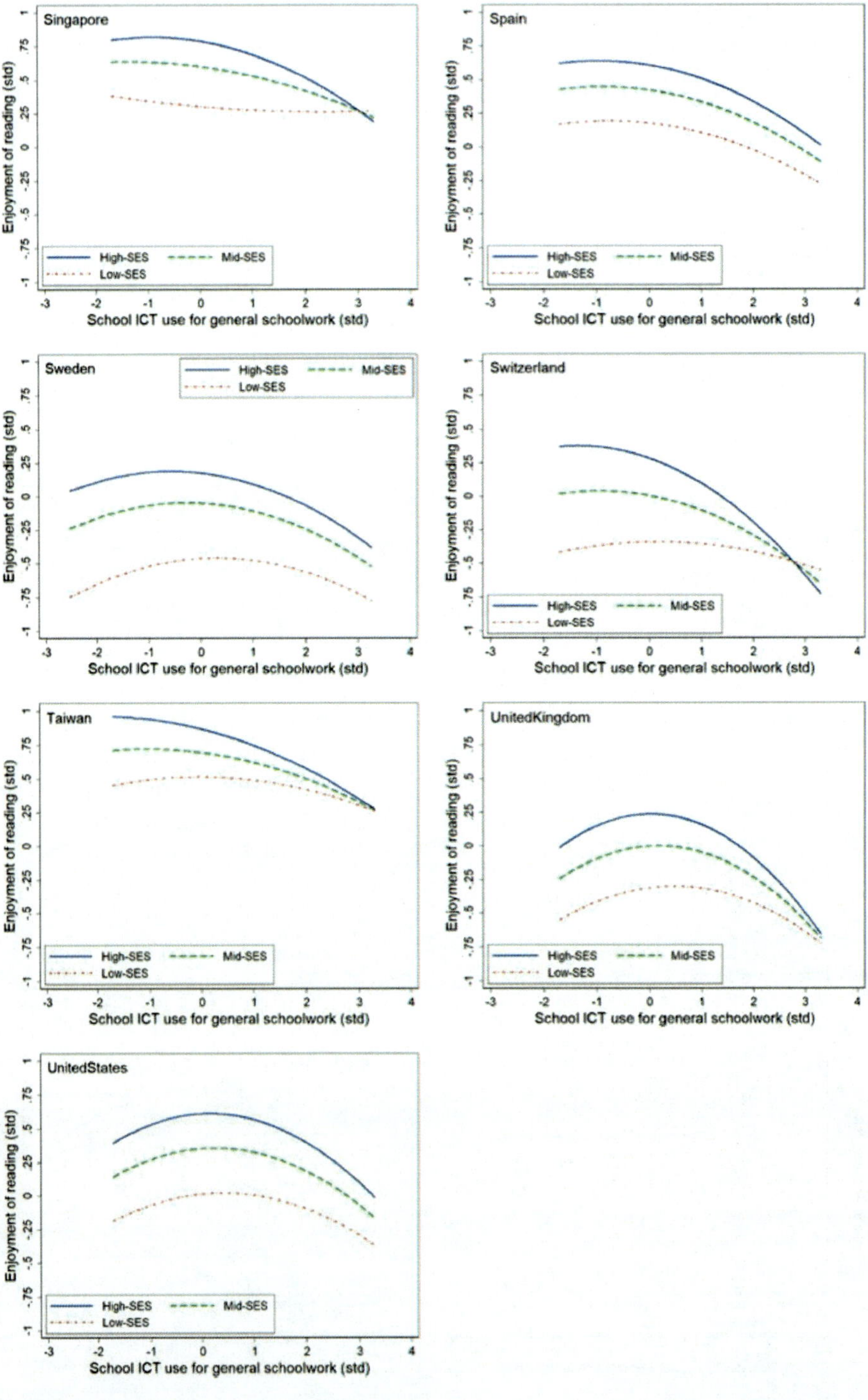

Fig. 5.3 (continued)

Table 5.3 Differences in predicted reading enjoyment between students who do not use ICT for schoolwork at school and students who moderately use ICT for schoolwork at school: Summary of 21 countries/societies in Fig. 5.3

	Low-SES student			High-SES student		
	No ICT use (1)[a]	Moderate ICT use (2)[b]	Difference (2)–(1)[c]	No ICT use (1)[a]	Moderate ICT use (2)[b]	Difference (2)–(1)[c]
North America						
United States	−0.19	0.02	0.21	0.39	0.61	0.22
Western and Southern Europe						
Belgium	−0.59	−0.21	**0.38**	Negative (or no positive) effect[d]		
United Kingdom	−0.55	−0.30	0.25	−0.01	0.23	0.25
France	−0.34	−0.17	0.17	0.27	0.47	0.20
Ireland	Negative (or no positive) effect[d]			Negative (or no positive) effect[d]		
Italy	Negative (or no positive) effect[d]			Negative (or no positive) effect[d]		
Luxembourg	Negative (or no positive) effect[d]			0.37	0.43	0.07
Spain	Negative (or no positive) effect[d]			Negative (or no positive) effect[d]		
Switzerland	−0.42	−0.34	0.08	Negative (or no positive) effect[d]		
Scandinavia						
Denmark	−0.65	−0.50	0.14	−0.33	0.08	**0.40**
Finland	Negative (or no positive) effect[d]			0.70	0.83	0.13
Iceland	−0.19	−0.04	0.15	0.39	0.48	0.09
Sweden	−0.75	−0.46	0.29	0.05	0.19	0.14
Pacific						
Australia	Negative (or no positive) effect[d]			0.13	0.40	0.27
New Zealand	−0.05	0.10	0.15	0.74	0.82	0.08
Asia						
Hong Kong	Negative (or no positive) effect[d]			Negative (or no positive) effect[d]		
Japan	0.16	0.22	0.06	0.40	0.56	0.16
Korea	Negative (or no positive) effect[d]			Negative (or no positive) effect[d]		
Macao	0.04	0.20	0.16	Negative (or no positive) effect[d]		
Singapore	Negative (or no positive) effect[d]			Negative (or no positive) effect[d]		
Taiwan	0.45	0.51	0.06	Negative (or no positive) effect[d]		

Data source The 2018 Programme for International Student Assessment (PISA) survey
Note Countries/societies in each geographical region are listed alphabetically. Low-SES students refer to those who are at the 10th percentile in family SES. High-SES students refer to those at the 90th percentile in family SES
[a]Predicted reading enjoyment for students who do not use ICT for schoolwork at school
[b]Predicted reading enjoyment for students who moderately use ICT for schoolwork at school
[c]Differences in gains of reading enjoyment between Columns 1 and 2. Scores that are above 30 (approximately 1/3 of a standard deviation in reading enjoyment) are highlighted in bold
[d]ICT use at school has no positive effect on reading enjoyment

5.4.2 The United States, the United Kingdom, Belgium, and Sweden

Table 5.3 shows that the use of digital technologies in school has similar effects on the level of reading enjoyment for students from different socioeconomic backgrounds in the United States and in the United Kingdom. For low-SES students, ICT use in school increases students' reading enjoyment by 0.21 and 0.25 standard deviations, respectively, in the United States and in the United Kingdom. For high-SES students in the two countries, the effects are 0.22 and 0.25 standard deviations. On the other hand, in Belgium and Sweden, we observe inverted U-shaped relationships between ICT use in school and students' reading enjoyment only for low-SES students but not for high-SES students.

5.4.3 Denmark and Australia

Data from Denmark and Australia indicate the problem of the third-level digital divide. In Denmark, ICT use in school increases high-SES students' reading enjoyment by 0.40 standard deviations, whereas the effect for low-SES students is only 0.14 standard deviations. In Australia, ICT use in school increases high-SES students' reading enjoyment by 0.27 standard deviations but has no positive effect on the reading enjoyment of low-SES students.

5.5 School ICT Use for General Schoolwork, Learning Attitudes in School, and Family SES

5.5.1 Overall Results

Figure 5.4 presents plots of the predicted values from multilevel regression analyses to illustrate the curvilinear relationship between school ICT use (x-axis) and students' learning attitudes (y-axis) for each country conditioned on family SES and controlling for individual-level and school-level characteristics. Table 5.4 summarizes and compares the effect size of school ICT use between low- and high-SES students.

As in the analyses of school ICT use on students' reading enjoyment, we find that using digital technologies in school is less important than home ICT use in promoting students' positive learning attitudes. Overall, we observe inverted U-shaped relationships between school ICT use and learning attitudes only in seven of the 21 countries/societies in the analyses. These seven countries are Australia, Denmark, France, Macao, New Zealand, Sweden, and the United Kingdom. For students in these countries, a moderate level of ICT use at school is associated with an increase

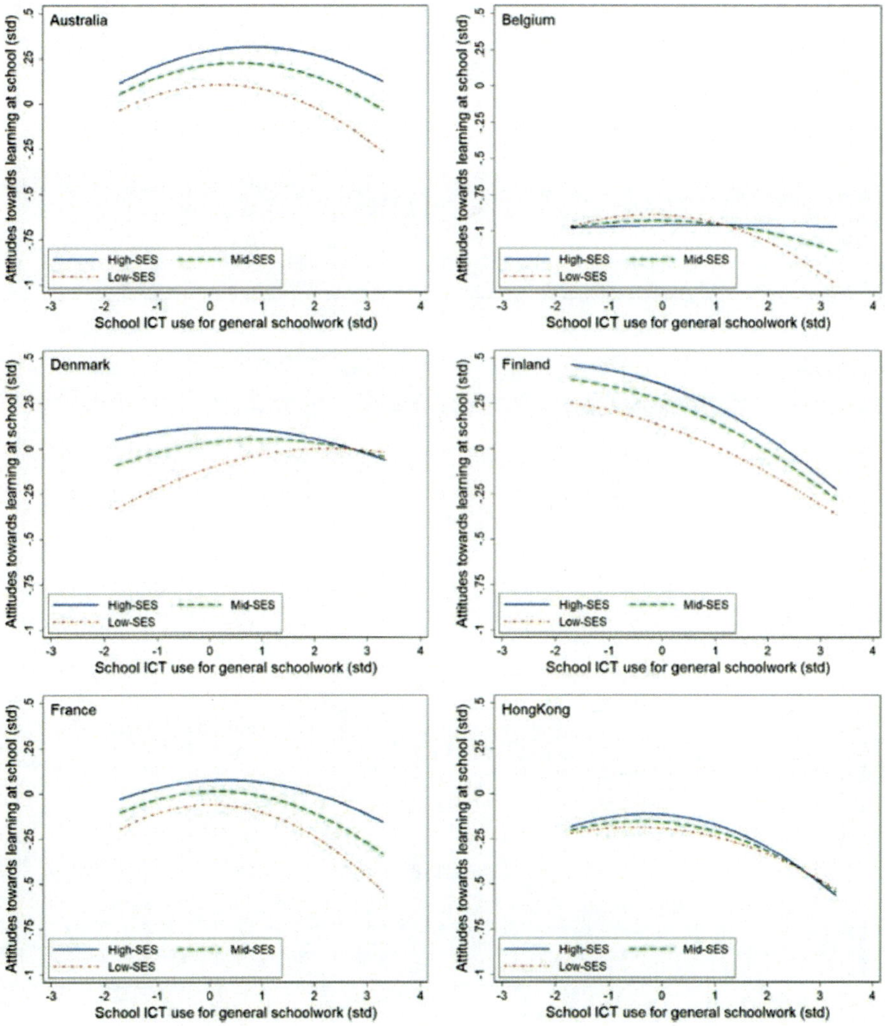

Fig. 5.4 Curvilinear effects of school ICT use for general schoolwork on learning attitudes in school by family SES (*Data source* The 2018 Programme for International Student Assessment [PISA] survey. *Note* Countries/societies are listed alphabetically. High-SES refers to students who are at the 90th percentile in family SES. Mid-SES and Low-SES refer to those at the 50th and 10th percentiles in family SES, respectively. Predicted values are calculated based on two-level multilevel models for each country, where student-level variables are used in the Level-1 equation and schools' characteristics are used in the Level-2 equation. All multilevel models include country-specific educational program, school grade, student age, gender, immigration status, foreign language use at home, ICT resources at home, home ICT use for general schoolwork, and perceived digital competence as Level-1 controls. School average SES, public/private school, rural/town/urban school, shortage of educational staff, and shortage of educational material are Level-2 control variables. All Level-1 equations include the interaction effects between family SES and school ICT use for general schoolwork, and between family SES and the squared term of school ICT use for general schoolwork. The following countries are not included in these analyses because key independent or dependent variables are unavailable from the country's PISA data: Canada, Austria, Germany, the Netherlands, Portugal, Norway, and China)

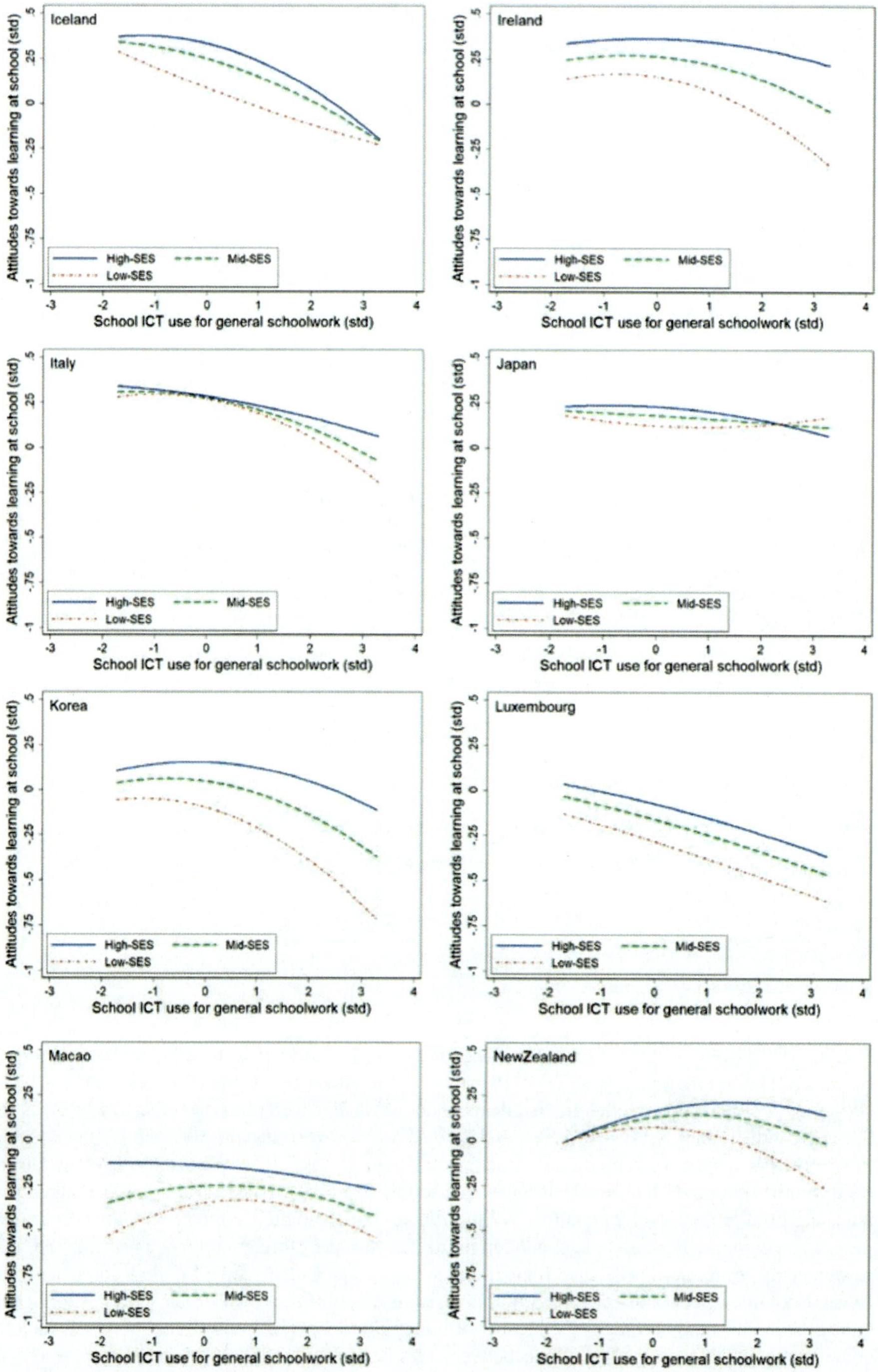

Fig. 5.4 (continued)

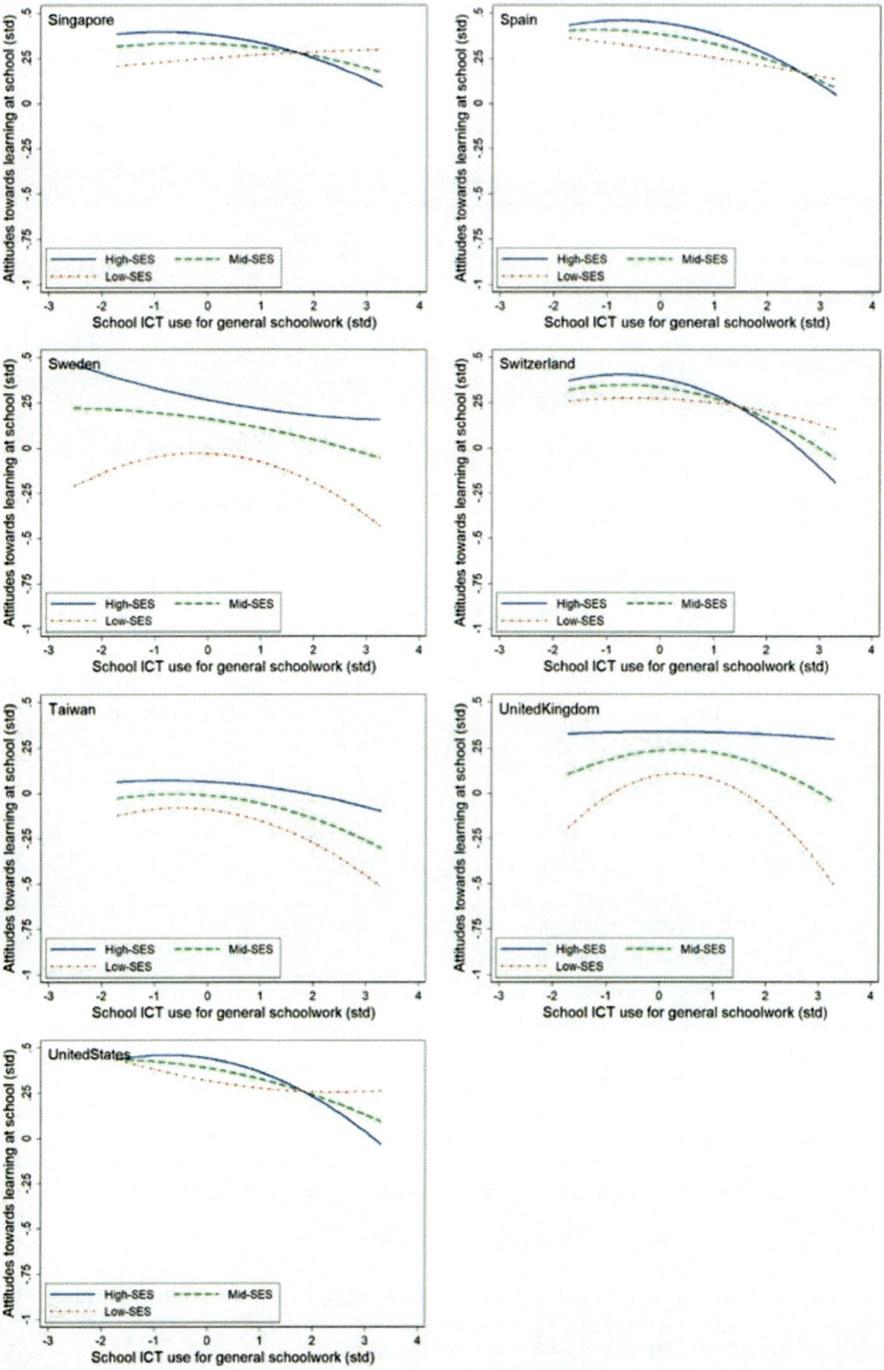

Fig. 5.4 (continued)

Table 5.4 Differences in predicted learning attitudes between students who do not use ICT for schoolwork at school and students who moderately use ICT for schoolwork at school: Summary of 21 countries/societies in Fig. 5.4

	Low-SES student			High-SES student		
	No ICT use (1)[a]	Moderate ICT use (2)[b]	Difference (2)–(1)[c]	No ICT use (1)[a]	Moderate ICT use (2)[b]	Difference (2)–(1)[c]
North America						
United States	Negative (or no positive) effect[d]			Negative (or no positive) effect[d]		
Western and Southern Europe						
Belgium	−0.97	−0.88	0.09	Negative (or no positive) effect[d]		
United Kingdom	−0.19	0.11	**0.30**	Negative (or no positive) effect[d]		
France	−0.20	−0.06	0.13	−0.03	0.07	0.10
Ireland	Negative (or no positive) effect[d]			Negative (or no positive) effect[d]		
Italy	Negative (or no positive) effect[d]			Negative (or no positive) effect[d]		
Luxembourg	Negative (or no positive) effect[d]			Negative (or no positive) effect[d]		
Spain	Negative (or no positive) effect[d]			Negative (or no positive) effect[d]		
Switzerland	Negative (or no positive) effect[d]			Negative (or no positive) effect[d]		
Scandinavia						
Denmark	−0.34	0.00	**0.34**	0.05	0.11	0.06
Finland	Negative (or no positive) effect[d]			Negative (or no positive) effect[d]		
Iceland	Negative (or no positive) effect[d]			Negative (or no positive) effect[d]		
Sweden	−0.21	−0.03	0.18	Negative (or no positive) effect[d]		
Pacific						
Australia	−0.04	0.10	0.14	0.11	0.31	0.20
New Zealand	−0.01	0.08	0.09	−0.01	0.21	0.23
Asia						
Hong Kong	Negative (or no positive) effect[d]			−0.19	−0.11	0.07
Japan	Negative (or no positive) effect[d]			Negative (or no positive) effect[d]		
Korea	Negative (or no positive) effect[d]			0.11	0.15	0.05
Macao	−0.53	−0.34	0.20	Negative (or no positive) effect[d]		
Singapore	0.21	0.30	0.09	Negative (or no positive) effect[d]		
Taiwan	−0.12	−0.08	0.04	Negative (or no positive) effect[d]		

Data source The 2018 Programme for International Student Assessment (PISA) survey
Note Countries/societies in each geographical region are listed alphabetically. Low-SES students refer to those who are at the 10th percentile in family SES. High-SES students refer to those at the 90th percentile in family SES
[a]Predicted learning attitudes for students who do not use ICT for schoolwork at school
[b]Predicted learning attitudes for students who moderately use ICT for schoolwork at school
[c]Differences in improvement of learning attitudes between Columns 1 and 2. Scores that are above 30 (approximately 1/3 of a standard deviation in learning attitudes) are highlighted in bold
[d]ICT use at school has no positive effect on learning attitudes

in students' learning attitudes, but the size of the effect is again modest. In other countries, such as the United States, Finland, and South Korea, ICT use in school has a consistently negative effect on learning attitudes. Table 5.4 further suggests that this pattern also applies to most of the Western European, Southern European, and Asian developed countries.

5.5.2 *The United Kingdom, Denmark, Sweden, and Macao*

Figure 5.4 shows that in the United Kingdom, Denmark, Sweden, and Macao, ICT use in school and students' learning attitudes have an inverted U-shaped relationship for low-SES students, but not for high-SES students. In the United Kingdom, for example, ICT use in school increases low-SES students' positive learning attitudes by 0.30 standard deviations. In Denmark, ICT use in school increases low-SES students' positive learning attitudes by 0.34 standard deviations. For high-SES students, the effects are either small or nonexistent.

5.5.3 *New Zealand*

Finally, we find that in New Zealand, ICT use in school increases high-SES students' positive learning attitudes by 0.23 standard deviations, whereas it increases low-SES students' positive learning attitudes only by 0.09 standard deviations. These unequal returns of school ICT use may further increase the disparities between socially advantaged and disadvantaged students in New Zealand.

5.6 Summary and Conclusion

Using 2018 PISA data, this chapter analyzes the effects of ICT use at home and in school on adolescents' learning attitudes and enjoyment of reading. Learning attitudes are a complex construct composed of elements such as feelings or beliefs that efforts on schoolwork are important for future academic and career development. Reading enjoyment is the satisfaction that adolescents derive from reading in their daily lives. Despite the close relationship between reading enjoyment, learning attitudes, and academic performance, empirical studies on the effects of ICT use tend to focus on academic achievement, which often overlook learning attitudes.

The results of our multilevel analyses confirm that disparities in students' learning attitudes may widen as a result of the digital divide. Although adolescents may participate in digital activities in school and at home, our findings suggest that home environments are more important than schools in shaping adolescents' learning attitudes and reading enjoyment. In virtually all developed countries and societies, we have found clear inverted U-shaped relationships between digital inclusion at home, learning attitudes, and reading enjoyment. In contrast, school ICT use is less important in changing students' learning attitudes and reading enjoyment, with substantial effects in fewer than half of the 21 countries. This is not surprising, since K-12 schools often teach only basic digital skills and knowledge. This said, our findings caution that intensive ICT use at home may still yield diminishing returns or even have negative effects on students' learning attitudes and enjoyment of reading.

As in Chapter 4, our analyses suggest that ICT effects vary by students' socioeconomic background and across countries. In the United Kingdom and Scandinavian countries, ICT use tends to narrow the digital gaps in learning attitudes and reading enjoyment between low- and high-SES students. However, in most other Western and Asian societies (except for Belgium and Macao), the positive effects of ICT use are greater for high-SES students than for low-SES students. The unequal returns of ICT use thus increase the disparities between socially advantaged and disadvantaged students. These findings suggest that ICT policy in education in most developed countries should be revised to accommodate students from socially disadvantaged backgrounds.

Reference

OECD. (2021). *PISA 2018 technical report*. PISA, OECD Publishing. https://www.oecd.org/pisa/data/pisa2018technicalreport/

Chapter 6
Digital Inclusion, Psychological Well-Being, and Digital Competence

Abstract Although a large proportion of adolescent students regularly use digital devices and the internet, the effects of digital technology on psychological health and digital competence are still a matter of policy and scholarly debates. Using 2018 PISA data, this chapter examines the influences of ICT use at home and in school on adolescents' sense of belonging at school, positive psychological feelings, sense of purpose and meaning in life, and perceived ICT competence. Results of multilevel analyses across 22 developed countries suggest that ICT use for schoolwork both at home and in school increases adolescents' perceived ICT competence. Although school ICT use has minimal positive effects on students' psychological well-being in a few countries, the benefits of home ICT use are substantial. ICT use has equal or greater positive effects on perceived ICT competence and psychological well-being for low-SES students in half of the developed countries (e.g., the United Kingdom and Iceland), and greater positive effects for high-SES students in the other half. This suggests that some countries are more capable than others in implementing ICT use in education, which may mitigate some of the disparities in adolescent students' psychological well-being.

Keywords Digital inclusion · Psychological well-being · School belonging · Digital competence · Home vs. school · Curvilinear relationship

DIGITAL technologies have all-encompassing effects on people's lives. Adolescents and young adults are developing innovative ways of navigating this new technological age, such as virtual learning, maintaining social networking with friends old and new, finding and buying merchandise, and entertaining themselves in the cyber world. While many of these changes are beneficial, there are increasing concerns about the drawbacks of these technologies. ICT use in the information society has doubtless created a new source of inequality in social and psychological well-being.

In this chapter, we examine the influence of digital inclusion at home and in school on adolescent students' psychological well-being. Psychological well-being

J. K.-H. Ma and S. Cheng, *Adolescent Well-being and ICT UseX*,
Human Well-Being Research and Policy Making,
https://doi.org/10.1007/978-3-031-04412-0_6

should be taken as an important addition to the academic outcome measures typically included in digital inequality research on adolescents because of the growing role of ICT use in adolescent life. Moreover, because students' knowledge, skills, and confidence in digital technologies affect their academic and personal success, this chapter examines whether and how ICT use at home and in school influences adolescents' perceived digital competence.

6.1 Methodology

Using data from the 2018 Programme for International Student Assessment (PISA) survey and the same multilevel analyses as in Chaps. 4 and 5, this chapter has three goals: (1) To examine the differences in the effects of digital inclusion at home versus digital inclusion in school on both subjective and psychological well-being and digital competence, (2) to address cross-national variations in the effects of educational technology, and (3) to examine whether the magnitude and the direction of these effects vary by students' socioeconomic background. Digital inclusion is broadly defined as the use of digital technologies for learning-related activities and school-related work.

6.1.1 Outcome Variables

This chapter focuses on four outcome variables that measure adolescent students' psychological well-being and ICT competence: (1) Perceived sense of belonging at school, (2) perceived positive psychological feelings, (3) perceived sense of positive meaning and purpose in life, and (4) perceived ICT competence. The first outcome variable, *adolescents' perceived sense of belonging at school*, is a PISA-created IRT index *(BELONG)* standardized to an OECD mean of 0 and an OECD standard deviation of 1. In the questionnaire, student respondents were asked "Thinking about your school: to what extent do you agree with the following statements?" The response categories from lower to higher values are "Strongly disagree," "Disagree," "Agree," and "Strongly agree." This index is based on the following six statements.

- I feel like an outsider (or left out of things) at school (reverse coding).
- I make friends easily at school.
- I feel like I belong at school.
- I feel awkward and out of place in my school (reverse coding).
- Other students seem to like me.
- I feel lonely at school (reverse coding).

The second outcome variable, *perceived positive psychological feelings*, is also a PISA-created IRT index *(SWBP)* standardized to an OECD mean of 0 and an OECD standard deviation of 1. In the questionnaire, student respondents were asked

"Thinking about yourself and how you normally feel: how often do you feel as described below?" The response categories from lower to higher values are "Never," "Rarely," "Sometimes," and "Always." This index is based on students' responses to three feelings.

- Joyful.
- Cheerful.
- Happy.

The third outcome variable, *perceived sense of positive meaning (and positive purpose) in life*, is another PISA-created IRT index *(EUDMO)* with an OECD mean of 0 and an OECD standard deviation of 1. In the questionnaire, student respondents were asked "How much do you agree with the following statements?" The response categories from lower to higher values are "Strongly disagree," "Disagree," "Agree," and "Strongly agree." The index is based on students' responses to the following three statements.

- My life has a clear meaning or purpose.
- I have discovered a satisfactory meaning in life.
- I have a clear sense of what gives meaning to my life.

The fourth outcome variable is *perceived ICT competence*, a PISA-created IRT index (*COMPICT*) with an OECD mean of 0 and an OECD standard deviation of 1. In the questionnaire, student respondents were asked "Thinking about your experience with digital media and digital devices: to what extent do you disagree or agree with the following statements?" The response categories from lower to higher values were: "Strongly disagree," "Disagree," "Agree," and "Strongly agree." This index is based on the following five statements.

- I feel comfortable using digital devices that I am less familiar with.
- If my friends and relatives want to buy new digital devices or applications, I can give them advice.
- I feel comfortable using my digital devices at home.
- When I come across problems with digital devices, I think I can solve them.
- If my friends and relatives have a problem with digital devices, I can help them.

6.1.2 Explanatory Variables, Family SES, and Control Variables

As in Chaps. 4 and 5, we use two explanatory variables to measure the extent to which students use ICT for school activities at home and in school: (1) Home ICT use for general schoolwork and (2) school ICT use for general schoolwork (OECD, 2021). Both variables are standardized to have an OECD mean of 0 and an OECD standard deviation of 1. We use family SES to measure students' social class backgrounds and include the following control variables in the analyses: *country-specific program, school grade, student age, gender, immigration status, foreign language use at home, available ICT resources at home* (student-level), *school average SES*; *public or private school*; *rural, town, or urban school*; *shortage of educational staff*; and *shortage of educational material* (school-level). Moreover, *perceived digital competence* is included as an additional control in the analyses of the first three outcome variables. Analyses of the effect of home ICT use control for *school ICT use for general schoolwork*. Analyses of the effect of school ICT use control for *home ICT use for general schoolwork*. Please see the variable descriptions in Chaps. 4 and 5 for more details.

6.2 Predicting Students' Perceived Sense of Belonging in School

6.2.1 The Effect of Home ICT Use

Figure 6.1 presents the plots from multilevel regression analyses to illustrate the curvilinear relationship between home ICT use for general schoolwork (*x*-axis) and perceived sense of belonging at school (*y*-axis) conditioned on family SES and controlling for individual- and school-level characteristics. Table 6.1 summarizes the effects of home ICT use on perceived sense of belonging at school for low- and high-SES students.

In Fig. 6.1, we observe some extent of inverted U-shaped or linear relationships between home ICT use and adolescents' perceived sense of belonging at school for 13 of the 22 countries and societies in the analyses, but the effect size is small. For example, we appear to see linear relationships in Hong Kong, South Korea, Taiwan, and the United Kingdom, which suggest that home ICT use for school-related activities at home is positively associated with the sense of belonging in school perceived by students. On the other hand, an inverted U-shaped relationship suggests that a moderate level of home ICT use for school-related activities at home may increase students' perceived sense of belonging in school, but intensive home use of ICT for school-related activities may decrease students' perceived sense of belonging in school.

It is worth noting that for low-SES students, ICT use at home for schoolwork has almost no positive effect on their perceived senses of school belonging, except for low-SES students living in the United States, Hong Kong, Japan, and Macao. In the United States, home use of ICT for school-related work may increase low-SES students' sense of school belonging by 0.41 standard deviations (0.43 standard deviations for high-SES students). In Hong Kong, Japan, and Macao, the sizes of the positive effect of home ICT use for low-SES students are approximately 0.28, 0.32, and 0.44 standard deviations, respectively.

Home ICT use for schoolwork has more substantial positive effects for high-SES student in many developed nations. Coupled with the small effects of home ICT use

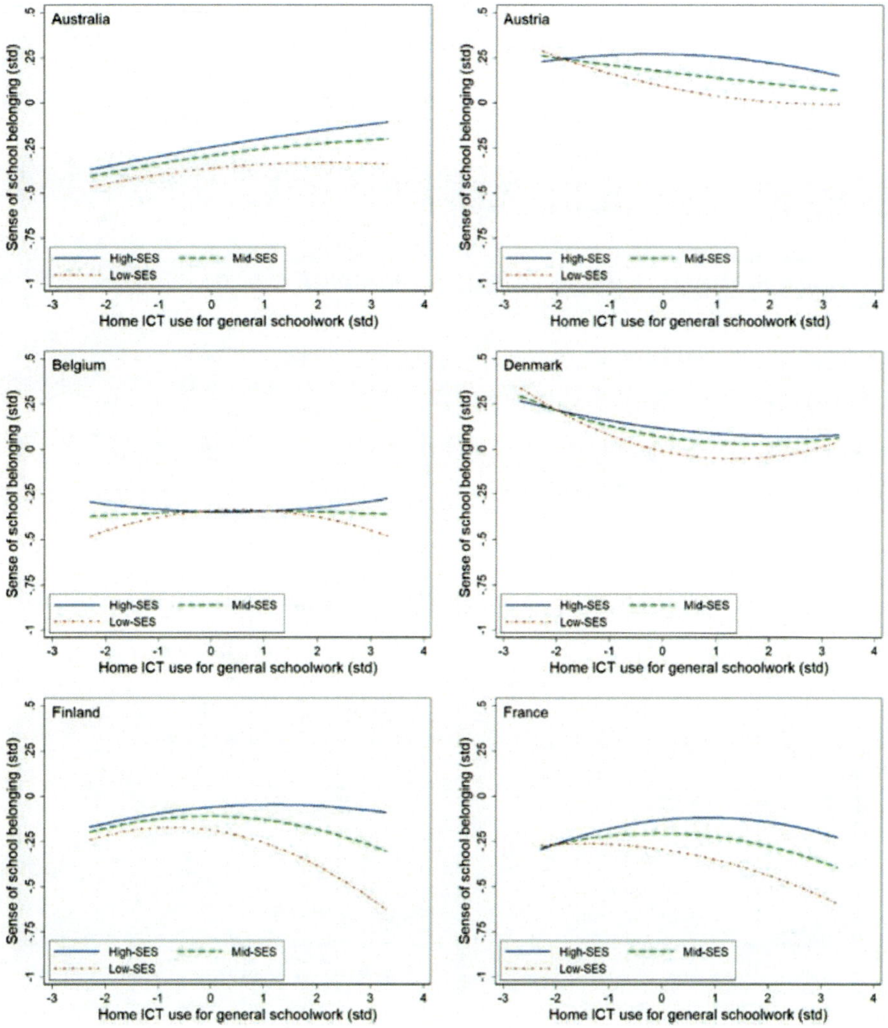

Fig. 6.1 Curvilinear effects of home ICT use for general schoolwork on perceived sense of belonging in school by family SES (*Data source* The 2018 Programme for International Student Assessment [PISA] survey. *Note* Countries/societies are listed alphabetically. High-SES refers to students who are at the 90th percentile in family SES. Mid-SES and Low-SES refer to those at the 50th and 10th percentiles in family SES, respectively. Predicted values are calculated based on two-level multilevel models for each country, where student-level variables are used in the Level-1 equation and schools' characteristics are used in the Level-2 equation. All multilevel models include country-specific educational program, school grade, student age, gender, immigration status, foreign language use at home, ICT resources at home, school ICT use for general schoolwork, and perceived digital competence as Level-1 controls. School average SES, public/private school, rural/town/urban school, shortage of educational staff, and shortage of educational material are Level-2 control variables. All Level-1 equations include the interaction effects between family SES and home ICT use for general schoolwork and between family SES and the squared term of home ICT use for general schoolwork. The following countries are not included in these analyses because key independent or dependent variables are unavailable from the country's PISA data: Canada, Germany, the Netherlands, Portugal, Norway, and China)

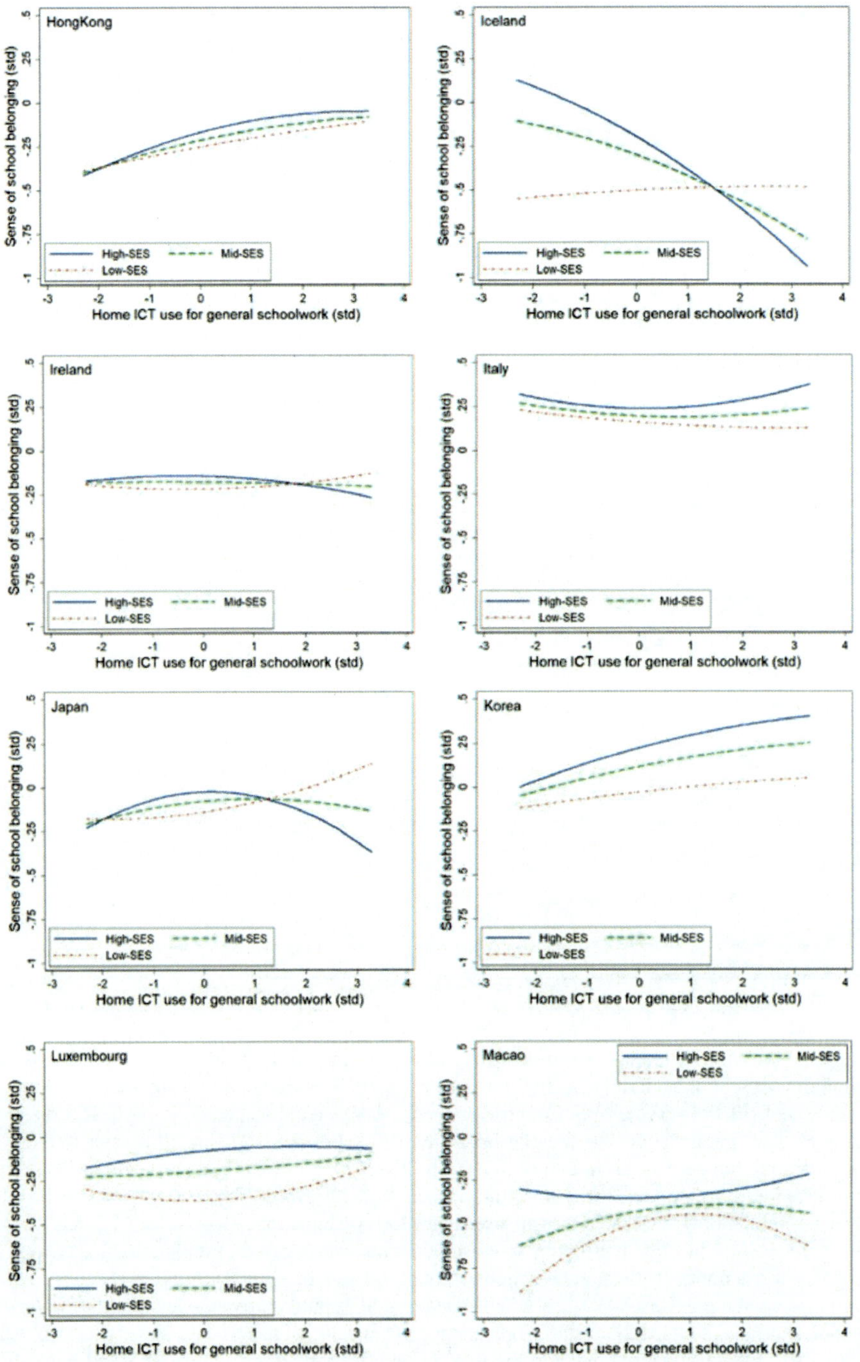

Fig. 6.1 (continued)

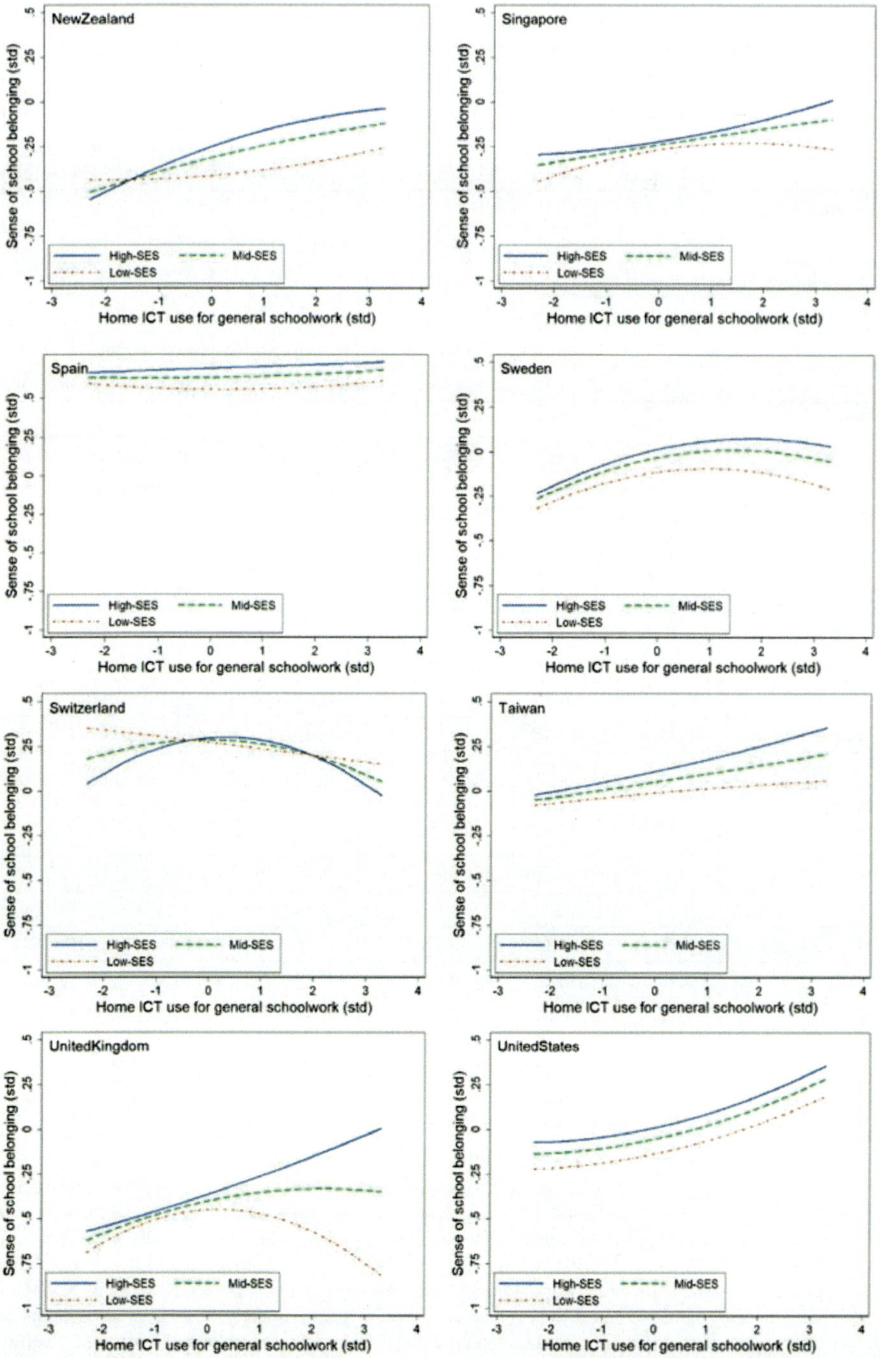

Fig. 6.1 (continued)

Table 6.1 Differences in predicted sense of belonging in school between students who do not use ICT for schoolwork at home and students who moderately use ICT for schoolwork at home: Summary of 22 countries/societies in Fig. 6.1

	Low-SES student			High-SES student		
	No ICT use (1)[a]	Moderate ICT use (2)[b]	Difference (2) − (1)[c]	No ICT use (1)[a]	Moderate ICT use (2)[b]	Difference (2) − (1)[c]
North America:						
United States	−0.22	0.19	**0.41**	−0.07	0.36	**0.43**
Western and Southern Europe:						
Austria	negative (or no positive) effect[d]			negative (or no positive) effect[d]		
Belgium	−0.48	−0.34	0.14	negative (or no positive) effect[d]		
United Kingdom	−0.69	−0.45	0.24	−0.57	0.01	**0.58**
France	negative (or no positive) effect[d]			−0.30	−0.12	0.18
Ireland	negative (or no positive) effect[d]			negative (or no positive) effect[d]		
Italy	negative (or no positive) effect[d]			negative (or no positive) effect[d]		
Luxembourg	negative (or no positive) effect[d]			−0.17	−0.05	0.12
Spain	negative (or no positive) effect[d]			0.66	0.73	0.07
Switzerland	negative (or no positive) effect[d]			0.04	0.30	0.26
Scandinavia:						
Denmark	negative (or no positive) effect[d]			negative (or no positive) effected		
Finland	−0.24	−0.17	0.07	−0.17	−0.05	0.12
Iceland	−0.55	−0.48	0.07	negative (or no positive) effected		
Sweden	−0.32	−0.09	0.22	−0.23	0.07	**0.31**
Pacific:						
Australia	−0.47	−0.33	0.13	−0.37	−0.11	0.26
New Zealand	negative (or no positive) effected			−0.55	−0.04	**0.51**
Asia:						
Hong Kong	−0.39	−0.11	0.28	−0.41	−0.05	**0.37**
Japan	−0.18	0.14	**0.32**	−0.23	−0.02	0.20
Korea	−0.12	0.05	0.17	0.00	0.41	**0.40**
Macao	−0.89	−0.45	**0.44**	negative (or no positive) effect[d]		
Singapore	−0.44	−0.23	0.22	−0.29	0.01	**0.31**
Taiwan	−0.08	0.06	0.14	−0.02	0.36	**0.38**

Data source The 2018 Programme for International Student Assessment (PISA) survey
Note Countries/societies in each geographical region are listed alphabetically. Low-SES students refer to those who are at the 10th percentile in family SES. High-SES students refer to those at the 90th percentile in family SES. [a]Predicted values of perceived sense of belonging in school for students who do not use ICT for schoolwork at home. [b]Predicted values of perceived sense of belonging in school for students who moderately use ICT for schoolwork at home. [c]Differences in gains of perceived sense of belonging in school between Columns 1 and 2. Scores that are above 30 (approximately 1/3 of a standard deviation in perceived sense of belonging in school) are highlighted in bold. [d]ICT use at home has no positive effect on perceived sense of belonging in school

for low-SES students, this finding indicates the problem of the third-level digital divide in the United Kingdom, France, Switzerland, Sweden, New Zealand, South Korea, Singapore, and Taiwan. In the United Kingdom and South Korea, for example, the sizes of the positive effect of home ICT use on the sense of school belonging for high-SES students are 0.58 and 0.40 standard deviations, respectively, more than twice as large as the effects for low-SES students (0.24 and 0.17 standard deviations). In France, Switzerland, and New Zealand, home ICT use only has positive effects for high-SES students but not for low-SES students; this again indicates the problem of the third-level digital divide.

6.2.2 The Effect of School ICT Use

Figure 6.2 presents plots of multilevel regression analyses to illustrate the curvilinear relationship between school ICT use (x-axis) and adolescents' perceived sense of belonging in school (y-axis) conditioned on family SES and controlling for individual- and school-level characteristics. Table 6.2 summarizes the effects of school ICT use on perceived sense of belonging at school for low- and high-SES students.

The results in Fig. 6.2 and Table 6.2 suggest that ICT use in the classroom does *not* help promote students' perceived sense of school belonging for students in most of the countries and societies in our analyses. The exceptions are two countries in West Europe (i.e., the United Kingdom and Ireland) and three countries in Scandinavia (i.e., Denmark, Finland, and Iceland). Of these, the effect of school ICT use is greater for low-SES students than for high-SES students only in Iceland. Specifically, as shown in Table 6.2, school use of ICT increases low-SES students' sense of school belonging by 0.46 standard deviations but has no visible positive effect on high-SES students' sense of belonging in school. For the United Kingdom, Ireland, Denmark, and Finland, we see that ICT use in the classroom affects only the perceived sense of school belonging for socioeconomically advantaged students but not for low-SES students. In Denmark, for example, school ICT use increases high-SES students' sense of school belonging by 0.47 standard deviations. Taken together, these analyses suggest that ICT use in school has limited effects on students' perceived sense of belonging in school among most countries. In the rare cases that positive effects exist, the positive effects are limited only to high-SES students and thus further expand the educational disparities between socially advantaged and disadvantaged students.

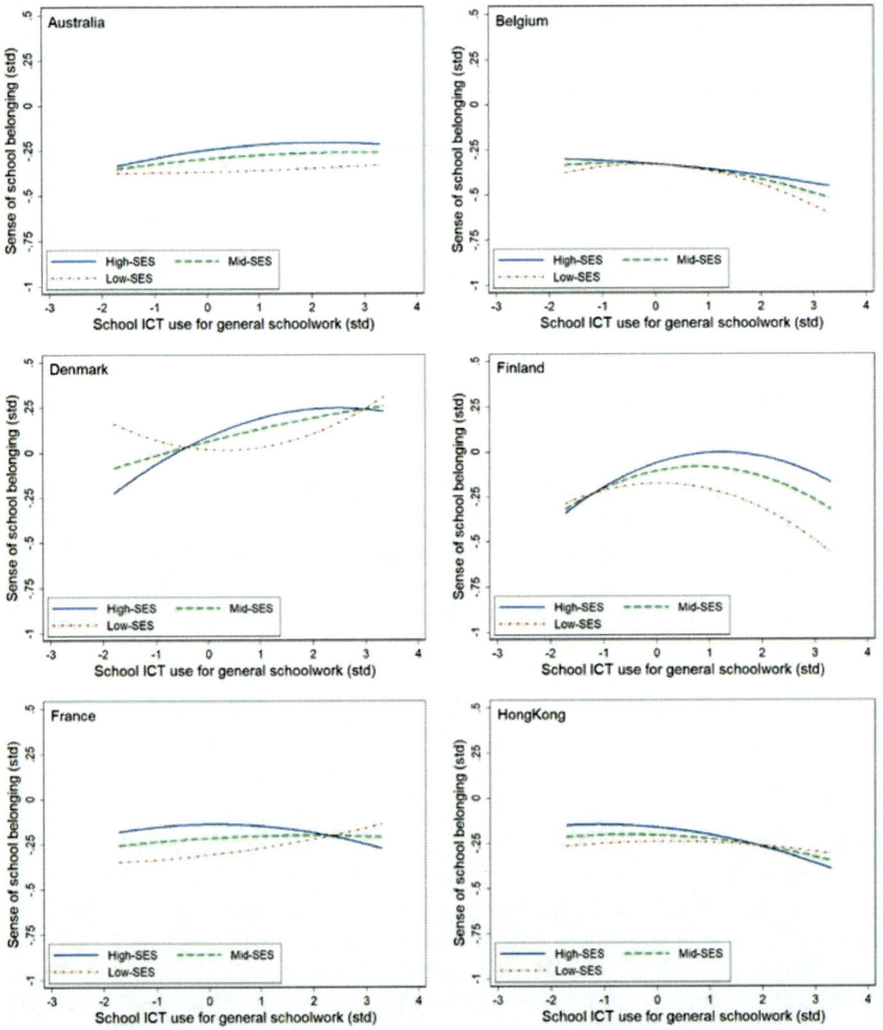

Fig. 6.2 Curvilinear effects of school ICT use for general schoolwork on perceived sense of belonging in school by family SES (*Data source* The 2018 Programme for International Student Assessment [PISA] survey. *Note* Countries/societies are listed alphabetically. High-SES refers to students who are at the 90th percentile in family SES. Mid-SES and Low-SES refer to those at the 50th and 10th percentiles in family SES, respectively. Predicted values are calculated based on two-level multilevel models for each country, where student-level variables are used in the Level-1 equation and schools' characteristics are used in the Level-2 equation. All multilevel models include country-specific educational program, school grade, student age, gender, immigration status, foreign language use at home, ICT resources at home, home ICT use for general schoolwork, and perceived digital competence as Level-1 controls. School average SES, public/private school, rural/town/urban school, shortage of educational staff, and shortage of educational material are Level-2 control variables. All Level-1 equations include the interaction effects between family SES and school ICT use for general schoolwork and between family SES and the squared term of school ICT use for general schoolwork. The following countries are not included in these analyses because key independent or dependent variables are unavailable from the country's PISA data: Canada, Austria, Germany, the Netherlands, Portugal, Norway, and China)

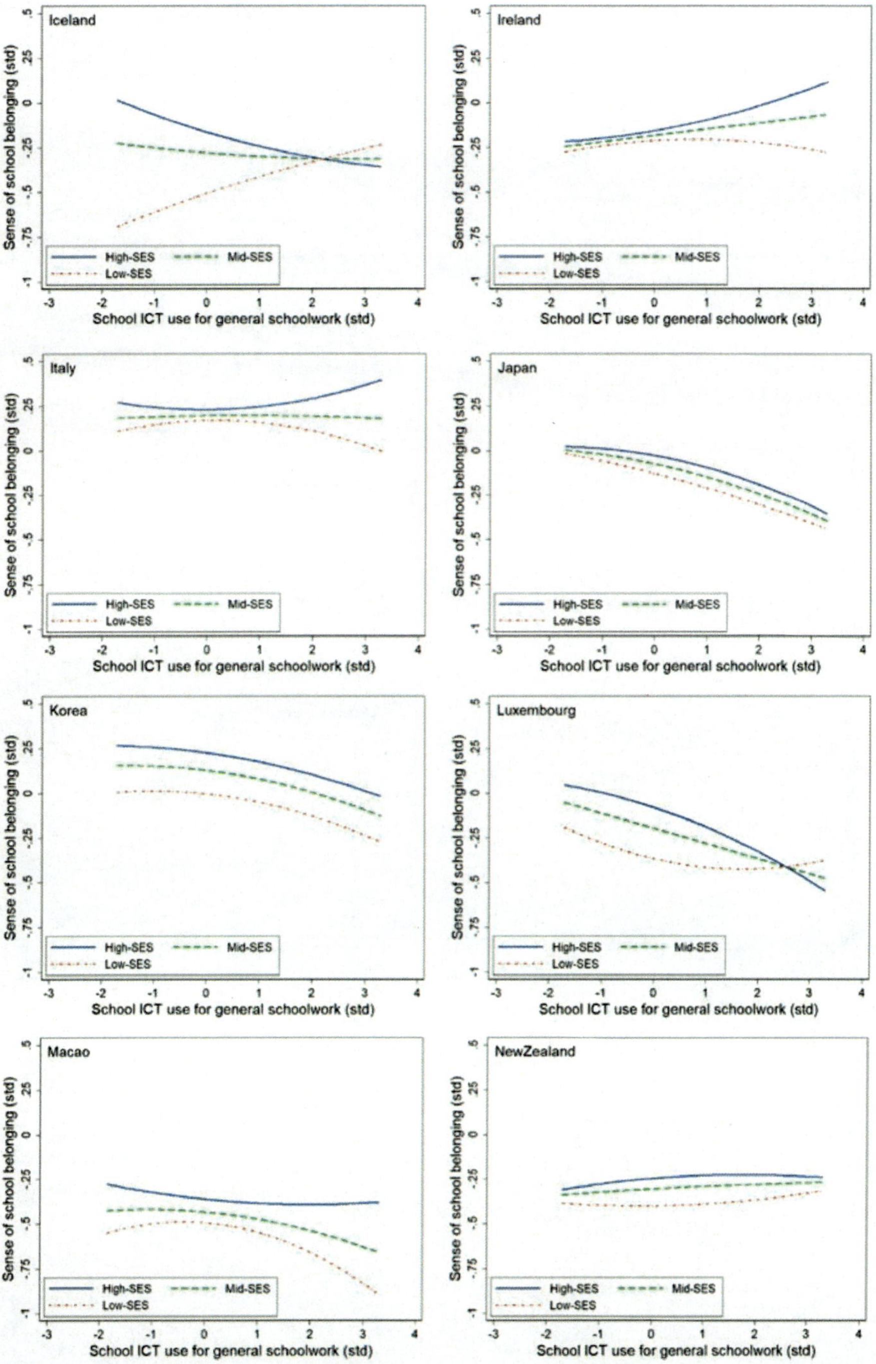

Fig. 6.2 (continued)

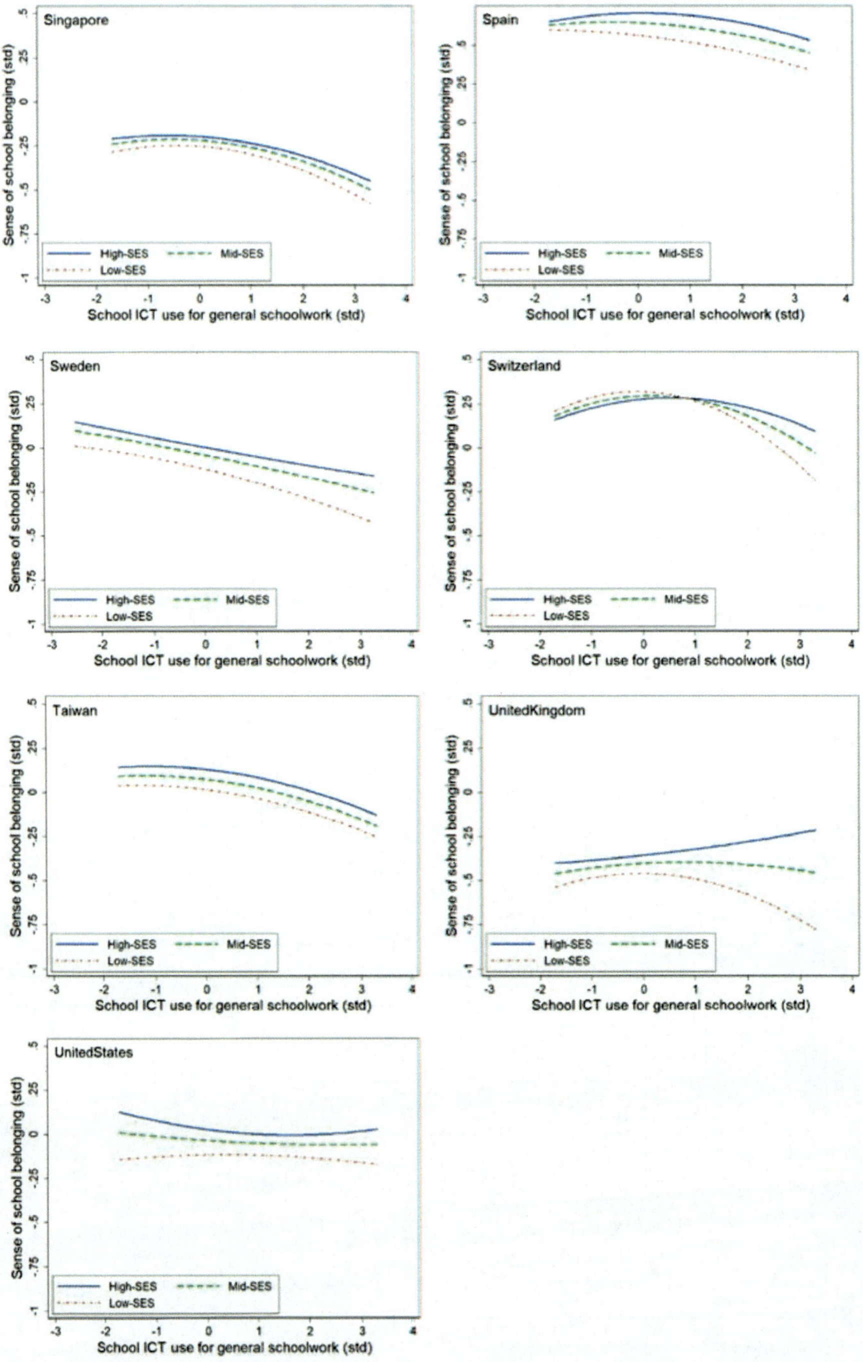

Fig. 6.2 (continued)

Table 6.2 Differences in predicted sense of belonging in school between students who do not use ICT for schoolwork at school and students who moderately use ICT for schoolwork at school: Summary of 21 countries/societies in Fig. 6.2

	Low-SES student			High-SES student		
	No ICT use (1)[a]	Moderate ICT use (2)[b]	Difference (2) – (1)[c]	No ICT use (1)[a]	Moderate ICT use (2)[b]	Difference (2) – (1)[c]
North America:						
United States	negative (or no positive) effect[d]			negative (or no positive) effect[d]		
Western and Southern Europe:						
Belgium	−0.38	−0.33	0.05	negative (or no positive) effect[d]		
United Kingdom	−0.54	−0.46	0.08	−0.40	−0.21	0.19
France	−0.35	−0.14	0.21	negative (or no positive) effect[d]		
Ireland	−0.28	−0.20	0.07	−0.22	0.12	**0.33**
Italy	0.11	0.17	0.06	negative (or no positive) effect[d]		
Luxembourg	negative (or no positive) effect[d]			negative (or no positive) effect[d]		
Spain	negative (or no positive) effect[d]			0.60	0.71	0.11
Switzerland	0.21	0.32	0.11	0.16	0.28	0.12
Scandinavia:						
Denmark	negative (or no positive) effect[d]			−0.22	0.25	**0.47**
Finland	−0.29	−0.18	0.11	−0.34	0.00	**0.34**
Iceland	−0.69	−0.23	**0.46**	negative (or no positive) effect[d]		
Sweden	negative (or no positive) effect[d]			negative (or no positive) effect[d]		
Pacific:						
Australia	negative (or no positive) effect[d]			−0.34	−0.21	0.13
New Zealand	−0.39	−0.32	0.07	−0.31	−0.23	0.09
Asia:						
Hong Kong	negative (or no positive) effect[d]			negative (or no positive) effect[d]		
Japan	negative (or no positive) effect[d]			negative (or no positive) effect[d]		
Korea	negative (or no positive) effect[d]			negative (or no positive) effect[d]		
Macao	−0.55	−0.49	0.06	negative (or no positive) effect[d]		
Singapore	negative (or no positive) effect[d]			negative (or no positive) effect[d]		
Taiwan	negative (or no positive) effect[d]			negative (or no positive) effect[d]		

Data source The 2018 Programme for International Student Assessment (PISA) survey
Note Countries/societies in each geographical region are listed alphabetically. Low-SES students refer to those who are at the 10th percentile in family SES. High-SES students refer to those at the 90th percentile in family SES. [a]Predicted values of perceived sense of belonging in school for students who do not use ICT for schoolwork at school. [b]Predicted values of perceived sense of belonging in school for students who moderately use in ICT for schoolwork at school. [c]Differences in gains of perceived sense of belonging in school between Columns 1 and 2. Scores that are above 30 (approximately 1/3 of a standard deviation in perceived sense of belonging in school) are highlighted in bold. [d]ICT use at school has no positive effect on perceived sense of belonging in school

6.3 Predicting Students' Perceived Positive Psychological Feelings

6.3.1 The Effect of Home ICT Use

Figure 6.3 presents plots of multilevel regression analyses to illustrate the curvilinear relationship between home ICT use for general schoolwork (*x*-axis) and adolescents' perceived positive psychological feelings, such as feeling joyful, cheerful, and happy (*y*-axis) conditioned on family SES and controlling for individual- and school-level characteristics. Table 6.3 summarizes the effects of home ICT use on perceived positive psychological feelings for low- and high-SES students.

The results in Fig. 6.3 and Table 6.3 suggest home ICT use for schoolwork has substantial positive effects on adolescents' psychological well-being at least for some students in almost all countries and societies in our analyses. In some countries, this relationship is either inverted U-shaped (e.g., Austria) or curvilinear (e.g., Denmark). In other countries and societies, such as Finland, Ireland, Japan, Luxembourg, Taiwan, the United Kingdom, and the United States, the relationship is linear.

The effects of home ICT use on adolescents' psychological well-being are equally or more important for socioeconomically disadvantaged students than for socioeconomically advantaged students in the United States, the United Kingdom, Iceland, Sweden, and Japan. In Iceland, for example, home ICT use increases the positive psychological feelings for low-SES students by 0.70 standard deviations, but only 0.17 standard deviations for high-SES students. In Sweden and Japan, home ICT use increases the positive psychological feelings for low-SES students by 0.46 and 0.53 standard deviations, but only 0.35 and 0.34 standard deviations for high-SES students, respectively.

In contrast, home ICT use for schoolwork has greater positive effects on adolescents' psychological well-being for high-SES students than for low-SES students in Austria, Ireland, Denmark, Hong Kong, and South Korea. These greater positive effects for high-SES students indicate the persistence of the third-level digital divide in these developed societies. Taking Austria as an example, the size of the positive effect of home ICT use is 0.37 standard deviations for high-SES students, approximately three times as large as the effect for low-SES students. In Ireland and Denmark, home ICT use for schoolwork has positive effects on perceived psychological feelings only for high-SES students, but not for low-SES students.

6.3.2 The Effect of School ICT Use

Figure 6.4 presents plots of multilevel regression analyses to illustrate the curvilinear relationship between school ICT use (*x*-axis) and adolescents' perceived positive psychological feelings (e.g., the feelings of joyful, cheerful, and happy) (*y*-axis)

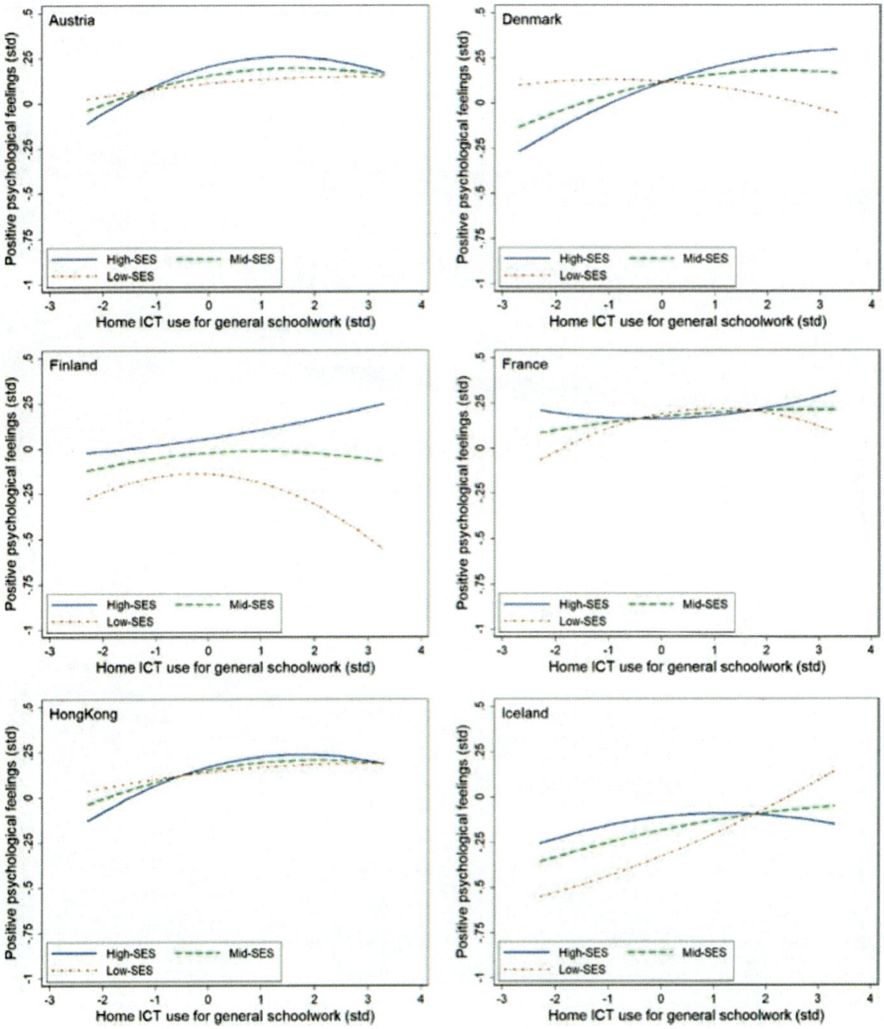

Fig. 6.3 Curvilinear effects of home ICT use for general schoolwork on perceived positive psychological feelings by family SES (*Data source* The 2018 Programme for International Student Assessment [PISA] survey. *Note* Countries/societies are listed alphabetically. High-SES refers to students who are at the 90th percentile in family SES. Mid-SES and Low-SES refer to those at the 50th and 10th percentiles in family SES, respectively. Predicted values are calculated based on two-level multilevel models for each country, where student-level variables are used in the Level-1 equation and schools' characteristics are used in the Level-2 equation. All multilevel models include country-specific educational program, school grade, student age, gender, immigration status, foreign language use at home, ICT resources at home, school ICT use for general schoolwork, and perceived digital competence as Level-1 controls. School average SES, public/private school, rural/town/urban school, shortage of educational staff, and shortage of educational material are Level-2 control variables. All Level-1 equations include the interaction effects between family SES and home ICT use for general schoolwork and between family SES and the squared term of home ICT use for general schoolwork. The following countries are not included in these analyses because key independent or dependent variables are unavailable from the country's PISA data: Canada, Belgium, Germany, Italy, the Netherlands, Portugal, Norway, Australia, New Zealand, China, and Singapore)

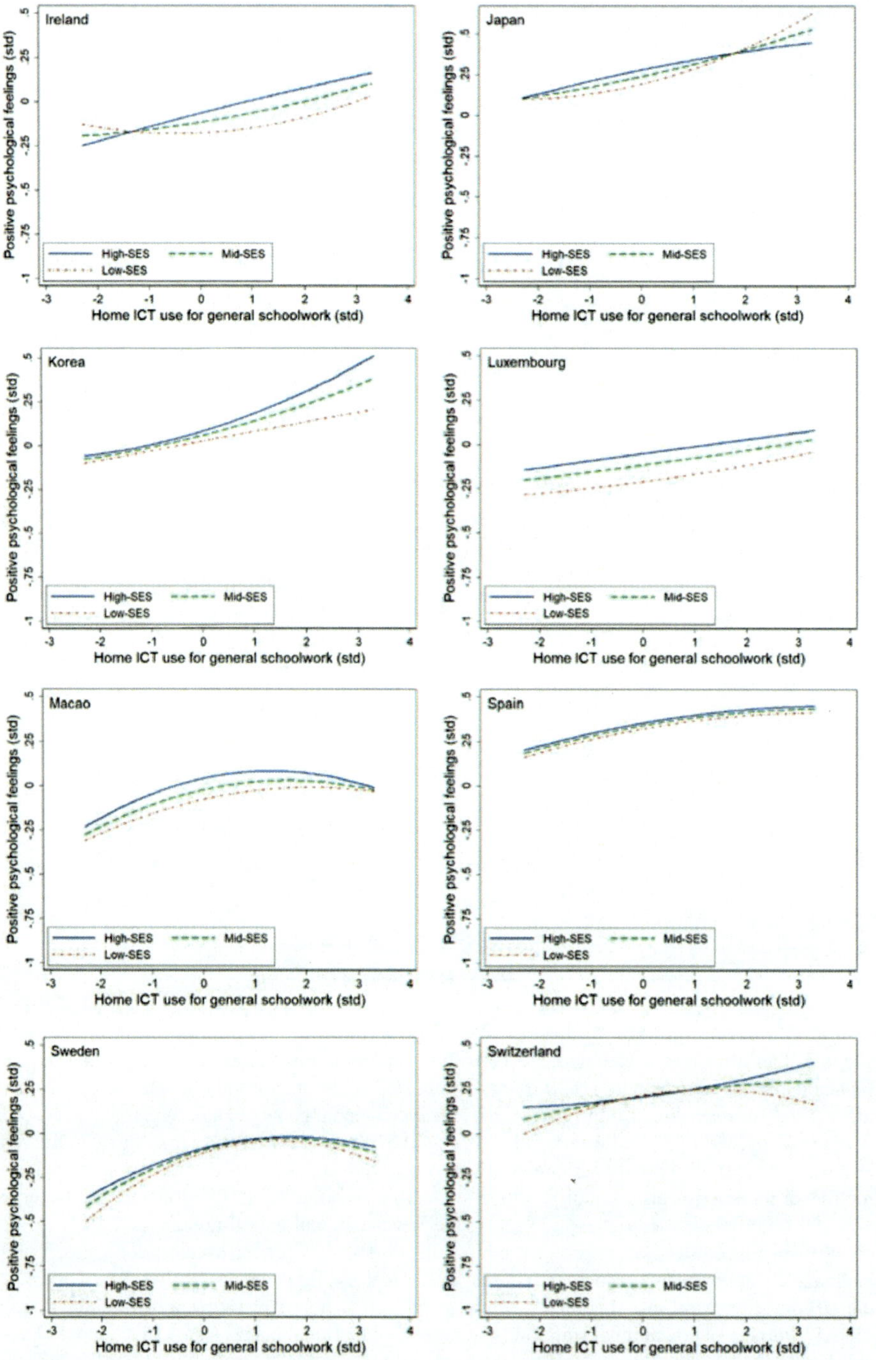

Fig. 6.3 (continued)

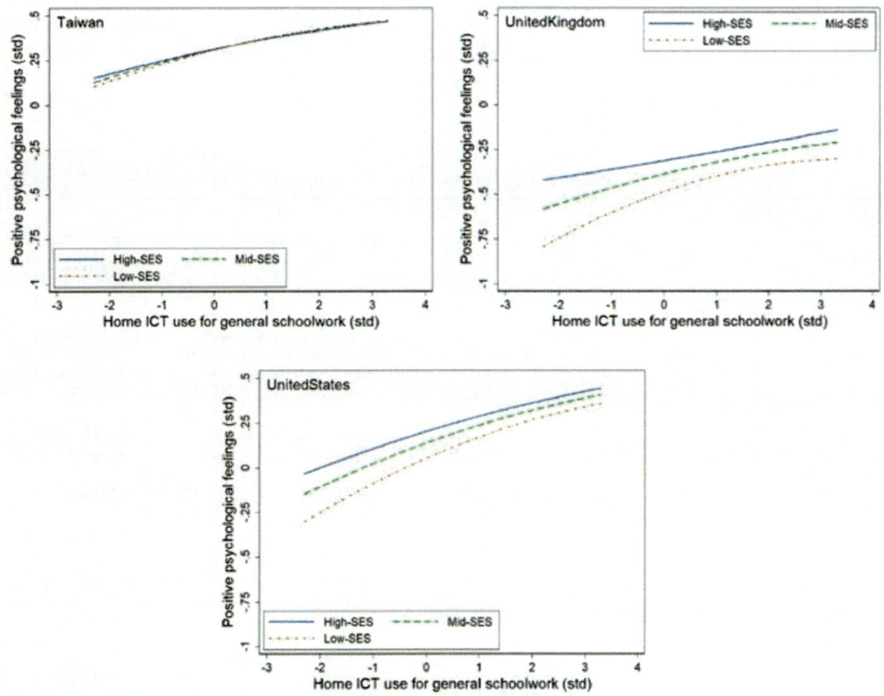

Fig. 6.3 (continued)

conditioned on family SES and controlling for individual- and school-level characteristics. Table 6.4 summarizes the effects of school ICT use on perceived positive psychological feelings for low- and high-SES students.

Of the 16 countries and societies in the analyses, we observe positive associations between ICT use in the classroom and perceived positive psychological feelings in eight countries. Of these, six are in Europe (the United Kingdom, France, Ireland, Denmark, Iceland, and Sweden) and two are in Asia (Japan and South Korea). Unlike the U-shaped relationships between ICT use and student outcomes that have been found in previous analyses, the effects of school ICT on adolescents' psychological feelings are relatively linear, but the effect sizes are small. In comparison with the patterns shown in Fig. 6.3, the results in Fig. 6.4 suggest that home ICT use for schoolwork is more important in shaping adolescent students' psychological well-being than use of digital technologies in classrooms.

The exceptions are the United Kingdom and Ireland, whereas school ICT use has visible effects on adolescents' perceived psychological feelings. In the United Kingdom, ICT use in school increases low-SES students' positive psychological feelings by 0.37 standard deviations, compared to an increase in positive psychological feelings by 0.11 standard deviations for high-SES students. In Ireland, ICT use in school increases low- and high-SES students' positive psychological feelings by 0.30 and 0.34 standard deviations, respectively.

Table 6.3 Differences in predicted sense of positive psychological feelings between students who do not use ICT for schoolwork at home and students who moderately use ICT for schoolwork at home: Summary of 17 countries/societies in Fig. 6.3

	Low-SES student			High-SES student		
	No ICT use (1)[a]	Moderate ICT use (2)[b]	Difference (2) − (1)[c]	No ICT use (1)[a]	Moderate ICT use (2)[b]	Difference (2) − (1)[c]
North America:						
United States	−0.30	0.36	**0.66**	−0.03	0.44	**0.48**
Western and Southern Europe:						
Austria	0.02	0.15	0.12	−0.11	0.26	**0.37**
United Kingdom	−0.79	−0.30	**0.49**	−0.42	−0.14	0.28
France	−0.07	0.22	0.28	negative (or no positive) effect[d]		
Ireland	negative (or no positive) effect[d]			−0.25	0.16	**0.41**
Luxembourg	−0.29	−0.04	0.24	−0.14	0.08	0.23
Spain	0.16	0.41	0.25	0.20	0.45	0.25
Switzerland	0.00	0.25	0.25	0.15	0.40	0.25
Scandinavia:						
Denmark	negative (or no positive) effect[d]			−0.27	0.30	**0.56**
Finland	−0.28	−0.14	0.14	−0.02	0.25	0.27
Iceland	−0.55	0.15	**0.70**	−0.26	−0.09	0.17
Sweden	−0.50	−0.04	**0.46**	−0.37	−0.02	**0.35**
Asia:						
Hong Kong	0.04	0.19	0.15	−0.13	0.24	**0.36**
Japan	0.10	0.63	**0.53**	0.11	0.45	**0.34**
Korea	−0.10	0.21	**0.31**	−0.06	0.51	**0.57**
Macao	−0.31	−0.01	**0.30**	−0.23	0.08	**0.32**
Taiwan	0.10	0.47	**0.37**	0.15	0.47	**0.32**

Data source The 2018 Programme for International Student Assessment (PISA) survey
Note Countries/societies in each geographical region are listed alphabetically. Low-SES students refer to those who are at the 10th percentile in family SES. High-SES students refer to those at the 90th percentile in family SES. [a]Predicted values of perceived positive psychological feelings for students who do not use ICT for schoolwork at home. [b]Predicted values of perceived positive psychological feelings for students who moderately use ICT for schoolwork at home. [c]Differences in gains of perceived positive psychological feelings between Columns 1 and 2. Scores that are above 30 (approximately 1/3 of a standard deviation in perceived positive psychological feelings) are highlighted in bold. [d]ICT use at home has no positive effect on perceived positive psychological feelings

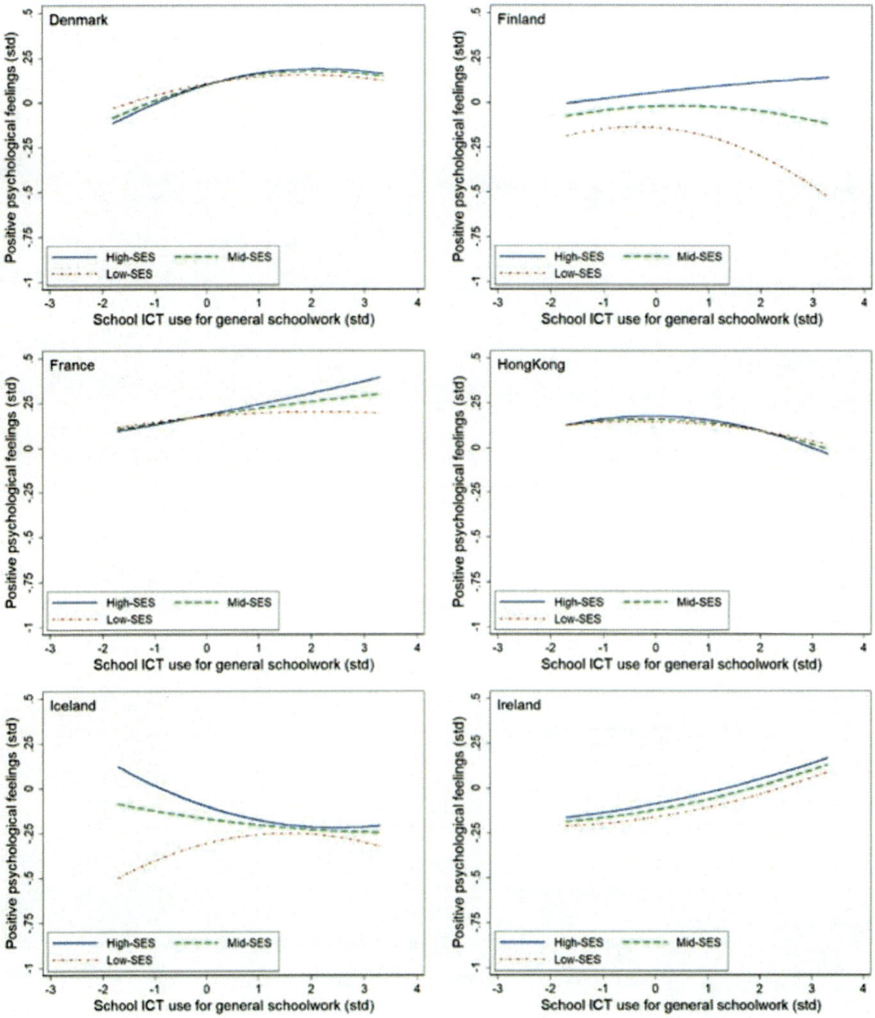

Fig. 6.4 Curvilinear effects of school ICT use for general schoolwork on perceived positive psychological feelings by family SES (*Data source* The 2018 Programme for International Student Assessment [PISA] survey. *Note* Countries/societies are listed alphabetically. High-SES refers to students who are at the 90th percentile in family SES. Mid-SES and Low-SES refer to those at the 50th and 10th percentiles in family SES, respectively. Predicted values are calculated based on two-level multilevel models for each country, where student-level variables are used in the Level-1 equation and schools' characteristics are used in the Level-2 equation. All multilevel models include country-specific educational program, school grade, student age, gender, immigration status, foreign language use at home, ICT resources at home, home ICT use for general schoolwork, and perceived digital competence as Level-1 controls. School average SES, public/private school, rural/town/urban school, shortage of educational staff, and shortage of educational material are Level-2 control variables. All Level-1 equations include the interaction effects between family SES and school ICT use for general schoolwork and between family SES and the squared term of school ICT use for general schoolwork. The following countries are not included in these analyses because key independent or dependent variables are unavailable from the country's PISA data: Canada, Austria, Belgium, Germany, Italy, the Netherlands, Portugal, Norway, Australia, New Zealand, China, and Singapore)

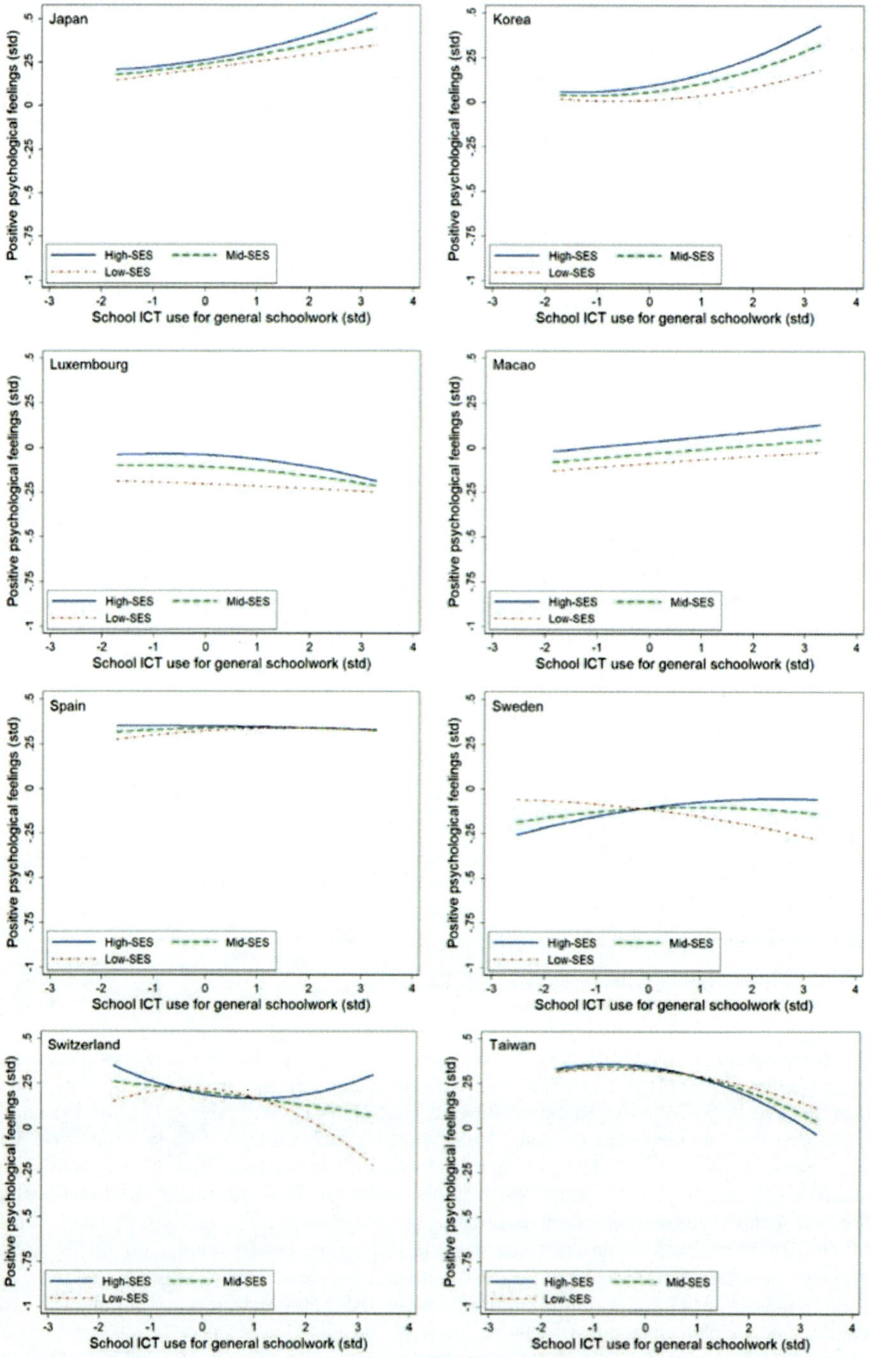

Fig. 6.4 (continued)

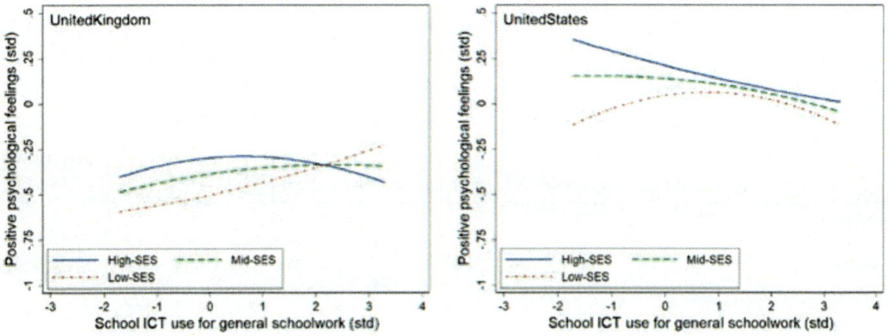

Fig. 6.4 (continued)

We find the third-level digital divide in France, Denmark, and South Korea. In both France and Denmark, school ICT use increases adolescents' perceived psychological feelings by 0.30 standard deviations for high-SES students, but only 0.09 and 0.18 standard deviations for low-SES students, respectively, in these two countries. In South Korea, school ICT use increases high-SES students' positive psychological feelings by 0.38 standard deviations but has no visible effect on low-SES students.

6.4 Predicting Students' Perceived Positive Meaning in Life

6.4.1 The Effect of Home ICT Use

Figure 6.5 presents plots of multilevel regression analyses to illustrate the curvilinear relationship between home ICT use (*x*-axis) and adolescents' perceived sense of positive meaning or positive purpose in life (*y*-axis) conditioned on family SES and controlling for individual- and school-level characteristics. Table 6.5 summarizes the effects of home ICT use on perceived sense of positive meaning (or positive purpose in life) for low- and high-SES students.

Overall, we see positive relationships between home ICT use and adolescents' perceived sense of positive meaning or positive purpose in life in all of the countries and societies in the analyses. In most cases, the positive effects are sizeable. In some countries/societies, the relationships are U-shaped; in others, the relationships are relatively linear.

Among 10 countries, ICT use for schoolwork at home has similar or greater positive effects on perceived sense of positive meaning or positive purpose in life for low-SES students than for high-SES students; these countries are the United States, the United Kingdom, Ireland, Italy, Luxembourg, Spain, Australia, Hong Kong, Japan, and Taiwan. In the United States and Italy, for example, home ICT use increases adolescents' positive perception of life meaning by 0.82 and 0.52 standard deviations for low-SES students, respectively, and by 0.39 and 0.21 standard

Table 6.4 Differences in predicted sense of positive psychological feelings between students who do not use ICT for schoolwork at school and students who moderately use ICT for schoolwork at school: Summary of 16 countries/societies in Fig. 6.4

	Low-SES student			High-SES student		
	No ICT use (1)[a]	Moderate ICT use (2)[b]	Difference (2) − (1)[c]	No ICT use (1)[a]	Moderate ICT use (2)[b]	Difference (2) − (1)[c]
North America:						
United States	−0.12	0.06	0.18	negative (or no positive) effect[d]		
Western and Southern Europe:						
United Kingdom	−0.60	−0.23	**0.37**	−0.40	−0.29	0.11
France	0.12	0.20	0.09	0.09	0.39	**0.30**
Ireland	−0.21	0.09	**0.30**	−0.17	0.17	**0.34**
Luxembourg	negative (or no positive) effect[d]			negative (or no positive) effect[d]		
Spain	0.28	0.34	0.06	negative (or no positive) effect[d]		
Switzerland	0.15	0.22	0.07	negative (or no positive) effect[d]		
Scandinavia:						
Denmark	−0.03	0.15	0.18	−0.12	0.19	**0.30**
Finland	−0.19	−0.14	0.05	−0.01	0.14	0.15
Iceland	−0.50	−0.25	0.25	negative (or no positive) effect[d]		
Sweden	negative (or no positive) effect[d]			−0.26	−0.05	0.20
Asia:						
Hong Kong	negative (or no positive) effect[d]			0.13	0.17	0.05
Japan	0.14	0.35	0.21	0.21	0.53	**0.33**
Korea	negative (or no positive) effect[d]			0.06	0.43	**0.38**
Macao	−0.13	−0.02	0.11	−0.02	0.13	0.15
Taiwan	negative (or no positive) effect[d]			negative (or no positive) effect[d]		

Data source The 2018 Programme for International Student Assessment (PISA) survey
Note Countries/societies in each geographical region are listed alphabetically. Low-SES students refer to those who are at the 10th percentile in family SES. High-SES students refer to those at the 90th percentile in family SES. [a]Predicted values of perceived positive psychological feelings for students who do not use ICT for schoolwork at school. [b]Predicted values of perceived positive psychological feelings for students who moderately use ICT for schoolwork at school. [c]Differences in gains of perceived positive psychological feelings between Columns 1 and 2. Scores that are above 30 (approximately 1/3 of a standard deviation in perceived positive psychological feelings) are highlighted in bold. [d]ICT use at school has no positive effect on perceived positive psychological feelings

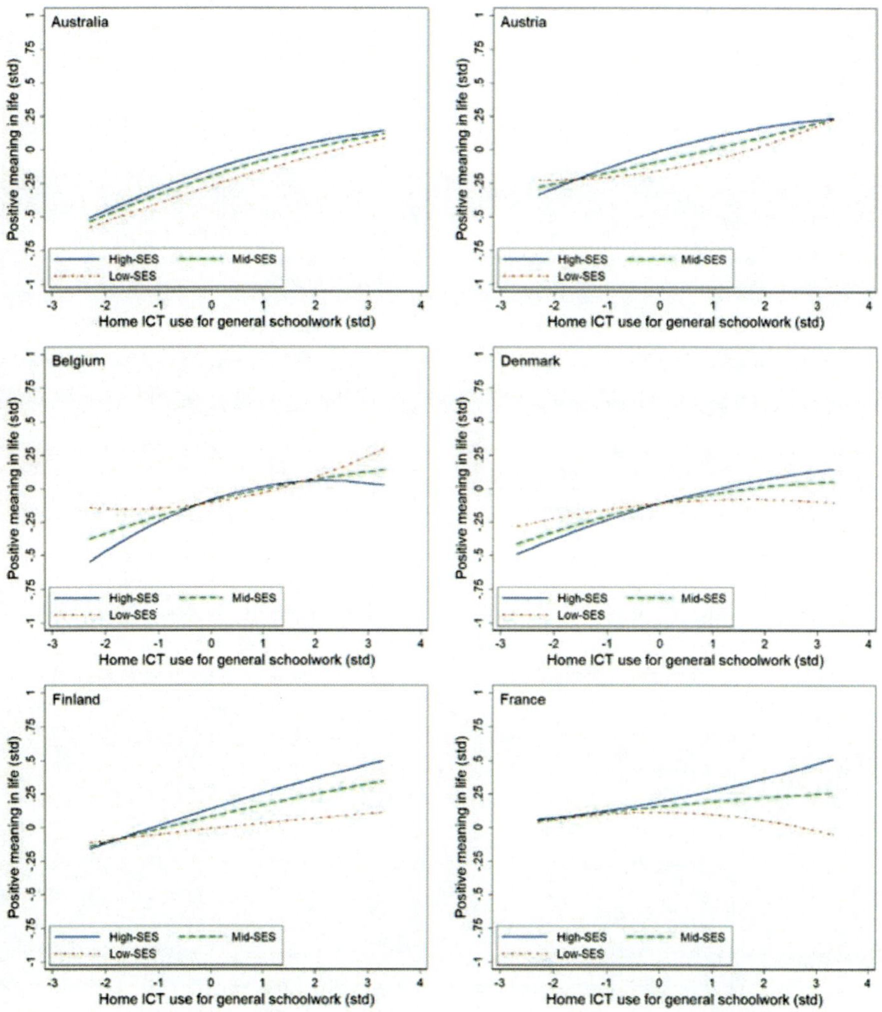

Fig. 6.5 Curvilinear effects of home ICT use for general schoolwork on perceived sense of positive meaning and positive purpose in life by family SES (*Data source* The 2018 Programme for International Student Assessment [PISA] survey. *Note* Countries/societies are listed alphabetically. High-SES refers to students who are at the 90th percentile in family SES. Mid-SES and Low-SES refer to those at the 50th and 10th percentiles in family SES, respectively. Predicted values are calculated based on two-level multilevel models for each country, where student-level variables are used in the Level-1 equation and schools' characteristics are used in the Level-2 equation. All multilevel models include country-specific educational program, school grade, student age, gender, immigration status, foreign language use at home, ICT resources at home, school ICT use for general schoolwork, and perceived digital competence as Level-1 controls. School average SES, public/private school, rural/town/urban school, shortage of educational staff, and shortage of educational material are Level-2 control variables. All Level-1 equations include the interaction effects between family SES and home ICT use for general schoolwork and between family SES and the squared term of home ICT use for general schoolwork. The following countries are not included in these analyses because key independent or dependent variables are unavailable from the country's PISA data: Canada, Germany, the Netherlands, Portugal, Norway, New Zealand, China, and Singapore)

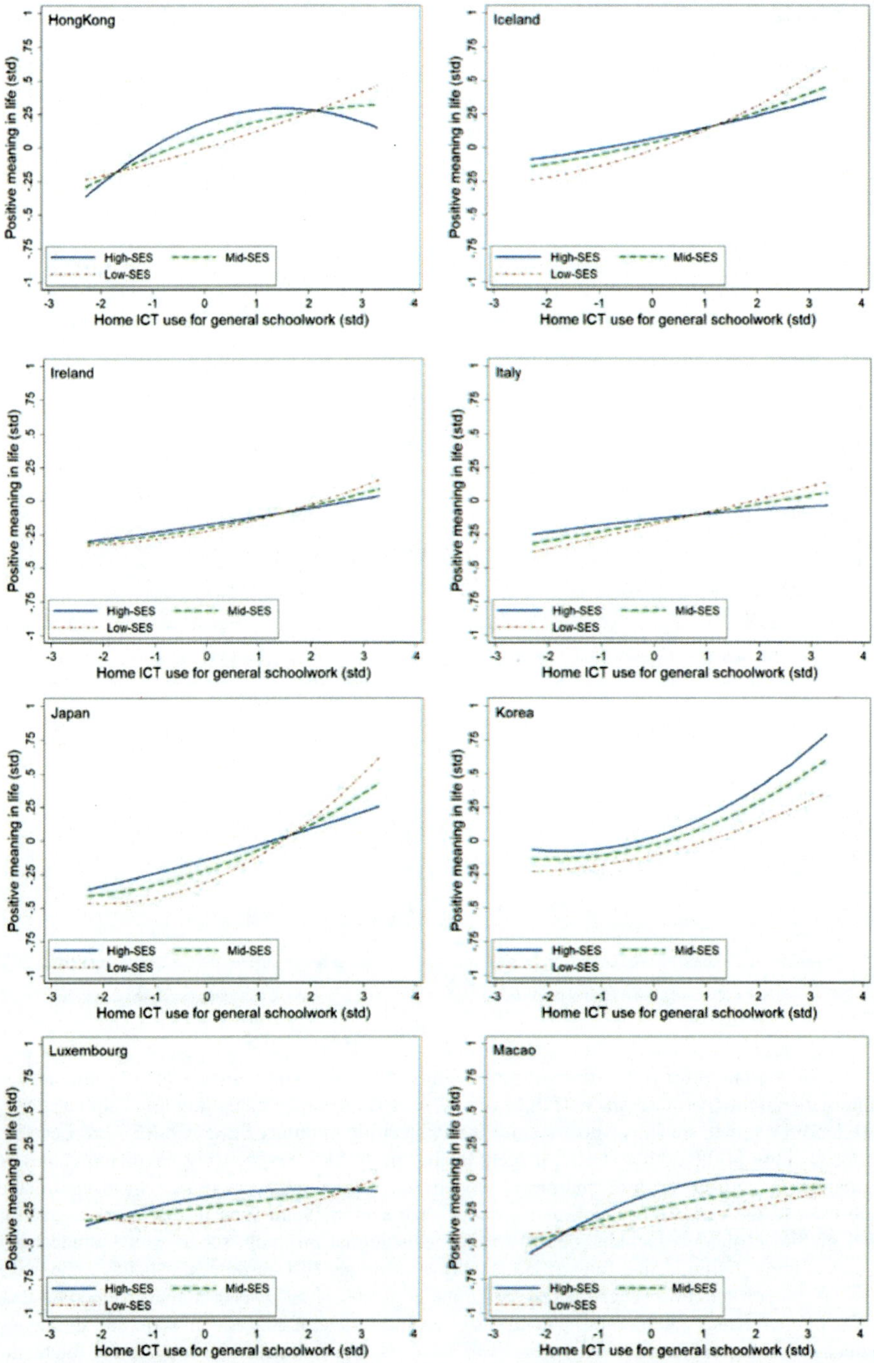

Fig. 6.5 (continued)

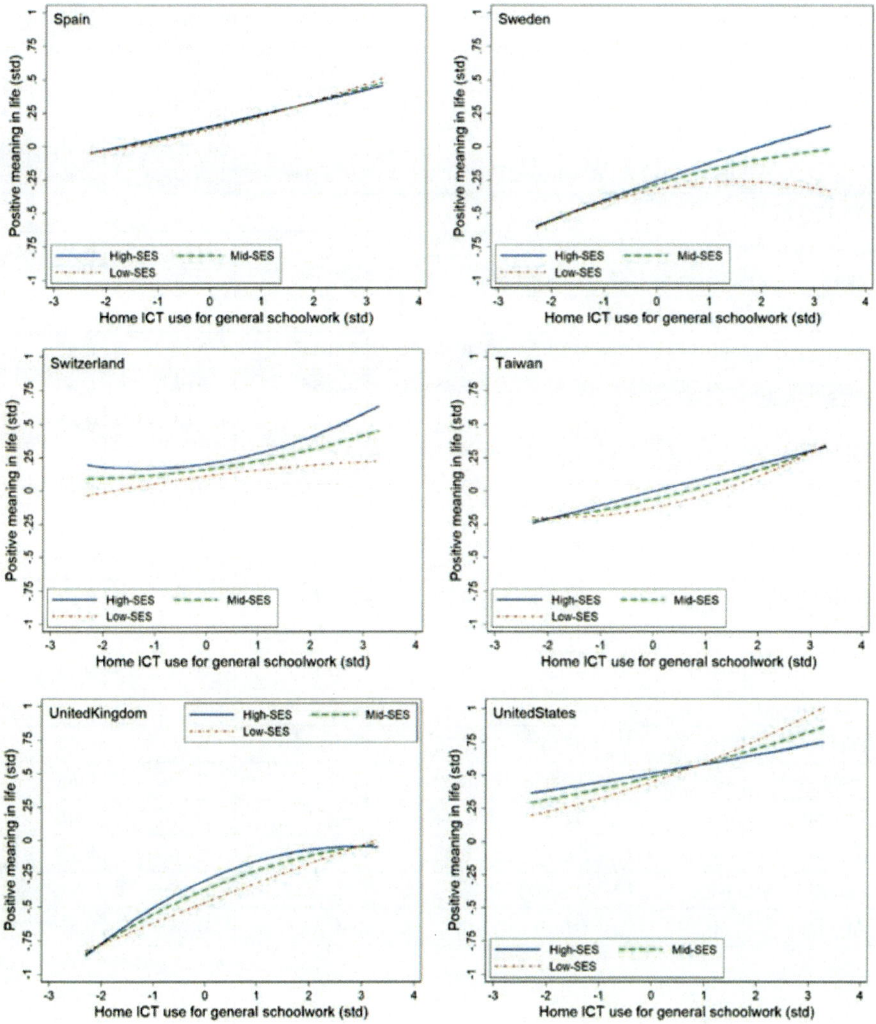

Fig. 6.5 (continued)

deviations for high-SES students. In the United Kingdom, home ICT use has similar positive effects for low-SES (0.83 standard deviations) and high-SES students (0.82 standard deviations). In Japan, the effect size is nearly two times greater for low-SES students (1.09 standard deviations) than for high-SES students (0.62 standard deviations).

In contrast, we see a notable third-level digital divide among nine countries. Of these, four are from Western Europe (Austria, Belgium, France, and Switzerland), three are from Northern Europe (Denmark, Finland, and Sweden), and two are from Asia (South Korea and Macao). In Austria, Belgium, France, and Switzerland, home ICT use for schoolwork increases positive perception of life meanings, respectively,

Table 6.5 Differences in predicted sense of positive meaning and positive purpose in life between students who do not use ICT for schoolwork at home and students who moderately use ICT for schoolwork at home: Summary of 20 countries/societies in Fig. 6.5

	Low-SES student			High-SES student		
	No ICT use (1)[a]	Moderate ICT use (2)[b]	Difference (2) − (1)[c]	No ICT use (1)[a]	Moderate ICT use (2)[b]	Difference (2) − (1)[c]
North America:						
United States	0.20	1.02	**0.82**	0.36	0.76	**0.39**
Western and Southern Europe:						
Austria	−0.23	0.23	**0.46**	−0.34	0.24	**0.57**
Belgium	−0.14	0.30	**0.45**	−0.55	0.06	**0.60**
United Kingdom	−0.83	0.01	**0.83**	−0.86	−0.05	**0.82**
France	0.04	0.11	0.07	0.06	0.51	**0.45**
Ireland	−0.33	0.16	**0.49**	−0.30	0.04	**0.34**
Italy	−0.38	0.14	**0.52**	−0.25	−0.04	0.21
Luxembourg	−0.27	0.00	0.27	−0.35	−0.08	0.27
Spain	−0.05	0.51	**0.56**	−0.05	0.45	**0.50**
Switzerland	−0.04	0.22	0.26	0.19	0.64	**0.44**
Scandinavia:						
Denmark	−0.28	−0.08	0.20	−0.49	0.15	**0.64**
Finland	−0.11	0.11	0.22	−0.16	0.50	**0.66**
Iceland	−0.24	0.60	**0.84**	−0.09	0.37	**0.46**
Sweden	−0.61	−0.26	**0.35**	−0.60	0.16	**0.75**
Pacific:						
Australia	−0.58	0.09	**0.67**	−0.51	0.14	**0.65**
Asia:						
Hong Kong	−0.23	0.46	**0.70**	−0.36	0.29	**0.65**
Japan	−0.47	0.62	**1.09**	−0.36	0.26	**0.62**
Korea	−0.23	0.36	**0.59**	−0.08	0.79	**0.87**
Macao	−0.42	−0.10	**0.31**	−0.56	0.02	**0.58**
Taiwan	−0.20	0.35	**0.56**	−0.24	0.33	**0.57**

Data source The 2018 Programme for International Student Assessment (PISA) survey
Note Countries/societies in each geographical region are listed alphabetically. Low-SES students refer to those who are at the 10th percentile in family SES. High-SES students refer to those at the 90th percentile in family SES. [a]Predicted values of perceived sense of positive meaning and positive purpose in life for students who do not use ICT for schoolwork at home. [b]Predicted values of perceived sense of positive meaning and positive purpose in life for students who moderately use ICT for schoolwork at home. [c]Differences in gains of perceived sense of positive meaning and positive purpose in life between Columns 1 and 2. Scores that are above 30 (approximately 1/3 of a standard deviation in perceived sense of positive meaning and positive purpose in life) are highlighted in bold. [d]ICT use at home has no positive effect on perceived sense of positive meaning and positive purpose in life

by 0.57, 0.60, 0.45, and 0.44 standard deviations, for high-SES students; for low-SES students, the effect sizes are 0.46, 0.45, 0.07, and 0.26 standard deviations, respectively. In Denmark, Finland, the positive effects of home ICT use on perceived sense of positive meaning in life are approximately three times greater for high-SES students (0.64 and 0.66 standard deviations) than for low-SES students (0.20 and 0.22 standard deviations, respectively). In Sweden, the effect size for high-SES students is about two times greater (0.75 standard deviations) than that for low-SES students (0.35 standard deviations).

6.4.2 *The Effect of School ICT Use*

Figure 6.6 presents plots of multilevel regression analyses to illustrate the curvilinear relationship between school ICT use (x-axis) and adolescents' perceived sense of positive meaning (or positive purpose) in life (y-axis) conditioned on family SES and controlling for individual- and school-level characteristics. Table 6.6 summarizes the effects of school ICT use on perceived sense of positive meaning (or positive purpose in life) for low- and high-SES students.

Among 10 developed countries or societies, there are positive associations between the use of digital technologies in classrooms and the perception of positive meaning in life; they are the United Kingdom, France, Ireland, Denmark, Finland, Sweden, Australia, Japan, South Korea, and Macao. While these associations are either linear or curvilinear, the sizes of the positive relationships are mostly small. A comparison of Figs. 6.5 and 6.6 again suggests that *home* ICT use is more influential than school ICT use for adolescents' perceived psychological well-being.

School ICT use has positive effects on perceived positive meaning in life for low-SES students only in the United Kingdom, Japan, and Ireland. In the United Kingdom, ICT use in school has similarly modest effects on both low- and high-SES students' perceived sense of positive meaning in life (0.34 standard deviations). In Japan, ICT use in school increases low-SES students' sense of positive meaning by 0.59 standard deviations. In Ireland, school ICT use is associated with an increase of positive meaning in life for low-SES students by 0.30 standard deviations, which is substantial but still smaller than the positive effect size for high-SES students (0.58 standard deviations).

We find the third-level digital divide among several affluent countries, including Ireland as noted above. In France, school ICT use increases high-SES students' perceived sense of positive meaning in life by 0.52 standard deviations, but it only increases low-SES students' perception of positive meaning in life by 0.12 standard deviations. Similar patterns are also found in Denmark, Finland, Sweden, South Korea, and Macao, where the positive effect of school ICT use is substantially greater for high-SES students than for low-SES students.

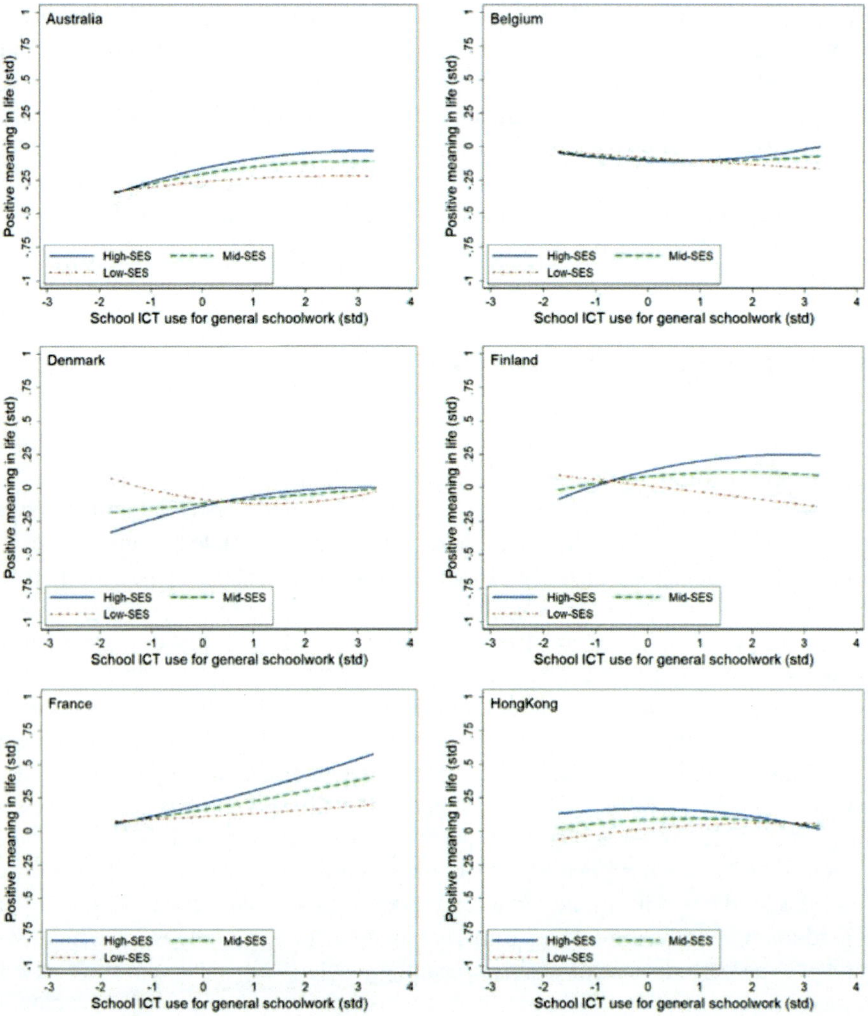

Fig. 6.6 Curvilinear effects of school ICT use for general schoolwork on perceived sense of positive meaning and positive purpose in life by family SES (*Data source* The 2018 Programme for International Student Assessment [PISA] survey. *Note* Countries/societies are listed alphabetically. High-SES refers to students who are at the 90th percentile in family SES. Mid-SES and Low-SES refer to those at the 50th and 10th percentiles in family SES, respectively. Predicted values are calculated based on two-level multilevel models for each country, where student-level variables are used in the Level-1 equation and schools' characteristics are used in the Level-2 equation. All multilevel models include country-specific educational program, school grade, student age, gender, immigration status, foreign language use at home, ICT resources at home, home ICT use for general schoolwork, and perceived digital competence as Level-1 controls. School average SES, public/private school, rural/town/urban school, shortage of educational staff, and shortage of educational material are Level-2 control variables. All Level-1 equations include the interaction effects between family SES and school ICT use for general schoolwork and between family SES and the squared term of school ICT use for general schoolwork. The following countries are not included in these analyses because key independent or dependent variables are unavailable from the country's PISA data: Canada, Austria, Germany, the Netherlands, Portugal, Norway, New Zealand, China, and Singapore)

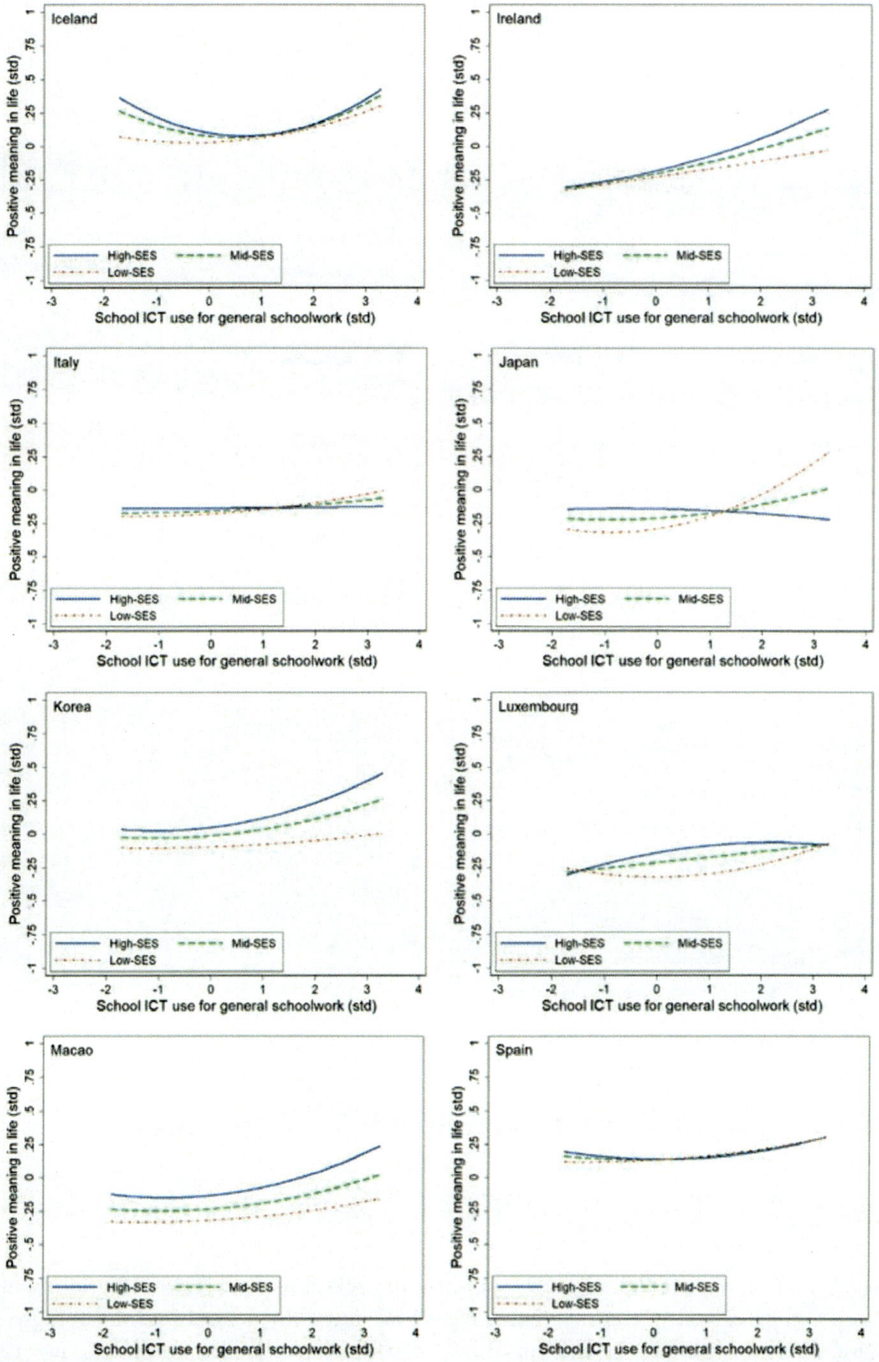

Fig. 6.6 (continued)

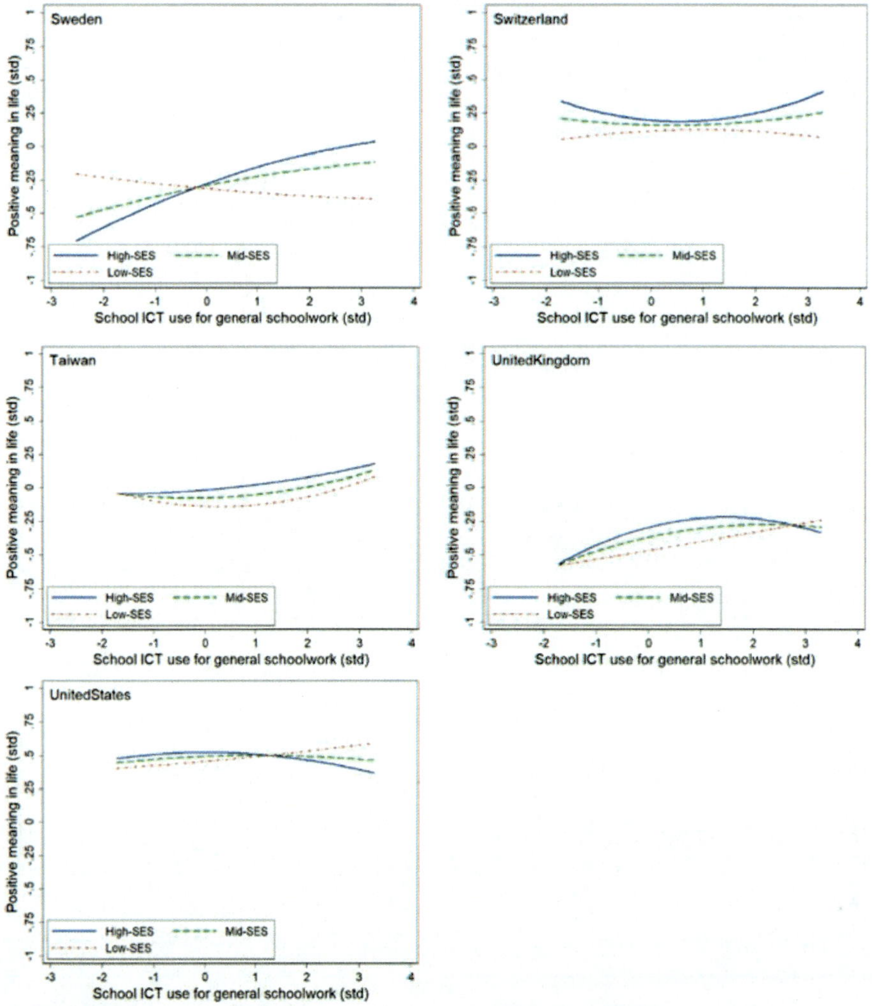

Fig. 6.6 (continued)

6.5 Predicting Students' Perceived ICT Competence

6.5.1 The Effect of Home ICT Use

The final section of this chapter examines the relationship between digital inclusion and perceived ICT competence. Figure 6.7 presents plots of multilevel regression analyses to illustrate the curvilinear relationship between home ICT use for general schoolwork (x-axis) and perceived ICT competence (y-axis) conditioned on family SES and controlling for individual- and school-level characteristics. Table 6.7

Table 6.6 Differences in predicted sense of positive meaning and positive purpose in life between students who do not use ICT for schoolwork at school and students who moderately use ICT for schoolwork at school: Summary of 19 countries/societies in Fig. 6.6

	Low-SES student			High-SES student		
	No ICT use (1)[a]	Moderate ICT use (2)[b]	Difference (2) − (1)[c]	No ICT use (1)[a]	Moderate ICT use (2)[b]	Difference (2) − (1)[c]
North America:						
United States	0.41	0.59	0.19	negative (or no positive) effect[d]		
Western and Southern Europe:						
Belgium	negative (or no positive) effect[d]			negative (or no positive) effect[d]		
United Kingdom	−0.58	−0.23	**0.34**	−0.56	−0.22	**0.34**
France	0.07	0.20	0.12	0.06	0.58	**0.52**
Ireland	−0.33	−0.03	**0.30**	−0.30	0.28	**0.58**
Italy	−0.20	−0.01	0.19	negative (or no positive) effect[d]		
Luxembourg	−0.26	−0.07	0.19	−0.30	−0.07	0.24
Spain	0.12	0.30	0.18	negative (or no positive) effect[d]		
Switzerland	0.05	0.12	0.07	negative (or no positive) effect[d]		
Scandinavia:						
Denmark	negative (or no positive) effect[d]			−0.33	0.00	**0.33**
Finland	negative (or no positive) effect[d]			−0.09	0.25	**0.34**
Iceland	0.07	0.30	0.23	negative (or no positive) effect[d]		
Sweden	negative (or no positive) effect[d]			−0.71	0.04	**0.74**
Pacific:						
Australia	−0.34	−0.22	0.12	−0.35	−0.03	**0.31**
Asia:						
Hong Kong	−0.06	0.06	0.13	negative (or no positive) effect[d]		
Japan	−0.30	0.29	**0.59**	negative (or no positive) effect[d]		
Korea	−0.10	0.01	0.11	0.03	0.45	**0.42**
Macao	−0.33	−0.16	0.17	−0.12	0.24	**0.36**
Taiwan	negative (or no positive) effect[d]			−0.05	0.18	0.23

Data source The 2018 Programme for International Student Assessment (PISA) survey
Note Countries/societies in each geographical region are listed alphabetically. Low-SES students refer to those who are at the 10th percentile in family SES. High-SES students refer to those at the 90th percentile in family SES. [a]Predicted values of perceived sense of positive meaning and positive purpose in life for students who do not use ICT for schoolwork at school. [b]Predicted values of perceived sense of positive meaning and positive purpose in life for students who moderately use ICT for schoolwork at school. [c]Differences in gains of perceived sense of positive meaning and positive purpose in life between Columns 1 and 2. Scores that are above 30 (approximately 1/3 of a standard deviation in perceived sense of positive meaning and positive purpose in life) are highlighted in bold. [d]ICT use at school has no positive effect on perceived sense of positive meaning and positive purpose in life

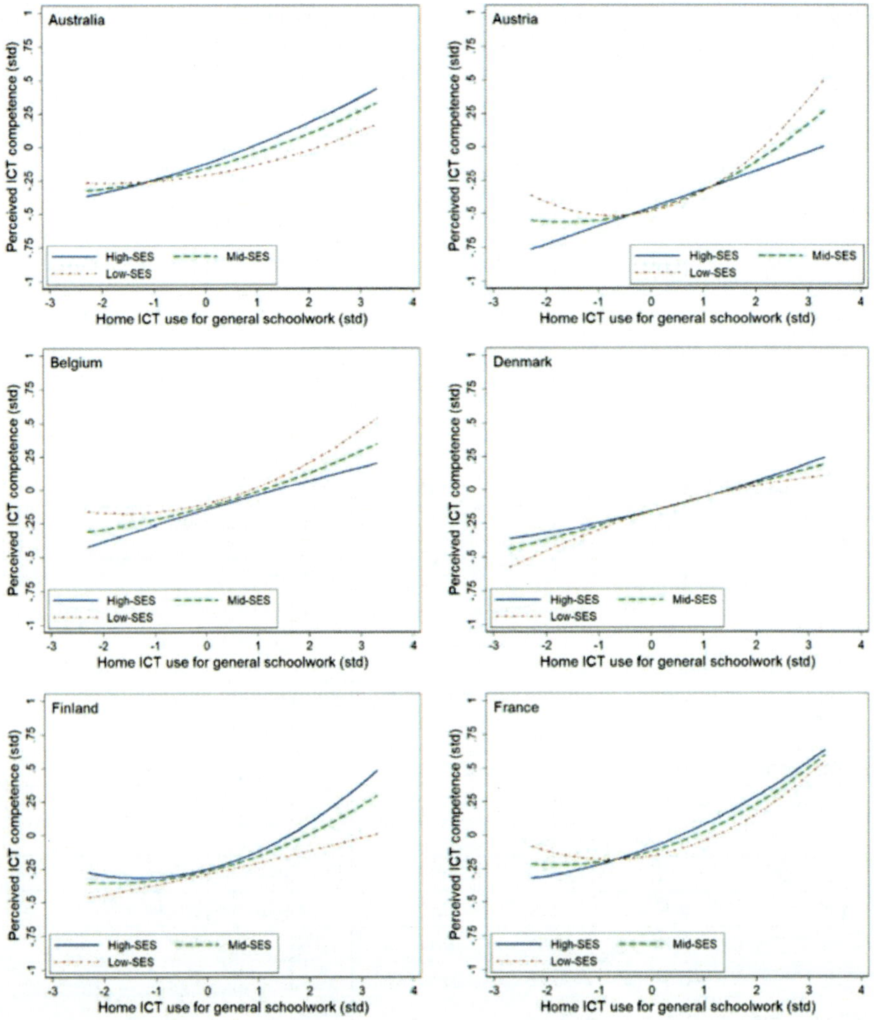

Fig. 6.7 Curvilinear effects of home ICT use for general schoolwork on perceived ICT competence by family SES (*Data source* The 2018 Programme for International Student Assessment [PISA] survey. *Note* Countries/societies are listed alphabetically. High-SES refers to students who are at the 90th percentile in family SES. Mid-SES and Low-SES refer to those at the 50th and 10th percentiles in family SES, respectively. Predicted values are calculated based on two-level multilevel models for each country, where student-level variables are used in the Level-1 equation and schools' characteristics are used in the Level-2 equation. All multilevel models include country-specific educational program, school grade, student age, gender, immigration status, foreign language use at home, ICT resources at home, and school ICT use for general schoolwork as Level-1 controls, and school average SES, public/private school, rural/town/urban school, shortage of educational staff, and shortage of educational material are Level-2 control variables. All Level-1 equations include the interaction effects between family SES and home ICT use for general schoolwork and between family SES and the squared term of home ICT use for general schoolwork. The following countries are not included in these analyses because key independent or dependent variables are unavailable from the country's PISA data: Canada, Germany, the Netherlands, Portugal, Norway, and China)

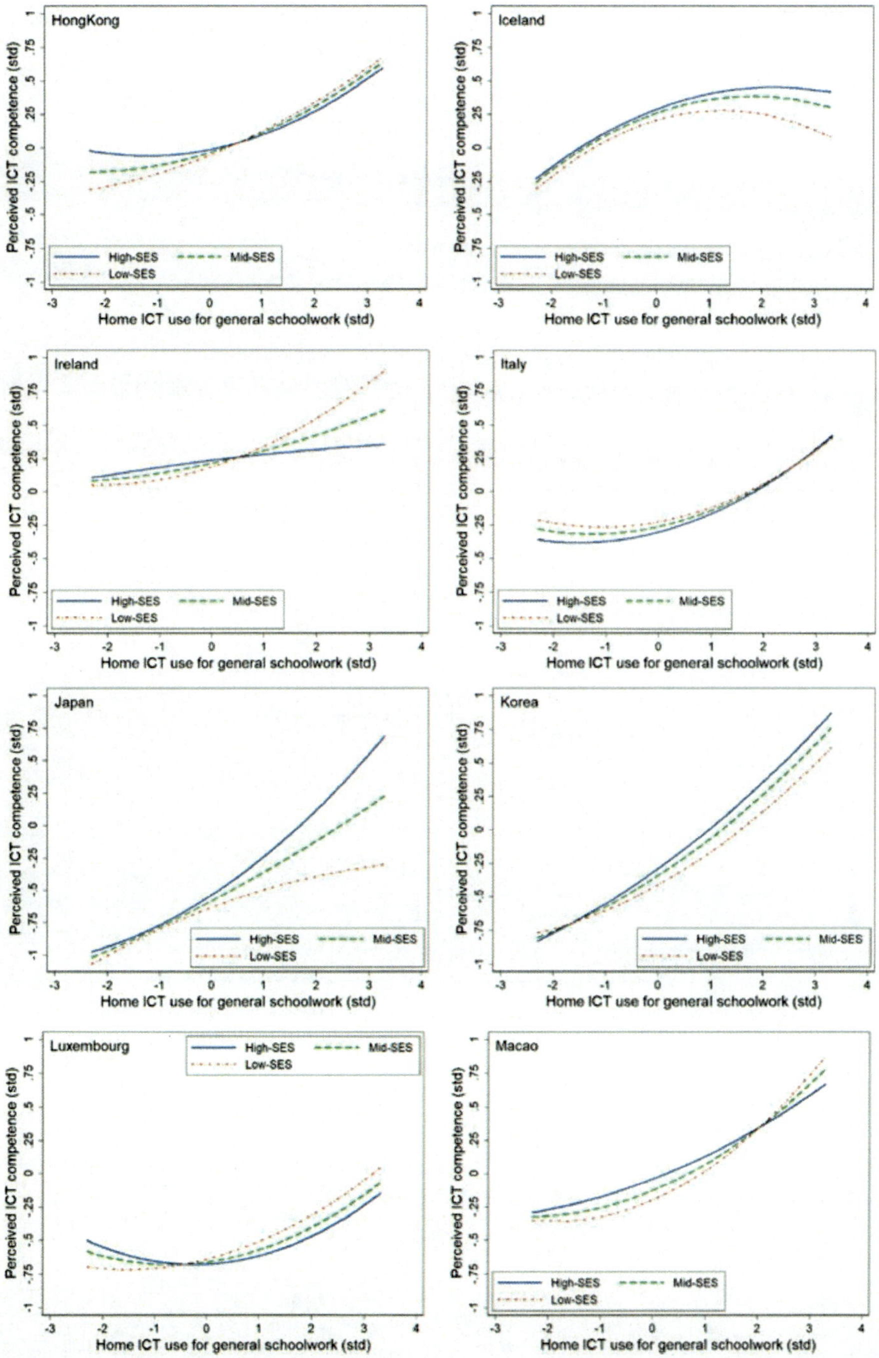

Fig. 6.7 (continued)

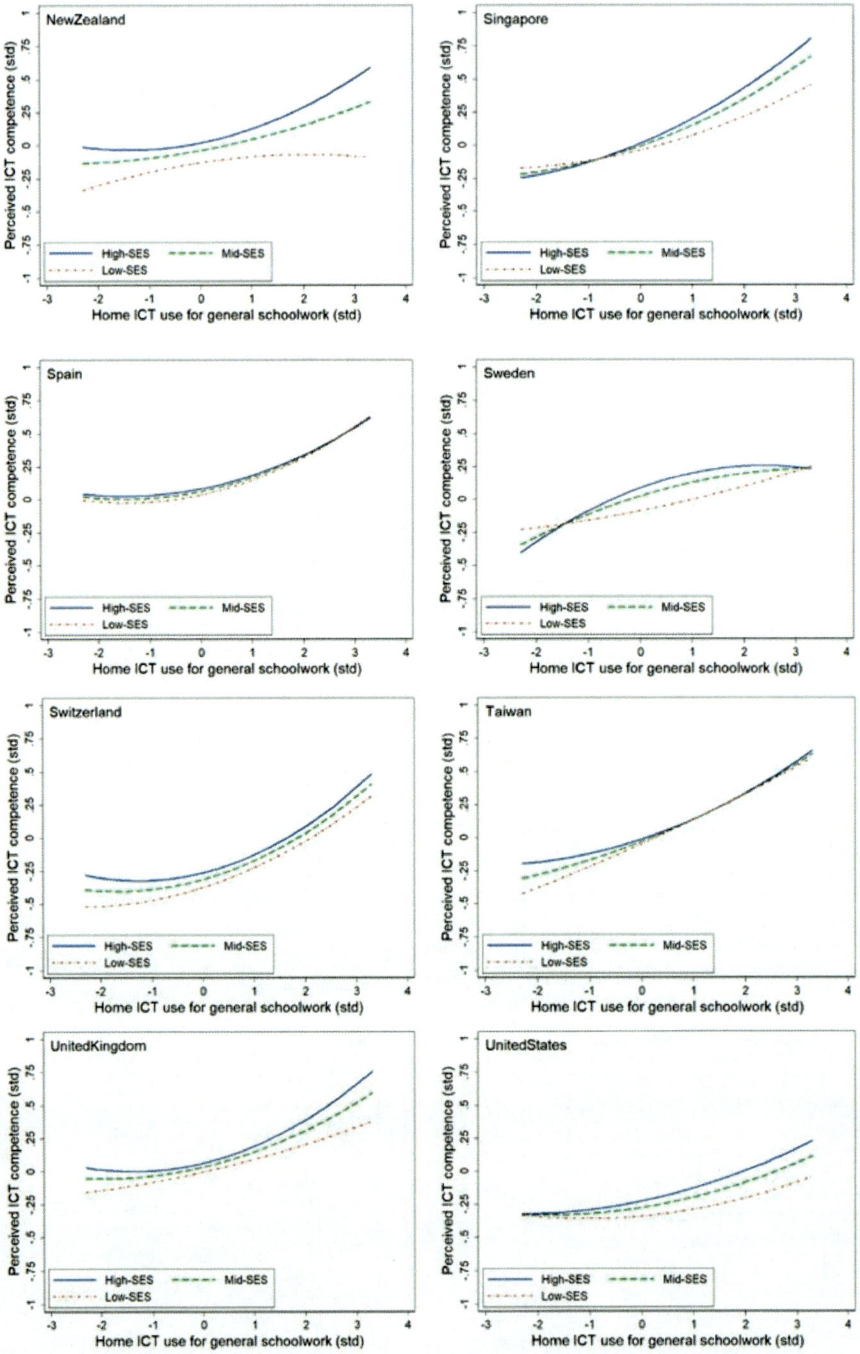

Fig. 6.7 (continued)

Table 6.7 Differences in predicted ICT competence between students who do not use ICT for schoolwork at home and students who moderately use ICT for schoolwork at home: Summary of 22 countries/societies in Fig. 6.7

	Low-SES student			High-SES student		
	No ICT use (1)[a]	Moderate ICT use (2)[b]	Difference (2) – (1)[c]	No ICT use (1)[a]	Moderate ICT use (2)[b]	Difference (2) – (1)[c]
North America:						
United States	−0.35	−0.04	**0.31**	−0.33	0.23	**0.56**
Western and Southern Europe:						
Austria	−0.36	0.50	**0.86**	−0.77	0.00	**0.77**
Belgium	−0.17	0.54	**0.71**	−0.42	0.20	**0.62**
United Kingdom	−0.16	0.38	**0.54**	0.03	0.76	**0.73**
France	−0.08	0.55	**0.63**	−0.32	0.63	**0.95**
Ireland	0.05	0.91	**0.87**	0.11	0.35	0.25
Italy	−0.21	0.40	**0.61**	−0.37	0.42	**0.79**
Luxembourg	−0.71	0.05	**0.76**	−0.50	−0.15	**0.35**
Spain	−0.02	0.63	**0.66**	0.03	0.62	**0.59**
Switzerland	−0.52	0.32	**0.84**	−0.28	0.48	**0.76**
Scandinavia:						
Denmark	−0.57	0.10	**0.67**	−0.36	0.24	**0.60**
Finland	−0.46	0.01	**0.47**	−0.28	0.48	**0.76**
Iceland	−0.31	0.28	**0.58**	−0.23	0.45	**0.68**
Sweden	−0.23	0.25	**0.48**	−0.40	0.25	**0.66**
Pacific:						
Australia	−0.27	0.17	**0.44**	−0.36	0.43	**0.80**
New Zealand	−0.34	−0.07	0.27	−0.01	0.59	**0.60**
Asia:						
Hong Kong	−0.31	0.68	**0.99**	−0.02	0.60	**0.62**
Japan	−1.07	−0.30	**0.77**	−0.97	0.69	**1.67**
Korea	−0.77	0.61	**1.39**	−0.83	0.87	**1.70**
Macao	−0.35	0.88	**1.23**	−0.29	0.67	**0.96**
Singapore	−0.18	0.45	**0.63**	−0.25	0.80	**1.05**
Taiwan	−0.42	0.60	**1.03**	−0.20	0.66	**0.85**

Data source The 2018 Programme for International Student Assessment (PISA) survey
Note Countries/societies in each geographical region are listed alphabetically. Low-SES students refer to those who are at the 10th percentile in family SES. High-SES students refer to those at the 90th percentile in family SES. [a]Predicted values of perceived ICT competence for students who do not use ICT for schoolwork at home. [b]Predicted values of perceived ICT competence for students who moderately use ICT for schoolwork at home. [c]Differences in gains of perceived ICT competence between Columns 1 and 2. Scores that are above 30 (approximately 1/3 of a standard deviation in perceived ICT competence) are highlighted in bold. [d]ICT use at home has no positive effect on perceived ICT competence

summarizes the effects of home ICT use on perceived ICT competence for low- and high-SES students.

Not surprisingly, Fig. 6.7 shows strong and positive relationships in the vast majority of developed countries and societies that are in our analyses. The sizes of the positive associations are notable in some countries. In South Korea, for example, home ICT use for schoolwork increases low- and high-SES students' perceived ICT competence, respectively, by 1.39 and 1.70 standard deviations. Unlike the effects of ICT use in previous analyses, we do not see any obvious inverted U-shaped effect of home ICT use on students' perceived ICT competence. Instead, the relationships are either relatively linear (e.g., Australia and Denmark) or curvilinear (e.g., Iceland and Ireland).

Table 6.7 indicates that home ICT use for schoolwork has either similar or greater effects on low-SES students' perceived ICT competence than that on high-SES students' ICT competence among 11 of the 22 countries/societies. They are Austria, Belgium, Ireland, Luxembourg, Spain, Switzerland, Denmark, Iceland, Hong Kong, Macao, and Taiwan. For example, home ICT use similarly increases low- and high-SES students' perceived ICT competence, respectively, by 0.86 and 0.77 standard deviations in Austria.

For the remaining 11 countries, however, the problem of the third-level digital divide is apparent, including the United States, the United Kingdom, France, Italy, Finland, Sweden, Australia, New Zealand, Japan, South Korea, and Singapore. In both Japan and Singapore, for example, the positive effects of home ICT use on ICT competence are approximately two times greater for high-SES students (1.67 and 1.05 standard deviations, respectively) than for low-SES students (0.77 and 0.63 standard deviations, respectively).

6.5.2 *The Effect of School ICT Use*

Figure 6.8 presents plots of multilevel regression analyses to illustrate the curvilinear relationship between school ICT use (x-axis) and predicted ICT competence (y-axis) conditioned on family SES and controlling for individual- and school-level characteristics. Table 6.8 summarizes the effects of school ICT use on perceived ICT competence for low- and high-SES students.

Overall, the results suggest that school ICT use has similar strong and positive effects on students' perceived ICT competence as home ICT use for schoolwork across all developed countries. The sizes of the positive effects are again notable in several countries such as the United States (0.83 standard deviations for low-SES students; 1.31 standard deviations for high-SES students) and Denmark (1.28 standard deviations for low-SES students; 0.95 standard deviations for high-SES students). As in the case of home ICT use, the effects of school ICT use on students' perceived ICT competence are relatively linear (e.g., Australia, Belgium, and Finland) or curvilinear (e.g., France, Hong Kong, and Iceland).

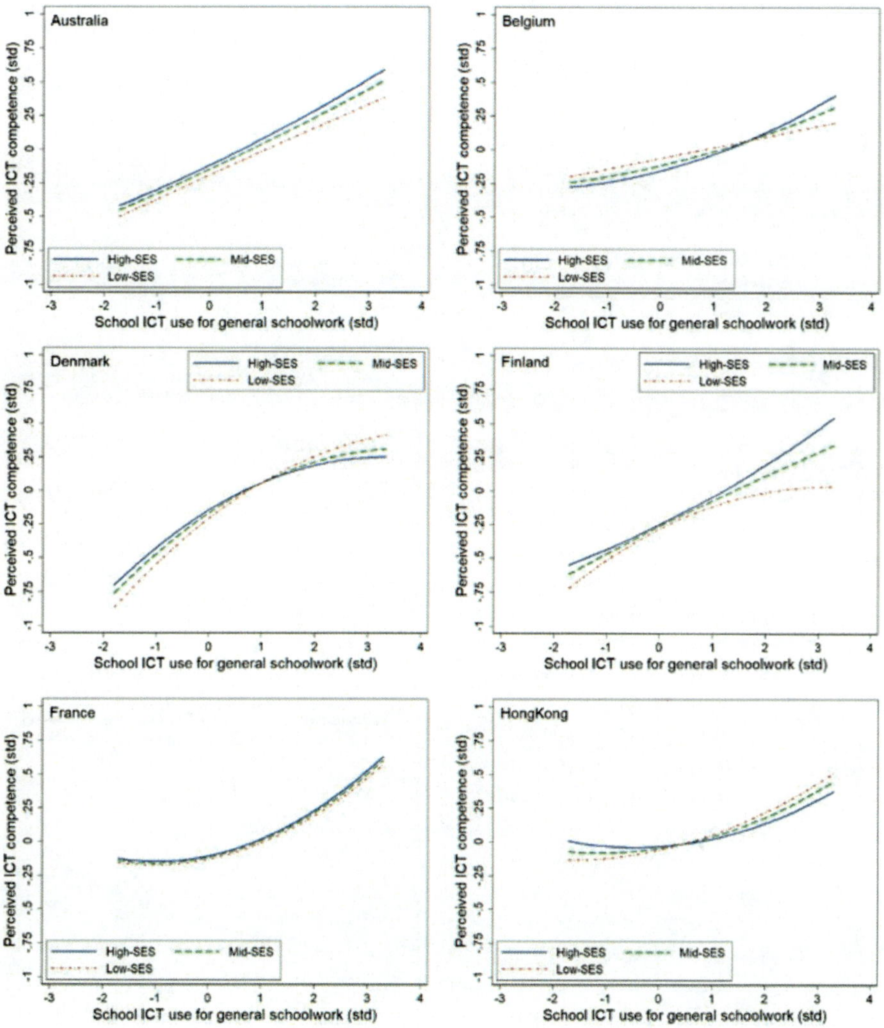

Fig. 6.8 Curvilinear effects of school ICT use for general schoolwork on perceived ICT competence by family SES (*Data source* The 2018 Programme for International Student Assessment [PISA] survey. *Note* Countries/societies are listed alphabetically. High-SES refers to students who are at the 90th percentile in family SES. Mid-SES and Low-SES refer to those at the 50th and 10th percentiles in family SES, respectively. Predicted values are calculated based on two-level multilevel models for each country, where student-level variables are used in the Level-1 equation and schools' characteristics are used in the Level-2 equation. All multilevel models include country-specific educational program, school grade, student age, gender, immigration status, foreign language use at home, ICT resources at home, and home ICT use for general schoolwork, as Level-1 controls, and school average SES, public/private school, rural/town/urban school, shortage of educational staff, and shortage of educational material are Level-2 control variables. All Level-1 equations include the interaction effects between family SES and school ICT use for general schoolwork and between family SES and the squared term of school ICT use for general schoolwork. The following countries are not included in these analyses because key independent or dependent variables are unavailable from the country's PISA data: Canada, Austria, Germany, the Netherlands, Portugal, Norway, and China)

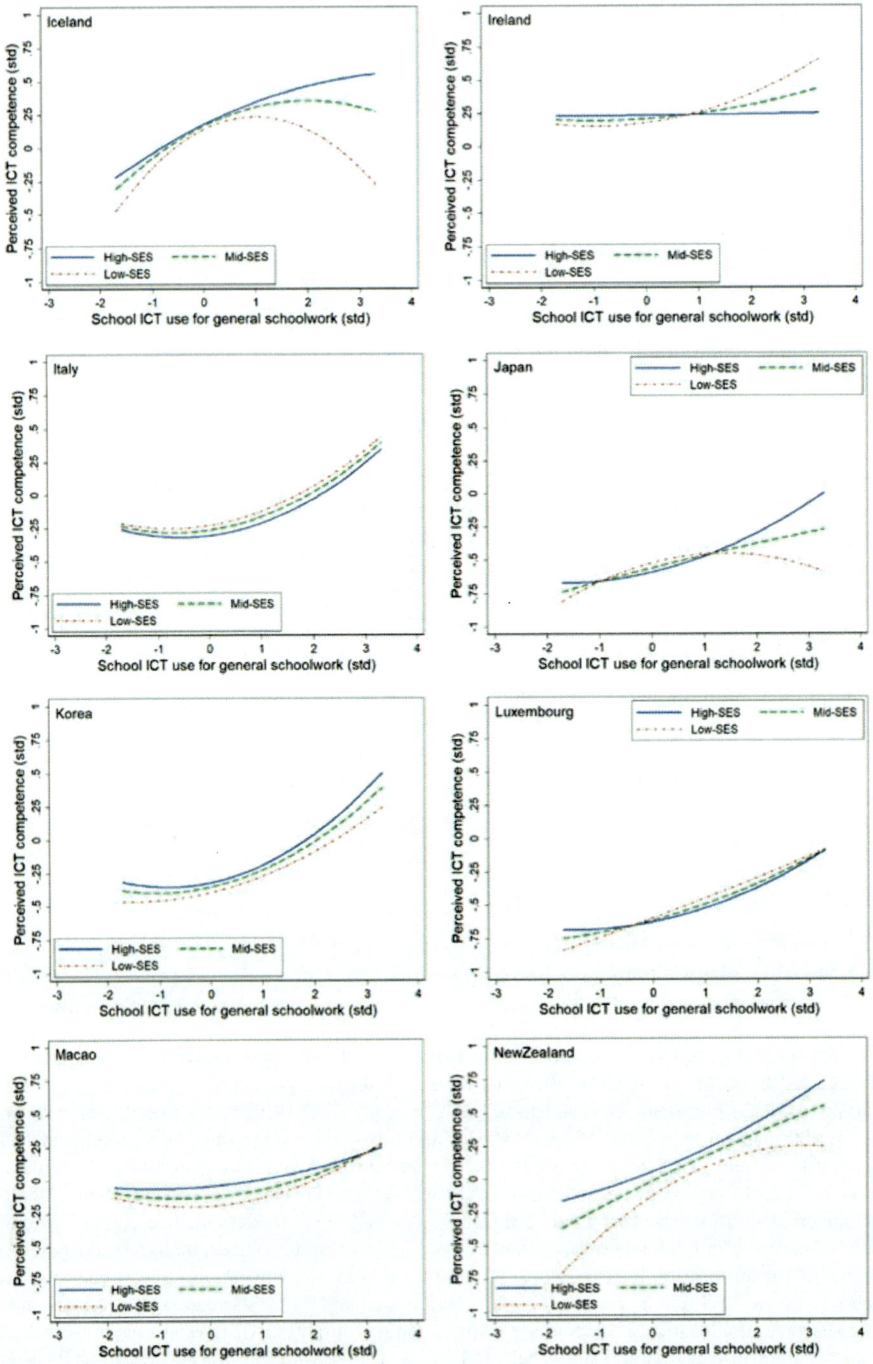

Fig. 6.8 (continued)

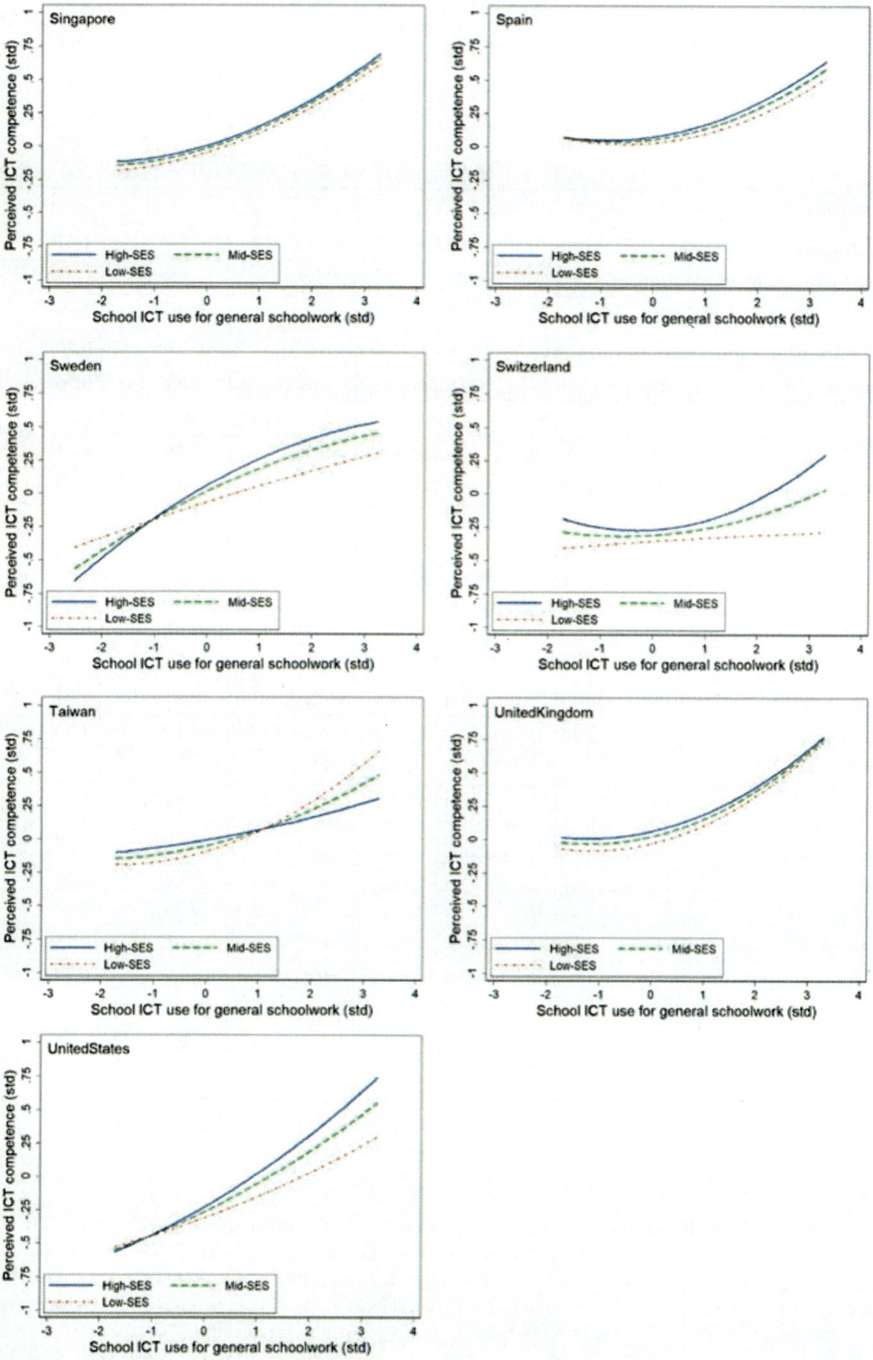

Fig. 6.8 (continued)

Table 6.8 Differences in predicted ICT competence between students who do not use ICT for schoolwork at school and students who moderately use ICT for schoolwork at school: Summary of 21 countries/societies in Fig. 6.8

	Low-SES student			High-SES student		
	No ICT use (1)[a]	Moderate ICT use (2)[b]	Difference (2) – (1)[c]	No ICT use (1)[a]	Moderate ICT use (2)[b]	Difference (2) – (1)[c]
North America:						
United States	−0.53	0.30	**0.83**	−0.57	0.74	**1.31**
Western and Southern Europe:						
Belgium	−0.20	0.20	**0.40**	−0.28	0.41	**0.68**
United Kingdom	−0.07	0.74	**0.81**	0.01	0.77	**0.76**
France	−0.16	0.57	**0.73**	−0.12	0.63	**0.76**
Ireland	0.16	0.66	**0.49**	negative (or no positive) effect[d]		
Italy	−0.22	0.44	**0.66**	−0.26	0.35	**0.61**
Luxembourg	−0.84	−0.08	**0.76**	−0.69	−0.09	**0.60**
Spain	0.07	0.52	**0.45**	0.07	0.65	**0.58**
Switzerland	−0.41	−0.29	0.12	−0.19	0.30	**0.49**
Scandinavia:						
Denmark	−0.87	0.41	**1.28**	−0.70	0.25	**0.95**
Finland	−0.72	0.03	**0.75**	−0.55	0.54	**1.09**
Iceland	−0.47	0.23	**0.71**	−0.22	0.55	**0.77**
Sweden	−0.41	0.31	**0.71**	−0.66	0.54	**1.19**
Pacific:						
Australia	−0.50	0.39	**0.89**	−0.42	0.59	**1.01**
New Zealand	−0.70	0.25	**0.95**	−0.16	0.74	**0.90**
Asia:						
Hong Kong	−0.13	0.51	**0.65**	0.01	0.38	**0.37**
Japan	−0.81	−0.45	**0.36**	−0.67	0.01	**0.68**
Korea	−0.47	0.24	**0.71**	−0.31	0.50	**0.82**
Macao	−0.13	0.28	**0.41**	−0.06	0.25	**0.31**
Singapore	−0.19	0.62	**0.81**	−0.12	0.69	**0.81**
Taiwan	−0.19	0.66	**0.86**	−0.10	0.30	**0.41**

Data source The 2018 Programme for International Student Assessment (PISA) survey*Data source* The 2018 Programme for International Student Assessment (PISA) survey

Note Countries/societies in each geographical region are listed alphabetically. Low-SES students refer to those who are at the 10th percentile in family SES. High-SES students refer to those at the 90th percentile in family SES. [a]Predicted values of perceived ICT competence for students who do not use ICT for schoolwork at school. [b]Predicted values of perceived ICT competence for students who moderately use ICT for schoolwork at school. [c]Differences in gains of perceived ICT competence between Columns 1 and 2. Scores that are above 30 (approximately 1/3 of a standard deviation in perceived ICT competence) are highlighted in bold. [d]ICT use at school has no positive effect on perceived ICT competence

When looking at results from Fig. 6.8 and Table 6.8, we find that school ICT use is likely to help enhance adolescent students' perceived digital competence (or their perceived ICT literacy). And this effect is large in size among students from various socioeconomic backgrounds. Figure 6.8 shows that using digital technologies in classrooms can help improve perceived digital competence of adolescent students of all backgrounds, but the effect sizes are either similar or greater for low-SES students than for high-SES students in 12 of the 21 countries/societies in the analyses, including the United Kingdom, France, Ireland, Italy, Luxembourg, Denmark, Iceland, New Zealand, Hong Kong, Macao, Singapore, and Taiwan. In France, for example, digital use in school similarly increases the perceived ICT competence by 0.73 standard deviations for low-SES students and by 0.76 standard deviations for high-SES students.

However, there remains the problem of the third-level digital divide among the remaining nine countries, including the United States, Belgium, Spain, Switzerland, Finland, Sweden, Australia, Japan, and South Korea. In the United States and Finland, for instance, school ICT use increases the perceived ICT competence for high-SES students by 1.31 and 1.09 standard deviations; these effects are greater than that for low-SES students (0.83 and 0.75 standard deviations, respectively).

6.6 Summary and Conclusion

The relationships between psychological health and the implementation and use of technology are matters of policy and scholarly debate. For the rising generation, ICT use promotes social interactions in virtual environments, allows young adults to keep in touch with their friends, increases the efficiency of learning, and thus may increase their sense of belonging, self-confidence, and life satisfaction. At the same time, the internet and digital technologies not only increase the possibility of cyberbullying but also reduce real-life communication and distract students from actual learning. The pressure to keep up with new technology and software may be a significant source of stress in itself.

In light of these debates, this chapter examines the influences of ICT use at home and in school on adolescent students' perceived ICT competence as well as their psychological well-being, using the 2018 PISA datasets. Students' perceived ICT competence is measured by an IRT index from five PISA survey questions (e.g., comfort with using digital devices and capability to solve problems with digital devices). We also include three additional composite variables to assess students' psychological well-being: (1) sense of belonging at school (e.g., the feeling like an outsider, the easiness to make friends, and the sense of loneliness); (2) positive psychological feelings (i.e., whether students feel joyful, cheerful, and happy); and (3) sense of purpose and meaning in life (e.g., "my life has a clear meaning or purpose" and "I have discovered a satisfactory meaning in life").

Our results confirm that ICT use increases adolescent students' perceived ICT competence in most developed countries. This suggests that to keep up with advancements in digital technologies and the widespread use of computer and mobile devices, education must incorporate ICT use in curriculum and in students' assignments. Educational policy in this direction will reduce adolescents' anxiety over the use and mastery of digital technology, increase their feelings of self-efficacy, and improve their psychological well-being.

According to the findings from this chapter, although using ICT at school has nearly little to no effects on students' sense of belonging at school and psychological well-being, the benefits of home ICT use on adolescents' psychological well-being are often quite substantial. In other words, the use of digital technologies for schoolwork at home can enhance adolescent students' psychological feelings and their sense of meaning in life. This pattern can be found in all affluent countries.

Our findings also suggest that when ICT use has visible effects on students' sense of belonging in school, the effects are likely to be greater for high- than for low-SES students. The exceptions are the United States, Iceland, Japan, and Macao. However, when assessing the effect of ICT use on psychological well-being and perceived ICT competence, ICT use seems to be more beneficial to low-SES students in half of the countries; and to higher SES students in the other half. This is not to say that the positive effects of ICT use on low- and high-SES students are random across developed countries. In fact, some countries or societies are doing well at implementing digital technologies in education, which helps reduce inequalities in adolescent students' psychological well-being and perceived ICT competence. For example, in the United Kingdom and Iceland (and to a lesser extent, the United States, Ireland, Luxembourg, Japan, Hong Kong, Macao, and Taiwan), ICT use for schoolwork tends to have more positive effects on low-SES students. In contrast, the use of ICT for schoolwork in countries like South Korea, France, Sweden, Denmark, and Finland may further exacerbate socioeconomic inequalities in adolescent students' psychological well-being and perceived ICT competence. Based on the cross-national comparative results, we suggest that governments can benefit from understanding how other countries adopt digital technologies and e-learning in school.

Reference

OECD. (2021). *PISA 2018 technical report*. PISA, OECD Publishing. https://www.oecd.org/pisa/data/pisa2018technicalreport/

Chapter 7
First- and Second-Level Digital Divides from 2009 to 2018

Abstract The third-level digital divide in outcomes and benefits of educational technology in the 2010s is associated with resurgent and more complex first- and second-level divides in ICT use and access. In this chapter, we return to a simple but important question: How did the digital divides in ICT use and access change from the late 2000s to late 2010s? We find that socioeconomic differences in internet access at home decreased substantially from 2009 to 2018 in developed countries. To our surprise, socioeconomic differences in *computer access at home* increased from 2009 to 2018, especially in Asia (with the exception of China). Furthermore, considerable percentages of low-SES students, especially in developed societies in Asia had no access to digital tablets. Although socioeconomic divides in home and school ICT use for schoolwork remained moderate and relatively stable from 2009 to 2018, we caution that the use of less functional digital devices for schoolwork at home by students of disadvantaged background may signal *increasing* (rather than decreasing) educational inequalities as a result of the resurgent first- and second-level digital divides.

Keywords Digital divide · Digital inequality · Internet access · Home computer · Digital tablet · Socioeconomic background · Asia

FOLLOWING the continuing development and worldwide diffusion of smartphones and new digital devices, ICT access and skills are no longer luxuries for students and teachers in the developed world. Schools make announcements to teachers, students, and parents by email and post important information on their websites. Teachers offer instruction in person, online, and hybrid modalities. Students register for classes using school websites, complete and submit assignments through the internet, and form online study groups. Some teachers and schools provide e-learning materials, but most are easy to find online and available to anyone who knows how to use a search engine. Educational activities now connect students and teachers in living rooms and bedrooms at home to schools, but these activities and resources are by no means equitably distributed.

J. K.-H. Ma and S. Cheng, *Adolescent Well-being and ICT UseX*,
Human Well-Being Research and Policy Making,
https://doi.org/10.1007/978-3-031-04412-0_7

As digital divides developed from the early 2000s to the 2020s, many researchers shifted their attention to differential learning outcomes by the use of ICT in education (i.e., the third-level digital divide) as we did in Chaps. 4–6. Acknowledging that the digital divide is now more complex than ever, this chapter returns to a simple yet important question: How did the digital divides in ICT use and access change from the late 2000s to the late 2010s? Using data from the 2009 and 2018 Programme for International Student Assessment (PISA) surveys, we analyze the inequalities in digital access (first-level digital divide) and ICT use (second-level digital divide) at home and in school and compare the data from 2009 and 2018. These analyses answer three research questions: Cross-nationally, how large is the first-level digital divide? How large is the second-level digital divide? And do these digital inequalities within and across countries change over time?

7.1 Methodology

7.1.1 Outcome Variables

To examine cross-national variations in the first-level digital divide, we analyze the extent to which family SES affects three measures of digital access: (1) *having internet access at home*, (2) *having access to a computer that can be used for school-related work at home*, and (3) *having access to a digital tablet at home*. The first two measures are available in both the 2009 and 2018 PISA datasets. The third measure is only available in the 2018 data. These measures are coded as dichotomous variables for whether adolescent students have internet access, computers, and digital tablets in their households (1 = yes, 0 = no).

To examine *cross*-national variations in the second-level digital divide, we analyze the extent to which family SES affects four measures for digital use. First, *home ICT use for general schoolwork* is a PISA-created IRT index (*HOMSCH in PISA 2009 and HOMESCH in PISA 2018*) with an OECD mean of 0 and an OECD standard deviation of 1. In the questionnaire, student respondents were asked "How often do you use digital devices for the following activities outside of school?" The response categories include "Never or hardly ever," "Once or twice a month," "Once or twice a week," "Almost every day," and "Every day." In PISA 2009, the index is based on the following five activities.

- Browsing the internet for schoolwork (e.g., preparing an essay or presentation).
- Using email for communication with other students about schoolwork.
- Using email for communication with teachers and submission of homework or other schoolwork.
- Downloading, uploading or browsing material from your school's website (e.g., time table or course materials).
- Checking the school's website for announcements (e.g., absence of teachers).

In PISA 2018, the index is based on the following 11 activities.

- Browsing the internet for schoolwork (e.g., for preparing an essay or presentation).
- Browsing the internet to follow up on lessons, e.g., for finding explanations.
- Using email for communication with other students about schoolwork.
- Using email for communication with teachers and submission of homework or other schoolwork.
- Using social networks for communication with teachers (e.g., Facebook and MySpace).
- Downloading, uploading, or browsing material from my school's website (e.g., timetable or course materials).
- Checking the school's website for announcements, e.g., absence of teachers.
- Doing homework on a computer.
- Doing homework on a mobile device.
- Using learning apps or learning websites on a computer.
- Using learning apps or learning websites on a mobile device.

Second, *home ICT use for core subjects* is also a PISA-created IRT index (*ICTOUTSIDE*) with an OECD standardized mean of 0 and an OECD standard deviation of 1. In the questionnaire, student respondents were asked "In a typical school week, how much time do you spend using digital devices outside of classroom lessons (regardless whether at home or in school) for the following subjects?" The response categories are "I do not study this subject," "No time," "1–30 minutes a week," "31–60 minutes a week," and "More than 60 minutes a week." This measure is not available in PISA 2009. In PISA 2018, the index is based on the following five subjects.

- Test language lessons.
- Mathematics.
- Science.
- Foreign language.
- Social sciences.

Third, *school ICT use for general schoolwork* is another PISA-created IRT index (*USESCH*) with an OECD mean of 0 and an OECD standard deviation of 1. In the questionnaire, student respondents were asked "How often do you use digital devices for the following activities at school?" The response categories are "Never or hardly ever," "Once or twice a month," "Once or twice a week," "Almost every day," and "Every day." In PISA 2009, the index is based on the following nine activities.

- Chating online at school.
- Using email at school.
- Browsing the internet for schoolwork.
- Downloading, uploading or browsing material from the school's website (e.g., intranet).
- Posting your work on the school's website.
- Playing simulations at school.

- Practicing and drilling, such as for foreign language learning or mathematics.
- Doing individual homework on a school computer.
- Using school computers for group work and communication with other students.

In PISA 2018, the index is based on the following 10 activities.

- Chatting online at school.
- Using email at school.
- Browsing the internet for schoolwork.
- Downloading, uploading, or browsing material from the school's website (e.g., intranet).
- Posting my work on the school's website.
- Playing simulations at school.
- Practicing and drilling, such as for foreign language learning or mathematics.
- Doing homework on a school computer.
- Using school computers for group work and communication with other students.
- Using learning apps or learning websites.

Fourth and finally, we include *school ICT use for core subjects*, a PISA-created IRT index (*ICTCLASS*) with an OECD mean of 0 and an OECD standard deviation of 1. In the questionnaire, student respondents were asked "In a typical school week, how much time do you spend using digital devices during classroom lessons?" The response categories are "I do not study this subject," "No time," "1–30 minutes a week," "31–60 minutes a week," and "More than 60 minutes a week." This measure is not available in PISA 2009. In PISA 2018, the index is based on the following five subjects.

- Test language lessons.
- Mathematics.
- Science.
- Foreign language.
- Social sciences.

7.1.2 Family SES and Other Control Variables

We use *family SES* to measure students' social class backgrounds. This variable is derived from the index of economic, social, and cultural status (*ESCS*) by PISA (OECD, 2012, 2021) as a composite of parental educational level, parental occupational status, and a set of household possessions. The index is standardized with an OECD mean of 0 and an OECD standard deviation of 1. Our analyses include the following student-level variables to control for students' personal and family background characteristics: *gender*, *student age*, *immigration status*, and *foreign language use at home*. Full descriptions of PISA variables are available in the OECD's official reports (OECD, 2012, 2021).

7.1.3 Analytical Strategies and Methods

To account for cross-national variations, we use the same analytical strategies as in Chaps. 4–6 by running separate multilevel models for *each* country using both the OECD PISA 2009 and 2018 data. Each multilevel model includes explanatory variables at the individual-student-level and accounts for the interdependent variations due to the clustering of students within schools. The general form of the model for a student i at school s can be written as,

$$Y_{is} = \beta_{0s} + \beta_{1s}(SES)_{is} + \sum_{2}^{k} \beta_{ks} x_{is} + e_{is} \tag{7.1}$$

At the individual-student-level (Eq. 7.1), Y_{is} is the dependent variable. β_{0s} represents the intercept, which is adjusted for other individual-student-level explanatory variables (i.e., family SES and β_{2s} to β_{ks}). As shown in Eq. 7.2 below, the intercept is assumed to vary randomly across schools (μ_{0s}).

$$\beta_{0s} = \gamma_{00} + \mu_{0s} \tag{7.2}$$

Because the three measures of digital access are coded as dichotomous variables and the four measures of digital use are coded as continuous variables, we use multilevel logit models for digital access outcomes and multilevel linear models for digital use outcomes. Our main goal is to compare the differences in digital access and digital use between high- and low-SES students for each of the countries/societies with available data in PISA 2009 and 2018. To ease the interpretation and presentation of the empirical findings, we use graphs to visualize cross-national variations in the effect of family SES on each of the digital access and digital use outcomes.

7.2 First-Level Digital Divide in 2009 and 2018

7.2.1 Access to the Internet at Home

Figure 7.1 presents cross-national variations in the first-level digital divide in internet access at home. For each country and society, the horizontal line indicates the size of the difference in the proportion of having internet access at home between high-SES students (students in the top decile of family SES mean) and low-SES students (students in the bottom decile of family SES mean). The left panel is the digital divide in 2009. The right panel is the digital divide in 2018.

The results in Fig. 7.1 suggest that the differences in internet access at home between high- and low-SES students decreased substantially from 2009 to 2018. In Australia, 82.6% of low-SES students and 99.6% of high-SES students had internet

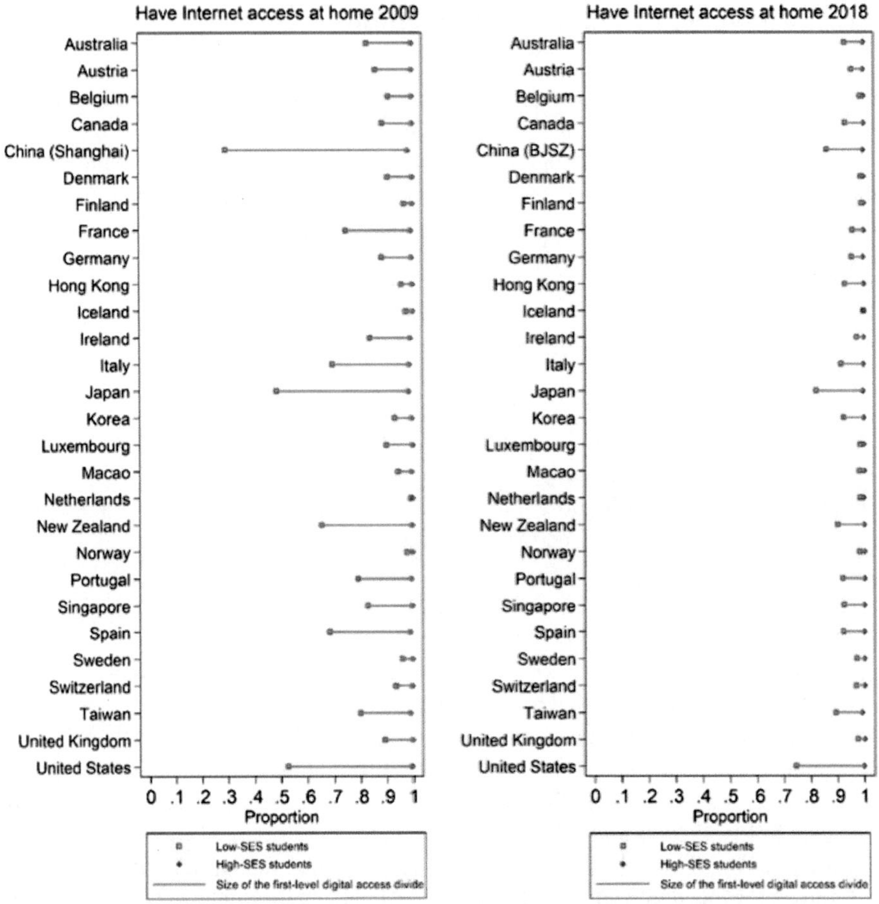

Fig. 7.1 The first-level digital divides in internet access at home: 2009 and 2018 (*Data source* The 2009 and 2018 Programme for International Student Assessment [PISA] surveys. *Note* The first-level digital divide is calculated based on two-level logit HLM for each country/society, where students are considered Level 1 and schools are considered Level 2. All models include the following Level 1 control variables: family SES, gender, student age, immigration status, and foreign language use at home. The line for each country indicates the difference between the average of high-SES students in the top decile of family SES mean and the average of low-SES students in the bottom decile of family SES mean. Countries/societies are listed alphabetically)

access at home in 2009, a difference of 17%. In 2018, the proportion of low-SES students with internet access at home rose to 93.0%, compared to 99.8% of high-SES students with internet access at home in the same year. This 6.8% difference in 2018 was much smaller than the 17% difference in 2009. In Austria, the proportions of low-SES students with internet access at home increased from 85.9% in 2009 to 95.5% in 2018, whereas the proportions of high-SES students with internet access at home remained high in both years. The substantial increase in digital access at home for low-SES students from 2009 to 2018 thus led to a much smaller digital divide between low- and high-SES students in Austria in 2018.

The pattern applies to all countries and societies in our analyses. In France, for example, the difference between high- and low-SES students in 2009 was 24.7% (74.6% for low-SES students and 99.3% for high-SES students). In 2018, the gap between high- and low-SES students decreased to 4.1%. In Italy, the digital divide decreased from 29.3% in 2009 to 8.2% in 2018. In New Zealand, the digital divide decreased from 34.4% in 2009 to 9.8% in 2018.

It is worth noting that home access to the internet for low-SES students was considerably lower in China, Japan, and the United States than in other developed countries in 2009. However, as a result of the rapid development of digital technology and its quick diffusion to poor and working-class families over the past 10 years, the large digital inequalities decreased significantly in these three countries in 2018. In 2009, only 29.3% of low-SES students in China had digital access at home. In 2018, 86.2% of low-SES students in China could access the internet at home. In Japan, only 48.6% of low-SES students were able to access the internet at home in 2009. 10 years later, in 2018, 82.1% of low-SES students had digital access at home. Similarly, in the United States, only 52.7% of low-SES students had internet access at home in 2009, compared to 74.4% of low-SES students with internet access at home in 2018. Despite such impressive improvements, the digital inequalities in these countries are still more visible than the smaller first-level digital divides in North European countries, Belgium, Ireland, Luxembourg, Macao, the Netherlands, Switzerland, and the United Kingdom. These stark differences highlight the possibility that lower-SES students may still experience an elevated level of digital inequalities even in some developed countries. In the next section, we present additional evidence that the digital disadvantages of low-SES students go beyond their internet access.

7.2.2 Access to Computers and Tablets for Schoolwork at Home

Students may access the internet using mobile phones, computers, or tablets. Although mobile phones provide easy and convenient access to the internet, computers are more multifunctional and allow students to conduct more intensive schoolwork. Therefore, internet access via mobile phones cannot replace computer access at home. In Fig. 7.2, we present cross-national variations in computer access for schoolwork at home and the digital divide between low- and high-SES students. Again, for each country, the horizontal line indicates the size of the difference in the proportion of computer access at home between high- and low-SES students. The left panel is the digital divide in 2009. The right panel is the digital divide in 2018.

The first unexpected pattern from Fig. 7.2 is that the differences in computer access at home by socioeconomic status *increased* from 2009 to 2018 in most developed countries and societies that we analyze. In Canada, 88.8% of low-SES students had

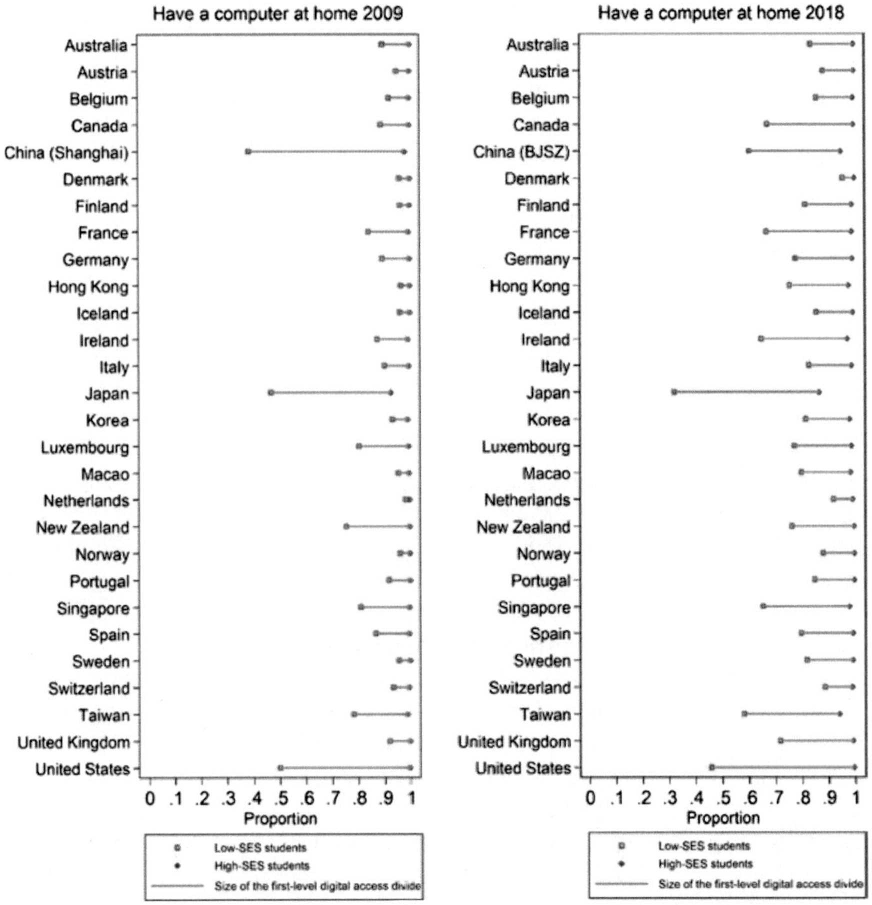

Fig. 7.2 The first-level digital divide in having a computer that can be used for schoolwork at home: 2009 and 2018 (*Data source* The 2009 and 2018 Programme for International Student Assessment [PISA] surveys. *Note* The first-level digital divide is calculated based on two-level logit HLM for each country/society, where students are considered Level 1 and schools are considered Level 2. All models include the following Level 1 control variables: family SES, gender, student age, immigration status, and foreign language use at home. The line for each country indicates the difference between the average of high-SES students in the top decile of family SES mean and the average of low-SES students in the bottom decile of family SES mean. Countries/societies are listed alphabetically)

computer access at home in 2009, but this percentage dropped to 66.9% in 2018. When considering the first digital divide based on computer access at home, the differences between high- and low-SES students in Canada increased from 11% in 2009 to 32.5% in 2018. The differences in computer access at home between low- and high-SES students were even more pronounced in the United States. Whereas almost all high-SES students had home computers to use for schoolwork in 2009, only 49.9% of low-SES students did. In 2018, 45.7% of low-SES students in the United States had access to a home computer for schoolwork.

The widening digital divide in computer access at home from 2009 to 2018 was not an isolated pattern in North America. In Finland, the difference in the rates of computer access at home between low- and high-SES students was 3.9% in 2009. In 2018, the difference rose to 17.6%. In France, the gap of computer access at home between low- and high-SES students was 15.4% in 2009. In 2018, the gap widened to 32.2%. In the United Kingdom, the disparity of computer access at home between low- and high-SES students was only 8.0% in 2009. From 2009 to 2018, the gap increased more than threefold, to 27.4%.

Although PISA has data only from the eastern coast of China, available data suggest that China is likely an exception. In 2009, 38.4% of low-SES students living along the eastern coast of China had computer access at home, compared to 98.0% of high-SES students. In 2018, the percentage of low-SES students with computer access at home rose to 60.2%, compared to 94.7% of high-SES students.

With the exception of China, the first-level digital divide widened from 2009 to 2018 in Asia. In Japan in 2009, 46.7% of low-SES students had computers at home. In 2018, the percentage dropped to 31.9%, leading to a 54.4% difference between high- and low-SES students. In Taiwan, the difference in computer access at home between low- and high-SES students was 20.8% in 2009 but rose to 35.9% in 2018. In Singapore, the disparity in computer access at home between low- and high-SES students was 18.7% in 2009. In 2018, the gap rose to 32.5%. If we consider only low-SES students in 2018, approximately 65.1% of low-SES students in Singapore could do their schoolwork on a home computer. In Taiwan, only 58.0% of low-SES students did.

One may speculate that low-SES students' decreasing access to computer at home in 2018 was partly attributable to the growing popularity of digital tablets. For example, instead of buying a computer, low-income and working-class families may buy a more affordable tablet for their children to do their homework. Therefore, without examining the socioeconomic differences in access to digital tablets at home, the analysis of the first digital divide would not be complete. In Fig. 7.3, we present cross-national variations in the first-level digital divide in access to digital tablets at home. Again, for each country, the horizontal line indicates the size of the difference in the proportion of access to digital tablets at home between high-SES students and low-SES students. Because questions about digital tablets were not available in PISA 2009, Fig. 7.3 presents only the analyses using the PISA 2018 data.

The results suggest large socioeconomic differences in access to digital tablets at home between high- and low-SES students, but the differences in Scandinavian nations, Ireland, the Netherlands, and the United Kingdom are smaller than the differences in other countries. Although still substantial, the differences in access to digital tablets at home between high- and low-SES students in Scandinavian countries are less than 20%. In the Netherlands, 86.5% of low-SES students have access to digital tablets at home, compared to 97.9% of high-SES students, a difference of 11.3%. In the United Kingdom, 85.4% of low-SES students and 98.8% of high-SES students have access to digital tablets at home, a difference of 13.4%.

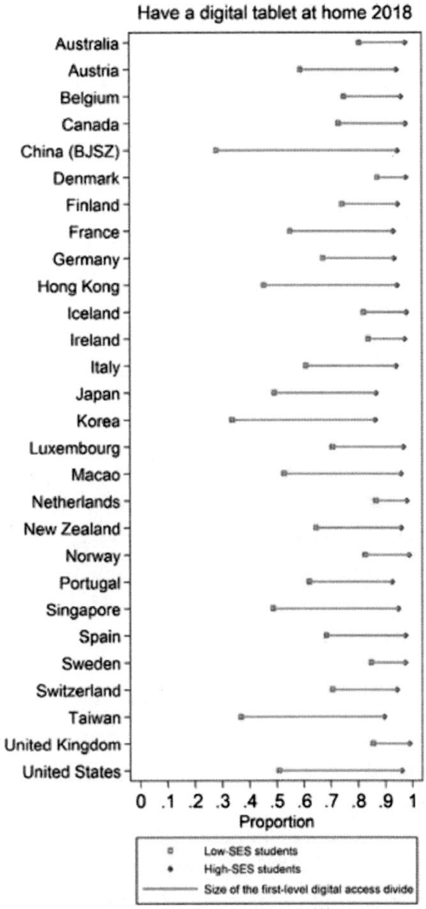

Fig. 7.3 The first-level digital divide in having a digital tablet at home: 2018 (*Data source* The 2018 Programme for International Student Assessment [PISA] survey. *Note* The first-level digital divide is calculated based on two-level logit HLM for each country/society, where students are considered Level 1 and schools are considered Level 2. All models include the following Level 1 control variables: family SES, gender, student age, immigration status, and foreign language use at home.The line for each country indicates the difference between the average of high-SES students in the top decile of family SES mean and the average of low-SES students in the bottom decile of family SES mean. Countries/societies are listed alphabetically)

Other Western countries have greater differences in home access to digital tablets between high- and low-SES students, particularly in Austria, France, Italy, New Zealand, and the United States. In Austria, France, and Italy, 94% of high-SES students had access to digital tablets at home. In contrast, just over half of the low-SES students in Austria (59.0%), France (55.1%), and Italy (60.8%) did. Similar patterns of the digital access gap apply to New Zealand and the United States.

The socioeconomic divide in home access to digital tablets was even greater in Asia. On China's eastern coast, we see that 94.6% of high-SES students had access to digital tables at home in 2018, whereas only 28.1% of low-SES students did. Similarly, in Hong Kong, Macao, Japan, South Korea, Singapore, and Taiwan, 80–90% of high-SES students were able to use digital tablets for schoolwork at home. When we focus on low-SES students, however, we see that the percentages were significantly lower—down to 45.4% in Hong Kong, 52.7% in Macao, 49.1% in Japan, 33.7% in South Korea, 48.6% in Singapore, and 36.8% in Taiwan. Overall, when access to both computers and digital tablets is taken into account, we conclude that the first-level digital divide is the largest in Asia, and the gaps between high-SES and low-SES students are the smallest in Scandinavian countries.

7.3 Second-Level Digital Divide in 2009 and 2018

7.3.1 ICT Use for School-Related Work at Home

Digital inequalities exist both in digital access (first-level digital divide) and ICT use (second-level digital divide). Indeed, even if high- and low-SES students have equal digital access, the former may still use digital devices and the internet for schoolwork more effectively than those from low-SES families. To assess the second-level digital divide, Figs. 7.4 and 7.5 present cross-national variations in home ICT use for general schoolwork and core subjects.

The results in Fig. 7.4 suggest a moderate socioeconomic divide in home ICT use for general schoolwork. In many developed countries, the differences between high- and low-SES students were stable from 2009 to 2018, around one-half standard deviations. In 2009 in Australia, ICT use for general schoolwork at home for low-SES students was 0.24 standard deviations lower than the OECD mean; for high-SES students, ICT use for schoolwork at home was 0.35 standard deviations above the OECD mean. These led to a difference of 0.59 standard deviations in home ICT use for general schoolwork between high- and low-SES students.

Beyond this pattern, we observe that the gaps in home ICT use for schoolwork increased slightly from 2009 to 2018 in Japan and South Korea. In Japan, the differences between low- and high-SES students grew from 0.37 standard deviations in 2009 to 0.49 in 2018. In South Korea, the difference was 0.41 standard deviations in 2009 and 0.54 in 2018. With the exceptions of Japan and South Korea, however, the socioeconomic divide in home ICT use for schoolwork decreased from 2009 to 2018 in most other countries, including Austria, Belgium, Denmark, Ireland, Italy, New Zealand, Singapore, and Spain. In Austria, the differences between high- and low-SES students was 0.51 standard deviations in 2009 (−0.26 standard deviations for low-SES students and 0.25 for high-SES students) and decreased by 0.25 standard deviations from 2009 to 2018. In Belgium, the socioeconomic gaps in home ICT use for schoolwork decreased from 0.36 standard deviations in 2009 to 0.24 in 2018. In New Zealand, the difference between high-SES and low-SES students was 0.76 standard deviations in 2009 and decreased to 0.45 in 2018.

Turning to Fig. 7.5, home ICT use for core subjects in 2018 also show similar patterns to those shown in Fig. 7.4. In 2018, the gaps in home ICT use for core subjects between low-SES and high-SES students were moderate. The gaps in home ICT use for core subjects seemed smaller than other measures of digital divide. The only two countries with large gaps in home ICT use for core subjects were Australia

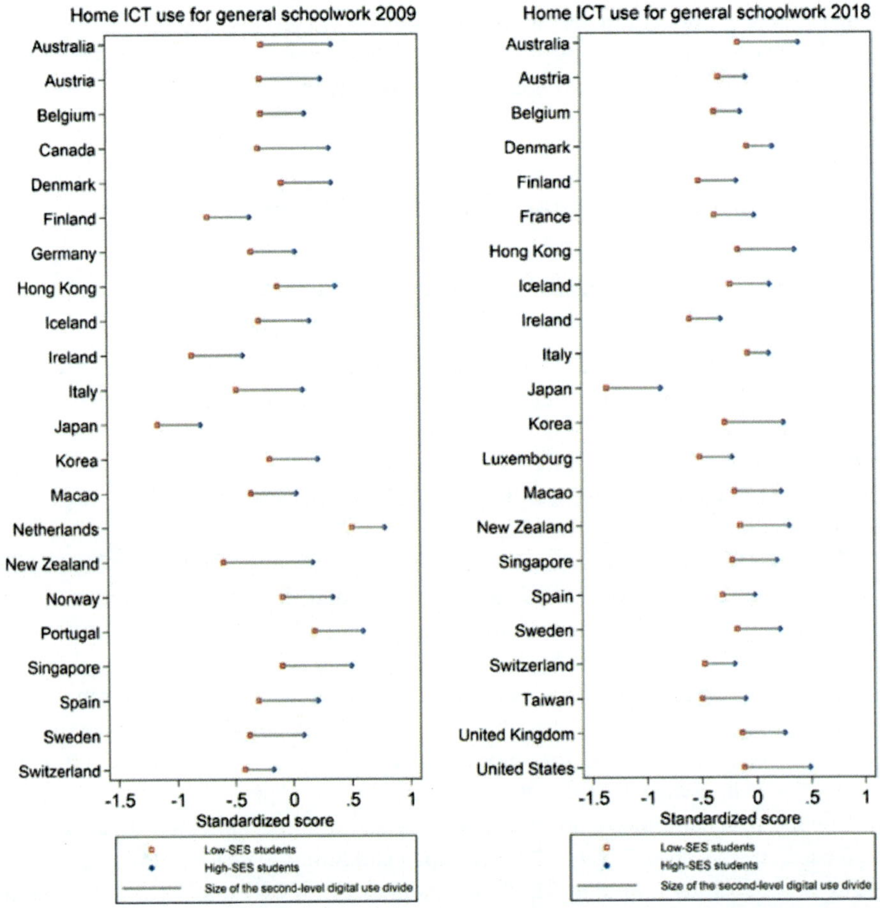

Fig. 7.4 The second-level digital divide in home ICT use for general schoolwork: 2009 and 2018 (*Data source* The 2009 and 2018 Programme for International Student Assessment [PISA] surveys. *Note* The second-level digital divide is calculated based on two-level logit HLM for each country/society, where students are considered Level 1 and schools are considered Level 2. All models include the following Level 1 control variables: family SES, gender, student age, immigration status, and foreign language use at home. The line for each country indicates the difference between the average of high-SES students in the top decile of family SES mean and the average of low-SES students in the bottom decile of family SES mean. Countries/societies are listed alphabetically)

and the United States. Even there, however, the digital gaps between high- and low-SES students were not severe: In Australia, the socioeconomic difference was 0.60 standard deviations. In the United States, the difference was 0.48. According to Figs. 7.4 and 7.5, we conclude that in 2009 and 2018, the second digital divide in home ICT use for schoolwork was moderate and relatively stable in most developed countries.

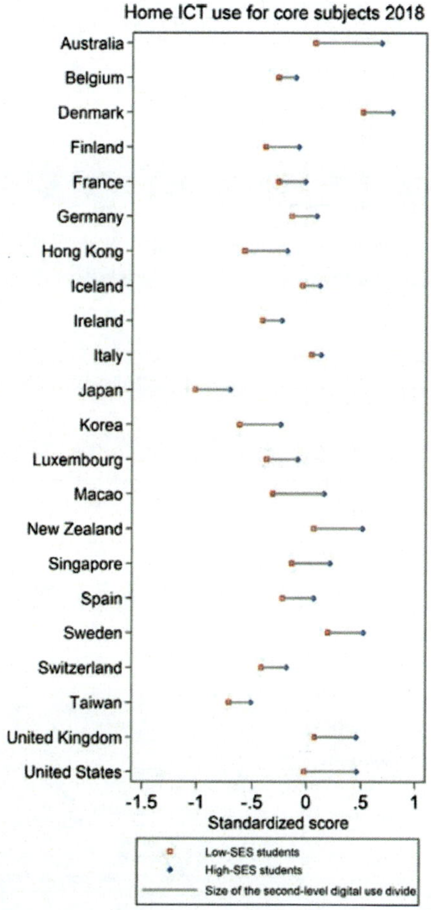

Fig. 7.5 The second-level digital divide in home ICT use for core subjects: 2018 (*Data source* The 2018 Programme for International Student Assessment [PISA] survey. *Note* The second-level digital divide is calculated based on two-level logit HLM for each country/society, where students are considered Level 1 and schools are considered Level 2. All models include the following Level 1 control variables: family SES, gender, student age, immigration status, and foreign language use at home. The line for each country indicates the difference between the average of high-SES students in the top decile of family SES mean and the average of low-SES students in the bottom decile of family SES mean. Countries/societies are listed alphabetically)

7.3.2 *ICT Use for Schoolwork at School*

Figures 7.6 and 7.7 present cross-national variations in the second-level digital divide in school ICT use for general schoolwork and for core subjects. Figure 7.6 suggests that in 2009 and 2018, the socioeconomic divide in school ICT use for general schoolwork was small in developed countries. The difference between high- and low-SES students was less than one-quarter of one standard deviation. In 2018, the ICT use for general schoolwork for low-SES students in Spain was 0.24 standard deviations lower than the OECD mean; the ICT use for general schoolwork at school for high-SES students in Spain was 0.12 standard deviations lower than the OECD mean. Together, the difference between high- and low-SES students in Spain was only 0.12 standard deviations.

The small digital divide at school notwithstanding, the digital gaps in school ICT use slightly increased from 2009 to 2018 in most of the countries in our analyses. In Scandinavia, the difference between high- and low-SES students in Denmark was

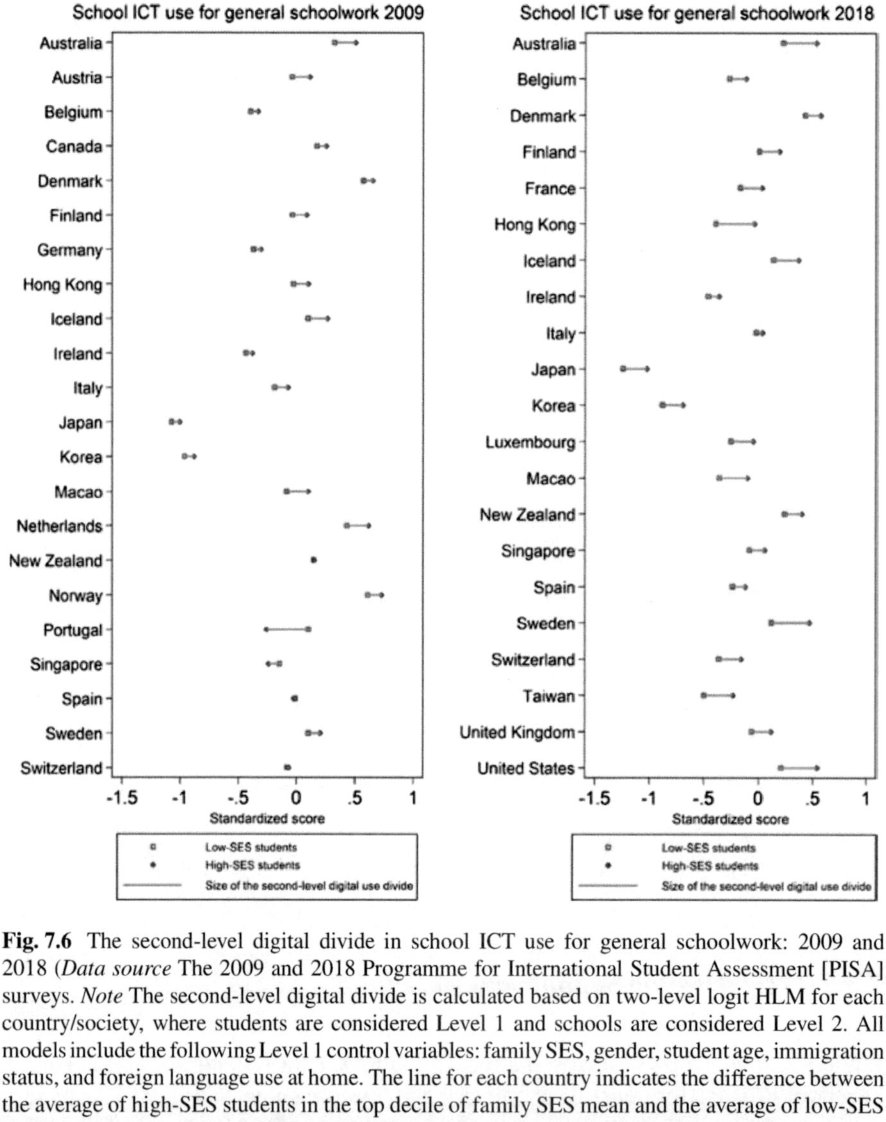

Fig. 7.6 The second-level digital divide in school ICT use for general schoolwork: 2009 and 2018 (*Data source* The 2009 and 2018 Programme for International Student Assessment [PISA] surveys. *Note* The second-level digital divide is calculated based on two-level logit HLM for each country/society, where students are considered Level 1 and schools are considered Level 2. All models include the following Level 1 control variables: family SES, gender, student age, immigration status, and foreign language use at home. The line for each country indicates the difference between the average of high-SES students in the top decile of family SES mean and the average of low-SES students in the bottom decile of family SES mean. Countries/societies are listed alphabetically)

0.08 standard deviations in 2009 (0.57 standard deviations for low-SES students and 0.65 for high-SES students), compared to 0.14 standard deviations in 2018. In Sweden, the socioeconomic gap widened from 0.10 standard deviations in 2009 to 0.35 in 2018.

The same pattern applies to other Western developed countries. In Australia, the socioeconomic gap increased from 0.18 standard deviations in 2009 to 0.31 in 2018. In New Zealand, the digital divide between high- and low-SES students was only

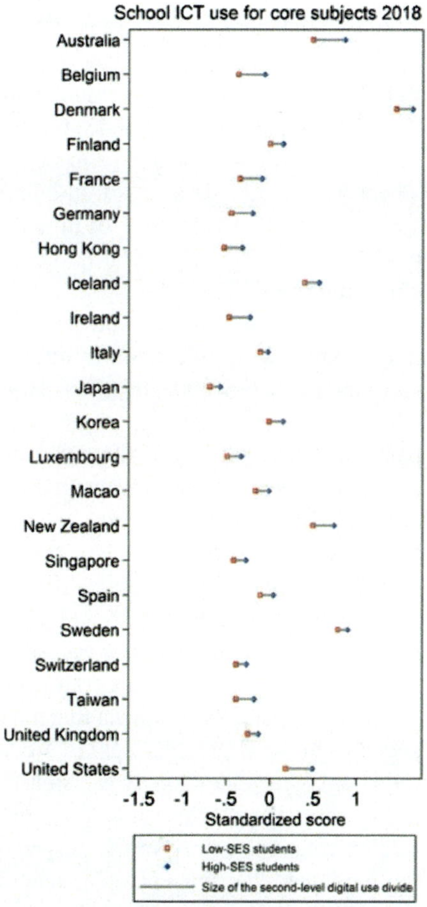

Fig. 7.7 The second-level digital divide in school ICT use for core subjects: 2018 (*Data source* The 2018 Programme for International Student Assessment [PISA] survey. *Note* The second-level digital divide is calculated based on two-level logit HLM for each country/society, where students are considered Level 1 and schools are considered Level 2. All models include the following Level 1 control variables: family SES, gender, student age, immigration status, and foreign language use at home. The line for each country indicates the difference between the average of high-SES students in the top decile of family SES mean and the average of low-SES students in the bottom decile of family SES mean. Countries/societies are listed alphabetically)

0.004 standard deviations in 2009. In 2018, however, the socioeconomic difference increased slightly to 0.16 standard deviations.

In Asia, the socioeconomic gap in Hong Kong increased from 0.13 standard deviations in 2009 to 0.35 in 2018. In Japan and South Korea, the socioeconomic differences were respectively 0.07 and 0.08 standard deviations in 2009 and increased slightly to 0.22 and 0.19 in 2018.

Finally, Fig. 7.7 shows cross-national variations in the second-level digital divide in school ICT use for core subjects in 2018. The patterns are similar to the results from Fig. 7.6. Across the board, the socioeconomic differences in school ICT use for core subjects were moderate. However, when we compare the results from Fig. 7.7 with those from Fig. 7.5 and the results of Fig. 7.6 with those from Fig. 7.4, the second-level digital divide in home ICT use is clearly greater than the second-level digital divide in school ICT use in these affluent societies.

7.4 Summary and Conclusion

In light of the resurgence and more complex first- and second-level digital divides in the 2010s, this chapter examines the 10-year changes of socioeconomic inequalities in ICT access and ICT use from 2009 to 2018. Considering the continuing diversification, we include access to the internet, computers, and digital tablets at home for schoolwork as measures of digital access. For second-level digital divides, we consider students' ICT use at home and in school for general schoolwork and for core subjects.

Analyses of PISA 2009 and 2018 using multilevel models suggest that in developed countries, socioeconomic differences in internet access at home decreased substantially from 2009 to 2018. Home internet access for low-SES students in China, Japan, and the United States was considerably lower in 2009. Despite significant improvements of ICT infrastructures over the past decade, differences in internet access between socially advantaged and disadvantaged students in these countries are still visible. These differences highlight the possibility that even in developed societies. socially disadvantaged students may still experience digital inequalities.

Surprisingly, socioeconomic differences in home computer access increased from 2009 to 2018, especially in Asia (with China as the exception). Some may suspect that this decreasing computer access at home was a function of low-income families replacing their children's computers with digital tablets for school use in 2018. However, our analyses suggest that many low-SES students, especially in developed societies in Asia, had no access to digital tablets. This may imply that many socially disadvantaged students only use smartphones to access the internet at home. This is not the most effective use of ICT for schoolwork, and may suggest the need for policy implementation to prevent the perpetuation of educational inequality as a result of the digital divide. For example, schools in some developed countries now assign a laptop to every student that they can use in the classroom and at home. Taking home access to the internet, computers, and tablets altogether, we conclude that the first-level digital divides are widest in Asia and narrower in Scandinavian countries.

Finally, our analyses of home and school ICT use for general schoolwork and core subjects indicate moderate and relatively stable socioeconomic divides from 2009 to 2018. As good news as this is for educators and policymakers in developed countries (and as suggested by our analyses), we caution that the use of less functional digital devices for schoolwork at home by students of disadvantaged background may signal increasing rather than decreasing educational inequalities as a result of the resurgent first- and second-level digital divides. This resurgence thus may require more aggressive government interventions during and after the COVID-19 pandemic.

References

OECD. (2012). *PISA 2009 technical report*. PISA, OECD Publishing. https://doi.org/10.1787/9789264167872-en

OECD. (2021). *PISA 2018 technical report*. PISA, OECD Publishing. https://www.oecd.org/pisa/data/pisa2018technicalreport/

Chapter 8
Concluding Thoughts and Policy Implications

Abstract In light of the increasing consensus that digital competence and digital literacy are important lifelong skills in the global and knowledge economy of the twenty-first century, this book examines the causes and consequences of digital inclusion and exclusion for students in secondary education. In this concluding chapter, we summarize the major findings of our empirical analyses and discuss their implications. The discussion highlights the challenges faced by policymakers and educators when addressing digital divides and the important questions scholars may consider when exploring the solutions for this persistent form of social inequality. We then provide policy recommendations for educators and governments to improve e-learning home environments and to integrate digital and internet technologies into education.

Keywords COVID-19 · Remote education · Digital divide · Digital inclusion · Twenty-first-century skills · Well-being · e-learning environment · Home vs. school · Policy implications

ICT has a profound effect on life in the twenty-first century. It has altered how educators teach in the classroom, how millennials do schoolwork, and how students today acquire skills and knowledge both inside and outside of school. With the new digital media (Warschauer & Matuchniak, 2010) and the readiness of ICT infrastructure (Cruz-Jesus et al., 2017; Robison & Crenshaw, 2010), e-learning technology has matured over recent years, especially in the developed countries. The COVID-19 pandemic unexpectedly forced schools to move many educational activities online, and accelerated the application of ICT in education, making digital technology and internet connection indispensable components of modern education. In this context, our book examines the causes and consequences of digital inclusion and exclusion for students in secondary education. In this concluding chapter, we summarize the major findings of our empirical analyses, discuss their implications, and derive policy recommendations from the discussion.

J. K.-H. Ma and S. Cheng, *Adolescent Well-being and ICT UseX*,
Human Well-Being Research and Policy Making,
https://doi.org/10.1007/978-3-031-04412-0_8

How does the use of digital technology influence well-being? To answer this question, we use the 2018 Programme for International Student Assessment (PISA) survey to examine the effects of digital inclusion on adolescent students' academic performance (Chap. 4) and learning attitudes (Chap. 5), and then assess the effects on adolescent students' subjective and psychological well-being and digital competence (Chap. 6). The findings suggest that home environments are more significant than schools in promoting adolescents' e-learning experiences and in shaping their digital competencies, even though students engage in a variety of digital activities in schools. To understand the third-level digital divide literature and to answer the classic question of how digital technology may generate new forms of social exclusion, we explore whether and how the potential benefits of digital inclusion vary among students based on their family socioeconomic status (SES). The results suggest that variations in home learning environments explain most of digital inequalities in adolescent students' e-learning experiences (see 8.2 for more details).

Who are excluded from ICT? In what way(s)? In Chap. 7, we illustrate the patterns and trends of digital learning inequalities according to students' socioeconomic background in 2009 and 2018, and examine the first-level digital divide (differences in digital access; see Attewell & Battle, 1999; van Deursen & van Dijk, 2019) and the second-level digital divide (variations in digital use; see Hargittai & Hinnant, 2008; Leu et al., 2015).

Our mission in the book is to discuss how educational inequality is amplified and shaped by socioeconomic inequalities in access, skills, and uses of digital technologies—commonly known as the "digital divide." Taken together, our findings challenge the belief that ICT use in schools compensates for the digital gap in home environments and thus reduces educational inequalities between socially disadvantaged and advantaged students (Gamoran, 2001; Warschauer & Matuchniak, 2010). Because new media technologies present both opportunities and challenges for youth development, there is a need to develop new theoretical frameworks to "[better make] sense of this new and fast-changing communications landscape" (Sefton-Green et al., 2016, p. 4). Based on our examination of the research literature in Chaps. 2 and 3 and the empirical analyses from Chaps. 4 to 7, we identify explanations, concepts, and analytical approaches that can help educators and researchers to understand how ICT use can be optimized to enhance adolescent students' learning experiences, improve their academic performance, promote their well-being, and develop their digital skills and knowledge.

This book takes an international and comparative approach to analyze digital divides and their consequences. A clear advantage of conducting large-scale and cross-national analyses is that this method avoids overreliance on small and non-representative samples. Warschauer and Matuchniak (2010, p. 204) point out that the findings of previous studies on the influence of ICT on educational outcomes are often inconclusive and mixed because many of these studies "are based on very small sample sizes and take place in schools or classrooms where individual educators are highly expert in particular uses of technology, and thus these studies may not be generalizable to other contexts." Equally important, findings from cross-national analyses can help policymakers, educators, and scholars identify effective e-learning strategies and ICT policies from other nations (OECD, 2020).

In the concluding remarks, we discuss the implications of the empirical findings from the literature and our analyses in this book, and provide useful recommendations for educators and policymakers. It is imperative for educators and policymakers to implement ICT policies and initiatives based on rigorous research. As suggested by Arnott (2016, p. 271), research can help us better understand how young people integrate digital technologies into their daily lives, given a "complex ecological system" that has shaped their e-learning and ICT use experiences from a very young age. Similarly, Livingstone (2012, p. 11) contends that "despite considerable evidence that teachers, along with parents, pupils and other stakeholders believe ICT to improve outcomes, few independent evaluations comparing educational settings with versus without an ICT intervention have been conducted, and those that exist are rather equivocal in their conclusions." Our book provides further evidence that empirical research should serve as the foundation of future policymaking of e-learning and ICT use in education.

8.1 Opportunities and Obstacles of Developing Adolescents' Twenty-First Century Skills

> *Consider the example of Max, a 14-year-old boy who hopes to be a director or filmmaker, and thus decides to set up a video-production company. Max and his friend produce humorous and dramatic videos that they post on YouTube, at least one of which has received 2 million views and more than 5,000 text comments and has been aired on ABC's Good Morning America. Max also regularly receives fan mail and has received offers to purchase some of his videos for online advertisements. Who would doubt that Max's use of digital media has enhanced the development of his media literacy, creativity and innovation, communication and collaboration, and initiative and self-direction?* (Warschauer & Matuchniak, 2010, p. 209)

Scholars suggest that digital competence and digital literacy are necessary lifelong skills in the global and knowledge economy of the twenty-first century (Livingstone et al., 2011; Warschauer & Matuchniak, 2010). According to Livingstone (2012), the adoption of ICT and the access to information resources can produce a new form of education that is more flexible and learner-centered, and promotes a constructive learning style that encourages peer collaboration and fosters learner motivation. Furthermore, ICT "may liberate teachers and pupils from the rigid hierarchies which have locked them to their desks, curricula and assessment straitjacket, mobilizing multiple activities as mediators of learning—not only reading and writing but also creating, designing, performing, searching and playing" (p. 17). Overall, there is a growing consensus that the rising generations must develop a set of learning skills closely tied with sophisticated ICT use in order to face the challenges of the twenty-first century, including information skills (e.g., information literacy and media literacy), learning and innovation skills (e.g., creativity, critical thinking, and problem solving), and life and career skills (flexibility and adaptability, social and cross-cultural skills, and leadership and responsibility) (Partnership for 21st Century Skills, 2009). Millennials and students should engage in more sophisticated digital media activities and learn a variety of ICT skills as soon as they enter secondary education.

8.1.1 The Influence of the COVID-19 Pandemic

Despite the availability of vaccines for COVID-19, medical scientists believe that variants may continue to exist and influence human life (The British Academy, 2021). The pandemic has transformed the educational landscape, and unexpectedly increased the role of ICT in teaching and learning activities. Educators and the public are concerned that the COVID-19 pandemic may exacerbate long-standing social inequalities because of the intersection of educational inequality and the digital divide (The British Academy, 2021). Because schools, on-site after-school programs, public libraries, and other local community services have restricted public access, many learning opportunities that had once been readily available to socially disadvantaged students are now less accessible. Students are more dependent than ever on the internet to learn and complete schoolwork.

Students of lower socioeconomic background are more likely than more privileged students to have difficulties with remote learning from home (Calarco, 2020; Palfrey, 2016). Socioeconomically disadvantaged students tend to receive less learning support at home (Calarco, 2020). In contrast, students from affluent families tend to have more offline and online resources that can enhance their e-learning experience, such as dedicated study spaces, learning tools, high-speed internet access, state-of-the-art computers, and most importantly, parental support (The British Academy, 2021). Overall, the changes of teaching and learning practices as the results of COVID-19 would lead to a significant loss in human capital development (OECD, 2020). This adverse impact is more pronounced for socially disadvantaged students who lack the e-learning tools and reliable internet access required to participate in online courses. They also are less likely to have their parents' assistance with their assignments.

8.1.2 The Three Problems that Should Be Addressed

There are several problems and questions that policymakers, scholars, and educators should address in order to bridge the digital learning divide. In their report based on the analyses of the 2010 EU Kids Online survey, Livingstone et al. (2011) identify three problems with the use of digital technologies by children and adolescents. The first is that it is a mistake to assume that children and adolescents know it all. Livingstone et al. (2011) argue that most people may overestimate these young people's digital skills. In reality, an overwhelming majority of children and adolescents do not equip with proper internet literacy and need support from parents, teachers, and peers in developing their ICT competency.

In addition, not all children gain the same benefits from ICT use. This variation is partially due to the socioeconomic inequalities in digital use and digital skills. According to Livingstone et al. (2011), only less than a quarter of children aged between 9 and 16 years old are able to reach the most creative and sophisticated steps of internet activities. There are a great deal of variations in how children and adolescents use ICT and what digital skills they possess, even if the majority of them have started using digital devices and appliances since a very young age (Marsh et al., 2015).

The third problem is particularly applicable to students from more affluent countries. Unlike people in the developing world, people in affluent countries are more likely to have easy access to high-speed internet and e-learning resources. They also enjoy more freedom in the use of the internet. However, Livingstone et al. (2011) contend that any efforts that increase online opportunities also may simultaneously increase online risks. For instance, social networking sites enable young people to connect easily with others, but they might not know how to protect themselves and their privacy online. It is also likely that they will use the internet exclusively for leisure activities and entertainment, not for education.

8.1.3 The Three Questions that Should Be Asked

Scholars and educators should bear in mind three questions about the educational use of ICT. First, there is no doubt that educational technology will continue to play a key role in the future. Therefore, the question is no longer whether or not we should incorporate ICT into education, but rather how to optimize the use of educational technology into the learning environment (Cheung & Slavin, 2013). Indeed, there are many new challenges as the world becomes more digitized. To meet these challenges, educators and policymakers must more clearly identify the goals that schools should pursue and the roles they should play in creating a better e-learning environment. These are pressing issues in light of the increasing importance of distant/online learning and "learning beyond school" in the post-COVID-19 era (Forkosh-Baruch & Erstad, 2018).

Second, although most digital natives have been immersed in the digital world since childhood, it is unclear where and how they may develop the kinds of digital skills that are keys for success in the twenty-first century. Because homes are a more natural site than schools for children to learn digital literacy, researchers and educators should consider how young people may practice their digital skills at homes and how the learning environment beyond the school campus may shape their experiences with digital technologies (Sefton-Green et al., 2016).

Finally, educational technology is not simply about transforming teaching materials from a physical classroom to a virtual, online classroom. ICT use in education is more than improving students' understanding of core subjects, teaching operational skills regarding how to use a computer, or making up the learning gap due to the COVID-19 pandemic. The implications of newly emerging technologies can be very different from what teachers and students could imagine. In line with these thoughts, educators and researchers should explore how we could better define and measure digital skills in education and what kinds of practices or exercises may help students acquire different types of digital skills that are important in education and in their future life (Sefton-Green et al., 2016). Taken together, by thinking more seriously about these problems and questions, educators and policymakers can identify strategies to ensure the benefits of digital inclusion, thereby reducing the adverse effects of improper use of digital technologies in education (Forkosh-Baruch & Erstad, 2018).

8.2 Implications for Adolescent Students' ICT Use

8.2.1 Digital Inclusion and Academic Performance

It is also necessary to summarize the major findings from our empirical analyses in Chaps. 4–7. Chap. 4 suggests that digital inclusion at home has an inverted U-shaped effect on reading performance in Australia, Finland, Ireland, Japan, South Korea, New Zealand, Singapore, Taiwan, the United Kingdom, and the United States. On one hand, the inverted U-shaped curvilinear relationship suggests that a moderate level of ICT use at home for school-related tasks, such as browsing the internet for lessons, using the internet to communicate with teachers, and doing homework on a computer, is associated with an improvement in reading performance; and the use of ICT at home for core subjects, such as language and mathematics, has a moderately positive effect on reading. On the other hand, a high level of ICT use for school-related tasks at home is negatively associated with reading performance. This suggests that students who are heavy ICT users perform less well academically than their counterparts who do not use it as much.

How does digital inclusion in the classroom affect academic performance? We find an inverted U-shaped effect of ICT use for language, mathematics, and science in Australia, South Korea, New Zealand, the United States, and most Scandinavian countries. In these countries, this U-shaped effect means that a moderate level of ICT use for core subjects in classrooms is associated with an increase in reading performance, but students who are heavy ICT users in classrooms have lower reading performance than students who use ICT at a low or moderate frequency. We find weak evidence that the use of ICT to browse the internet for schoolwork, download lecture material from websites, and practice and drill in foreign language or mathematics in classrooms improves students' reading performance.

For other countries, we find nearly zero or even negative relationships between digital inclusion at school and reading performance. This suggests that a general use of ICT in classrooms does not improve students' academic performance. Livingstone et al. (2011) posit that many schools in these countries may be still in the early phase of developing a digitized learning environment, with educational technology in the classroom but no significant change in pedagogy and curriculum design. Many teachers may assume that their students already learned digital skills at home and are digitally literate. Teachers also may believe that the computer skills required for ICT use in education are more difficult for older people to acquire than students (van Dijk & van Deursen, 2014). However, adolescent students may think that computer use at school is boring, not useful (Livingstone et al., 2011), and an "altogether different digital world" from what they experience outside of school (van Dijk & van Deursen, 2014). Another possibility is that schools' sociotechnical factors and other institutional characteristics may explain the widening e-learning divide. For example, well-resourced schools extensively use ICT in classrooms, but ICT use in under-resourced schools is limited (Warschauer & Matuchniak, 2010).

Chap. 4 presents statistical analyses of reading performance. The Appendix presents the results on mathematics and science. The patterns are similar across the three measures of student outcomes, but digital inclusion has a stronger effect on reading performance than on math or science. This difference is consistent with the findings from previous research that ICT tends to improve students' reading scores, but not their math scores. This also may explain why digital resources are more widely used in reading classes than in other academic subjects (Dynarski et al., 2007).

Research on seasonal learning suggests that students are likely to experience a "learning loss" and declines in academic achievements during off-seasons when schools are closed, such as summer vacations and the close-off due to the COVID-19 outbreak. That such declines are more pronounced for mathematics than for reading (Kuhfeld & Tarasawa, 2020) suggests that without proper guidance from schoolteachers, adolescent students are more likely to experience difficulties in mathematics learning. Following this, it is reasonable to argue that digital inclusion at home has a greater potential to enhance students' reading experience than their mathematics learning.

Last but not the least, we ask how digital inclusion at home and in school may differentially affect the academic performance of high-SES and low-SES students. In the United Kingdom, New Zealand, and Scandinavian countries, we find that the role of e-learning at home is at least as important for low-SES students than for socioeconomically advantaged students. By extension, this indicates that socially disadvantaged students in these countries can benefit from digital inclusion. At the same time, however, we see a pronounced third-level digital divide in the United States, Australia, and South Korea. Taken together, these findings suggest that the academic benefits of digital inclusion are greater for high-SES students than for their low-SES peers, leading to a persistent if not increasing digital learning divide.

8.2.2 Digital Inclusion and Learning Attitudes

Chap. 5 clearly shows substantial inverted U-shaped effects of digital inclusion at home on learning attitudes in most affluent countries. Again, the inverted U-shaped curvilinear effects suggest that, on one hand, moderate ICT use for schoolwork at home enhances students' reading enjoyment and also improves their general learning attitudes. On the other hand, intensive ICT use at home may reduce students' enjoyment of reading and their desire to work hard on their studies.

Digital inclusion at school plays a less important role in promoting students' reading enjoyment or enhancing their positive learning attitudes than digital inclusion at home. Indeed, with the exception of the United Kingdom, Sweden, Australia, and New Zealand, our analyses show a generally negative effect of school ICT use on students' learning attitudes.

More importantly, we examine whether digital inclusion differentially affects the learning attitudes of high- and low-SES students. The results show that the role of digital inclusion at home equally or more positively promotes the learning attitude of low-SES students than those of high-SES students in the United Kingdom, Denmark, Iceland, and Sweden. Along with Chap. 4, these findings suggest that in these countries, home ICT use for educational purposes not only improves the academic performance of socioeconomically disadvantaged students, but also enhances their learning attitudes. Additionally, school ICT use has a small positive effect on low-SES students' learning attitudes in the United Kingdom and Sweden. Taken as a whole, these findings suggest that disadvantaged students in these countries receive substantial academic benefits from home ICT use for educational activities.

At the same time, the positive effect of digital inclusion at home on learning attitudes is more pronounced for high-SES students than their low-SES peers in Australia, New Zealand, and most developed societies in Asia (e.g., Japan, South Korea, and Macao). The unequal returns of ICT use increase the educational disparities between socially advantaged and disadvantaged students, suggesting that ICT policy in education in these countries should be revisited to apply to students of socially disadvantaged background.

8.2.3 Digital Inclusion and Psychological Well-Being

The influence of digital technologies on students' psychological well-being has received considerable scholarly and public attention in recent years (Orben & Przybylski, 2019; Przybylski & Weinstein, 2017). Chap. 6 shows that in Ireland, Japan, and the United States, home ICT use has a positive and linear effect on students' psychological well-being. In most other affluent countries, however, digital inclusion at home has an inverted U-shaped curvilinear effect on perceived positive psychological feelings and perceived sense of positive meaning in life. This suggests that moderate ICT use at home improves students' psychological well-being, but intensive ICT use leads to worse psychological well-being and less satisfaction with life (OECD, 2019). We also find evidence that digital inclusion at home has an inverted U-shaped or a nearly linear effect on students' sense of belonging in school in approximately half of the countries we analyze, but the effect is small.

Regarding digital inclusion in classrooms, our analyses show that school ICT has a positive effect on psychological feelings and sense of meaning in life in half of the countries we analyze, such as the United Kingdom, France, Ireland, Denmark, and Sweden. With the exception of the United Kingdom, Ireland, Denmark, Finland, and Iceland, school ICT use does not promote students' sense of belonging in school. Given that the positive effects of ICT inclusion in school tend to be small, we conclude that home ICT use is more likely to improve adolescent students' psychological well-being than school ICT use (Yuen & Hew, 2018).

With the exception of the United Kingdom, Iceland, and Ireland, schools' digital inclusion has greater positive effects on the psychological well-being of high-SES students than on low-SES students. This suggests a third-level digital divide in the influences of digital inclusion on adolescent students' psychological well-being. This finding has important policy implications, because socioeconomically disadvantaged students on average have a weaker sense of belonging in school than students of higher socioeconomic background (OECD, 2019).

8.2.4 Digital Inclusion and Digital Competence

Results from Chap. 6 show strong positive effects of home and school ICT use on students' perceived ICT competence (e.g., feeling comfortable using digital devices, being able to solve problems with digital devices, and being able to help friends and relatives when they have problems with digital devices) in almost all developed countries that we analyze. These relationships are either quasilinear or curvilinear, suggesting that higher levels of ICT use almost always improve adolescent students' digital skills and knowledge. These consistent patterns lead us to conclude that both digital inclusion at home and in school is useful in developing students' digital skills. This finding suggests that educators and policymakers should incorporate ICT use in schools and also teach digital skills and knowledge in class. Integration of ICT in school can help enhance students' digital skills; teaching digital skills and knowledge in class helps reduce the potential risks that adolescent students may encounter in the cyber world (Livingstone et al., 2011).

8.2.5 Persistent Socioeconomic Digital Divide

The results from Chaps. 4 to 6 highlight the persistence of the third-level digital divide in secondary education. High-SES students are more likely than low-SES students to reap the academic and non-academic benefits from digital inclusion. This finding is in line with a large body of research literature that suggests a pronounced socioeconomic difference in the benefits accruing from digital inclusion (e.g., Scheerder et al., 2019; Warschauer & Matuchniak, 2010). Zillien and Marr (2013, p. 6) contend that higher-SES people are more likely to "succeed in utilizing the internet to increase existing resources." Similarly, Akiyoshi et al. (2013, p. 99) argue that lower-SES people "are less likely to be aware of new applications delivered by broadband technology," and further suggest that "[differential] use practices are produced by different levels of cultural capital as well as by socioeconomic status and demographic attributes." Moreover, people from high-SES households are more likely to consult formal sources (e.g., school personnel and experts) when they encounter problems with digital devices, whereas people from low-SES household are more likely to seek informal support from family and friends (Helsper & van Deursen, 2017; Scheerder et al., 2019).

In Chap. 7, we find a second-level socioeconomic divide in ICT use for schoolwork. Given the well-documented digital learning inequalities in developed countries in the research literature (Helsper & Reisdorf, 2016; Ma et al., 2019; van Deursen & van Dijk, 2014), this finding is hardly surprising. Our analysis further shows that socioeconomic inequality in school ICT use is small or nonexistent in affluent countries, a pattern that is likely different from the sizable socioeconomic divide in school ICT use in less-developed countries (Eickelmann, 2018; Ma, 2021; Ragnedda & Muschert, 2013). Outside of schools, however, high-SES students are more likely than low-SES students to use digital technologies for e-learning or school activities.

Earlier research predicts that the first-level socioeconomic divide in ICT access in the household may eventually disappear with the advancement of digital technologies and as governments continue to build digital infrastructures. However, our analyses in Chap. 7 show that inequalities in digital access at home continue to exist and may have even increased in affluent countries (van Deursen & van Dijk, 2019). First, the percentages of low-SES students who had computer access at home declined from 2009 to 2018. For example, 89 percent and 47 percent of low-SES students in Canada and Japan had access to a home computer in 2009. In 2018, however, only 67 percent of low-SES students in Canada and 32 percent of low-SES students in Japan had computer access at home. Second, a profound socioeconomic gap in home access to digital tablets was ubiquitous in affluent societies in 2018. Among the few exceptions were Denmark, Iceland, Norway, Sweden, Ireland, the Netherlands, and the United Kingdom, where the gaps between high- and low-SES students ranged from 10 to 20 percent. In the rest of the developed world, the gap in access to digital tablets between high- and low-SES students was at least 30 percent. In China, the difference was more than 50 percent.

Limited ICT access may impede students' learning opportunities at home. Digital access "is not [simply] a binary division between information haves and have-nots" (Warschauer & Matuchniak, 2010, p. 185). Although all parents want their children to succeed and accordingly provide ICT resources, such as computers and high-speed internet connections, to increase their children's chances of standing out from their peers, many "struggle just as much as teachers with the practical difficulties of going online, often lacking the necessary financial, social or technical resources"

(Livingstone, 2012, p. 15). Therefore, it is important for policymakers and educators to understand that the ability of parents to provide digital resources for their children often depends on a household's technical, economic, and social condition (Gonzales et al., 2020; Warschauer & Matuchniak, 2010).

8.3 Creating an Ideal e-Learning Environment at Home: Some Suggestions

Providing an ideal e-learning home environment for adolescents is not easy. Bridging the digital gaps for students from socioeconomically disadvantaged and advantaged background is even more difficult. Based on the findings of the empirical analyses in this book, and the suggestions from the research literature on digital divide, we discuss four recommendations for policymakers, scholars, and educators to consider.

8.3.1 Acknowledging the Importance of Home as a Key E-Learning Field in the Twenty-First Century

Many adolescents "make computers part of their personal space and tailor them to their needs" at home (Warschauer & Matuchniak, 2010, p. 201). Dede (1996, p. 65) states:

> *Information technologies are more like clothes than like fire. Fire is a wonderful technology because, without knowing anything about how it operates, you can get warm just standing close by. People sometimes find computers, televisions, and telecommunications frustrating because they expect these devices to radiate knowledge. But all information technologies are more like clothes; to get a benefit, you must make them a part of your personal space, tailored to your needs.*

First, we acknowledge that homes are as important as schools in developing youth's digital literacy and e-learning experience. Digital skills, habits, values, and attitudes toward the use of media technologies are passed on from parents to children (Yuen et al., 2018). Students learn how to use digital technologies rather naturally at home, but schools often fail to integrate students' ICT experiences at home into curriculum design (Forkosh-Baruch & Erstad, 2018).

In response to this problem, schools may consider working with parents in guiding children's e-learning experiences (Forkosh-Baruch & Erstad, 2018). This coordination between schools and parents should begin as soon as children enter school, because the use of ICT as a tool for learning or exploration can produce considerable benefits even for preschoolers (Plowman, 2015).

8.3.2 Supporting and Encouraging Parents to Assist Their Children with E-learning Activities

Second, empirical evidence derived both from our analyses and from previous studies (Attewell & Seel, 2003; Scheerder et al., 2019; Vigdor et al., 2014) indicates that parenting—what parents do and how they coach their children at home—is an important source of digital learning inequalities. Researchers find that high-SES parents are more likely than low-SES parents to apply active technical mediation strategies to their children (Livingstone & Helsper, 2008; Livingstone et al., 2011; Yuen et al., 2018). To reduce digital learning divides, parents should encourage their children to engage in e-learning, and regulate their children's online behavior to protect them from potential harm by using internet filters and setting time limits for internet use (Livingstone et al., 2011). Because parents play a key role in helping their children to connect with e-learning, educators and policymakers should support parents in assisting their children with e-learning activities, including helping them to steer their children away from inappropriate internet activities and from the overuse of ICT for gaming and social networking.

8.3.3 Balancing Online with Offline Activities

Third, a major finding from our data analyses in this book is that digital inclusion has an inverted U-shaped effect on the well-being of adolescent students, including their educational performance, learning attitudes, and mental health. This pattern is ubiquitous in most affluent countries.

The implication of this findings is that ICT can play a supplementary role in the learning process, to help enhance adolescent students' learning experiences and learning outcomes. Because moderate ICT use for learning purposes at home promotes students' academic and non-academic well-being, but intensive ICT use could produce negative effects, adolescent students should find a balance between their online and offline activities. This is especially important during the COVID-19 pandemic, when access to school campuses and outdoor facilities has been limited. According to the OECD (2020), simply replacing in-class activities with lengthy online lectures may deteriorate students' learning and mental health. Therefore, teachers and educators must work hard to help young people balance their digital life with screen-free activities in order to "keep a pulse" on their psychological health.

8.3.4 *Providing Material and Social Resources to Support Students' Digital Experiences*

Fourth, a substantial digital access divide at home persists between high- and low-SES families. Even in affluent societies, students from low-SES families may lack the reliable internet access to participate in virtual class. Instead, they must complete their homework on mobile phones or substandard digital devices. Governments could rectify this problem by helping these students to improve their digital access at home, for instance by lending them reliable laptops, subsidizing internet fees, and improving IT infrastructures. For example, schools in the United Kingdom and Japan provide students with low ICT access at home printed work booklets (OECD, 2020).

Educators and policymakers should also acknowledge that social resources—such as parental guidance, assistance from others, and a support network—may be particularly important for younger students who are more likely to need assistance with home ICT use than older students. Warschauer and Matuchniak (2010, p. 193) note that the social resources for e-learning include "a community that values and enables the sharing of media knowledge and interests, which can be found among family, friends, interest groups, or educational programs such as computer clubs and youth media centers."

8.4 Integrating ICT in Secondary Schools: Some Suggestions

Another major finding from our empirical analyses is that ICT inclusion in school does not have as large of an effect on adolescent students' well-being as might have been expected. This finding lays a basis for policymakers and educators to reconsider how schools may reduce the digital divides in contemporary education. In this section, we discuss policy recommendations about the integration of digital technologies in schools.

8.4.1 *Focus on Assisting Socioeconomically Disadvantaged Adolescents*

Like other scholars in our field, we contend that formal education remains an indispensable component for adolescent students to learn internet literacy and digital skills, especially if they do not have adequate digital resources at home (van Dijk & van Deursen, 2014). The problem is that the rapid development of digital technologies makes it as difficult for teachers to keep up as it is for students. As a result, teachers often feel unprepared to teach about digital knowledge and skills (Dolan, 2016; Rafalow, 2018).

In their study of 26 European countries, Livingstone et al. (2011) suggest that on average, 58 percent of students across European nations receive advice on internet safety from schoolteachers. Considering the other 42 percent, Livingstone et al. (2011) suggest that "since schools have the resources to reach all children, they should take the biggest share of the task of reaching the 'hard to reach'" (p. 37). They add that "reaching the 'hard to reach', while difficult, is a priority given that vulnerable children are particularly susceptible to online harm" (p. 44).

Livingstone et al. (2011) suggest that 85 percent of students in the United Kingdom receive teacher advice about internet safety; this is the highest percentage among European countries. This finding echoes our empirical analyses showing stronger positive relationships between students' digital inclusion in school and at home and adolescent students' well-being in the United Kingdom than in many other developed countries. Indeed, the United Kingdom is among the few affluent countries in our analyses that consistently show more positive effects of school digital inclusion on low-SES students than on high-SES students. The successful experiences in the United Kingdom suggest that governments in other developed countries can implement better ICT policies in schools to further improve adolescent students' well-being and reduce digital divides between socially disadvantaged and advantaged students.

For example, an ICT infrastructure that governments may consider investing even more is the ICT facilities in libraries and community centers. In supplementary analyses, we find that low-SES students in affluent countries visit school libraries more frequently than high-SES students. This pattern does not apply to less-developed countries, perhaps because libraries and community centers in these countries are not accessible and well-equipped. Warschauer and Matuchniak (2010) suggest that public libraries serve as "an alternative outlet" for students without a reliable internet connection or computer access at home, and that the provision of formal computer courses and informal e-support by community centers can improve the digital skills of disadvantaged people. Following this, policymakers may consider how publicly funded institutions, including schools, libraries, community centers, and subsidized housing can work together to reduce the digital divide (Livingstone, 2012).

8.4.2 A Blended Pedagogical Model that Combines Online with Face-to-Face Curricula

The institutional characteristics and academic climate of schools have strong effects on a classroom's media use and students' e-learning experiences (Ma, 2021; Warschauer et al., 2004). The e-learning divide between schools remains, however (Hughes et al., 2015; Leu et al., 2015). Warschauer and Matuchniak (2010, p. 208) suggest that "schools that are already focused on the kinds of information literacy, critical thinking, and self-direction associated with twenty-first-century learning skills will find new media a powerful way to achieve these, whereas schools that do not have such a focus will not likely suddenly discover it through a diffusion of computers." Resta et al. (2018, p. 13) note that on one hand, "teachers often use technology in accordance with old instructional practices, doing the same thing as before, but a little more quickly, a little more frequently, or a little better," rather than seeing the great potential of educational technology "to do things differently." On the other hand, "teachers who are transforming their primary or secondary classrooms into blended learning environments by combining onsite and online learning activities—the 'flipped classroom' is the buzzword—are beginning to see it as 'the new normal.'" Many schools serving a majority of low-income and disadvantaged students use educational technology only for drills, practice, and for remediation activities (Warschauer, 2016; Warschauer et al., 2004). This does not help adolescent students to develop twenty-first-century skills (Warschauer & Matuchniak, 2010).

In Italy, the integration of ICT in schools remains largely restricted. Teachers tend to use digital technologies for their own professional development rather than for teaching (Manca & Ranieri, 2016b). Many factors, such as cultural resistance, institutional constraints, and pedagogical practices, should be considered when policymakers explore solutions to these problems (Manca & Ranieri, 2016a).

Before the COVID-19 pandemic, most teachers had little to no experience in e-lecturing and online teaching. The pandemic forced many to learn these skills on the job through trial and error. Schools must invest in training their teachers in educational technologies and online information skills. At the minimum, teachers should learn how to create online educational materials appropriate for remote teaching (Attewell et al., 2009; Tondeur et al., 2007).

In sum, using PowerPoint, computer screens, and projectors in traditional lectures is one thing. Designing an e-classroom is quite another. Future scholars and educators should work on the integration of ICT into teaching and learning processes. Considering the inverted U-shaped and unequal effects of ICT use on students' outcomes, we should bear in mind that students of various backgrounds and different learning needs may have quite different responses to e-learning. It is important to think about how digital technology can be properly designed and used in order to better address different students' learning conditions. For example, teachers may consider a pedagogical model that combines online with face-to-face curricula. As Dede states, digital technologies can "complement existing approaches to widen our repertoire of communication [and broaden our vision]; properly designed, they do not eliminate choices or force us into high tech, low touch situations" (Dede, 1996, p. 65).

8.4.3 Developing Students' Online Information and Strategic Skills

In the United Kingdom and Scandinavian countries, we find more significant positive effects of digital inclusion on adolescent students' well-being; these positive relationships are even stronger for low-SES students than for high-SES students. Because greater proportions of the populations in these countries have basic digital skills than other countries (ITU, 2018), it is possible that students with more digital competence and internet literacy are more likely to benefit from digital inclusion. Following this, we suggest that schools may provide more resources and opportunities for students to develop digital skills and internet literacy.

van Dijk and van Deursen (2014) distinguish several types of digital skills, and suggest that schools incorporate learning of advanced digital skills in formal curricula. Specifically, van Dijk and van Deursen (2014) suggest that students acquire basic digital skills outside of schools through trial and error, but it is difficult to learn information and strategic internet skills—such as the effective use of internet search engines—by themselves. They advise schools to incorporate online information and strategic skills into course offerings on language, arts, and science, and teach online operational skills separately. Schools should also teach online communication skills and provide guidance on internet security, personal identity and privacy, and legacy in courses on media education. Designs of digital education curricula should also take into account educational levels. For example, Ofsted (2009) suggests that primary schools should focus on online communication skills and help children become confident in their ICT use. Secondary schools should emphasize ICT and online presentation skills instead of spreadsheets or programming.

8.4.4 Working Together with Business and IT Industry to Develop New E-Learning Materials

A comment from a UNESCO report is instructive:

> *All aspects of the ICT in education ecosystem, such as content (e.g., open educational resources (OER), free and open-source software (FOSS), and other open learning solutions), access to and use of hardware (e.g., new devices, including mobile technologies, one-to-one computing options etc.), connectivity, ICT issues related to pedagogy and learning (including digital literacy, and issues of assessment), as well as teacher training, need to be explored in greater detail to have a fuller picture of the contribution of ICT to quality teaching and learning.* (UNESCO-UIS, 2014, p. 40)

Not only teachers, educators, and schools must work together to implement ICT use in education; it is also important to encourage collaborations among social actors, public institutions, and the private sector to improve digital education and design better e-learning materials (Sefton-Green et al., 2016). In particular, the IT industry may also provide expertise for academics in the design of ICT curriculum and pedagogy.

Finally, the distribution of e-learning resources is often uneven across socioeconomic strata, with newer technologies going only to schools in the most affluent areas (Ma et al., 2019). Therefore, a national regulatory institution to monitor the progress of ICT integration in education is important (UNESCO-UIS, 2014). This government-led institution can redistribute educational resources to under-resourced areas and monitor the outcomes of digital use among socially disadvantaged and academically underperforming students.

Taking Australia as an example, we find a robust pattern pertaining to the third-level digital divide by family SES. While Australian parents, teachers, and policymakers have all been adopting positive strategies to promote students' use of ICT in the learning process (Education Services Australia, 2012; Livingstone et al., 2011; Starkey & Finger, 2018), it is possible that the lack of a national regulatory institution is a key factor in the widening digital learning divide.

8.5 Summary and Conclusion

The COVID-19 pandemic has unexpectedly accelerated the application of ICT in education. This book therefore examines the causes and consequences of digital inclusion and exclusion for students in secondary education. This chapter summarizes the findings of the empirical analyses using the PISA data and discusses their implications. The discussion highlights the challenges faced by policymakers and educators when addressing digital divides and the important questions scholars may consider when exploring the solutions for this new form of social inequality. We conclude that digital competence and digital literacy are important lifelong skills in the global and knowledge economy of the twenty-first century, and provide recommendations for educators and policymakers to improve e-learning home environments and to integrate digital and internet technologies in education.

References

Akiyoshi, M., Tsuchiya, M., & Sano, T. (2013). Missing in the midst of abundance: The case of broadband adoption in Japan. In M. Ragnedda & G. W. Muschert (Eds.), *The digital divide: The Internet and social inequality in international perspective* (pp. 85–104). Routledge.

Arnott, L. (2016). An ecological exploration of young children's digital play: Framing children's social experiences with technologies in early childhood. *Early Years: An International Research Journal, 36*(3), 271–288. https://doi.org/10.1080/09575146.2016.1181049

Attewell, J., Savill-Smith, C., Douch, R., Learning and Skills Network (Great Britain), MoLeNET (Initiative), & Learning and Skills Council (Great Britain). (2009). *The impact of mobile learning: Examining what it means for teaching and learning.* LSN.

Attewell, P. A., & Battle, J. (1999). Home computers and school performance. *The Information Society, 15*(1), 1–10.

Attewell, P. A., & Seel, N. M. (2003). *Disadvantaged teens and computer technologies.* Waxmann.

Calarco, J. M. (2020). Coronavirus and the inequity of accountability for at-home learning. *American Sociological Association Footnotes, 48*(3), 18.

Cheung, A. C. K., & Slavin, R. E. (2013). The effectiveness of educational technology applications for enhancing mathematics achievement in K-12 classrooms: A meta-analysis. *Educational Research Review, 9*, 88–113. https://doi.org/10.1016/j.edurev.2013.01.001

Cruz-Jesus, F., Oliveira, T., Bacao, F., & Irani, Z. (2017). Assessing the pattern between economic and digital development of countries. *Information Systems Frontiers, 19*(4), 835–854. https://doi.org/10.1007/s10796-016-9634-1

Dede, C. (1996). Testimony to the US Congress, House of Representatives, joint hearing on educational technology in the 21st century. In United States Congress House Committee (Ed.), *Educational technology in the 21st century: Joint hearing before the Committee on science and the committee on economic and educational opportunities* (pp. 56–65). U.S. Government Printing Office.

Dolan, J. E. (2016). Splicing the divide: A review of research on the evolving digital divide among K-12 students. *Journal of Research on Technology in Education, 48*(1), 16–37. https://doi.org/10.1080/15391523.2015.1103147

Dynarski, M., Agodini, R., Heaviside, S., Novak, T., Carey, N., Campuzano, L., Means, B., Murphy, R., Penuel, W., Javitz, H., Emery, D., & Sussex, W. (2007). *Effectiveness of reading and mathematics software products: Findings from the first student cohort*. US Department of Education, Institute of Education Sciences. https://files.eric.ed.gov/fulltext/ED496015.pdf

Education Services Australia. (2012). *National digital learning resources network*. http://www.ndlrn.edu.au/default.asp

Eickelmann, B. (2018). Cross-national policies on information and communication technology in primary and secondary schools: An international perspective. In J. Voogt, G. Knezek, R. Christensen, & K.-W. Lai (Eds.), *Second handbook of information technology in primary and secondary education* (pp. 1–12). Springer International Publishing. https://doi.org/10.1007/978-3-319-53803-7_84-1

Forkosh-Baruch, A., & Erstad, O. (2018). Upbringing in a digital world: Opportunities and possibilities. *Technology, Knowledge and Learning, 23*(3), 377–390. https://doi.org/10.1007/s10758-018-9386-8

Gamoran, A. (2001). American schooling and educational inequality: A forecast for the 21st century. *Sociology of Education, 74*, 135–153.

Gonzales, A. L., Calarco, J. M., & Lynch, T. (2020). Technology problems and student achievement gaps: A validation and extension of the technology maintenance construct. *Communication Research, 47*(5), 750–770. https://doi.org/10.1177/0093650218796366

Hargittai, E., & Hinnant, A. (2008). Digital inequality: Differences in young adults' use of the Internet. *Communication Research, 35*(5), 602–621.

Helsper, E. J., & Reisdorf, B. C. (2016). The emergence of a "digital underclass" in Great Britain and Sweden: Changing reasons for digital exclusion. *New Media & Society, 19*(8), 1253–1270. https://doi.org/10.1177/1461444816634676

Helsper, E. J., & van Deursen, A. J. (2017). Do the rich get digitally richer? Quantity and quality of support for digital engagement. *Information, Communication & Society, 20*(5), 700–714. https://doi.org/10.1080/1369118X.2016.1203454

Hughes, J. E., Read, M. F., Jones, S., & Mahometa, M. (2015). Predicting middle school students' use of web 2.0 technologies out of school using home and school technological variables. *Journal of Research on Technology in Education, 47*(4), 211–228. https://doi.org/10.1080/15391523.2015.1065156

ITU. (2018). *Measuring the information society*. ITU.

Kuhfeld, M., & Tarasawa, B. (2020). *The COVID-19 slide: What summer learning loss can tell us about the potential impact of school closures on student academic achievement*. NWEA. https://eric.ed.gov/?id=ED609141

Leu, D. J., Forzani, E., Rhoads, C., Maykel, C., Kennedy, C., & Timbrell, N. (2015). The new literacies of online research and comprehension: Rethinking the reading achievement gap. *Reading Research Quarterly, 50*(1), 37–59. https://doi.org/10.1002/rrq.85

Livingstone, S. (2012). Critical reflections on the benefits of ICT in education. *Oxford Review of Education, 38*(1), 9–24. https://www.tandfonline.com/doi/abs/10.1080/03054985.2011.577938

Livingstone, S., Haddon, L., Görzig, A., & Ólafsson, K. (2011). *EU kids online: Final report*. EU Kids Online, London School of Economics & Political Science. http://eprints.lse.ac.uk/39351/1/EU_kids_online_final_report_%5BLSERO%5D.pdf

Livingstone, S., & Helsper, E. J. (2008). Parental mediation and children's Internet use. *Journal of Broadcasting & Electronic Media, 52*(4), 581–599. https://doi.org/10.1080/08838150802437396

Ma, J. K.-H. (2021). The digital divide at school and at home: A comparison between schools by socioeconomic level across 47 countries. *International Journal of Comparative Sociology, 62*(2), 115–140. https://doi.org/10.1177/00207152211023540

Ma, J. K.-H., Vachon, T. E., & Cheng, S. (2019). National income, political freedom, and investments in R&D and education: A comparative analysis of the second digital divide among 15-year-old students. *Social Indicators Research, 144*(1), 133–166. https://doi.org/10.1007/s11205-018-2030-0

Manca, S., & Ranieri, M. (2016a). Facebook and the others: Potentials and obstacles of social media for teaching in higher education. *Computers & Education, 95*, 216–230. https://doi.org/10.1016/j.compedu.2016.01.012

Manca, S., & Ranieri, M. (2016b). "Yes for sharing, no for teaching!": Social media in academic practices. *The Internet and Higher Education, 29*, 63–74. https://doi.org/10.1016/j.iheduc.2015.12.004

Marsh, J., Plowman, L., Yamada-Rice, D., Bishop, J. C., Lahmar, J., Scott, F., Davenport, A., Davis, S., French, K., Piras, M., Thornhill, S., Robinson, P., & Winter, P. (2015). *Exploring play and creativity in pre-schoolers' use of apps: Final project report*. Technology and Play. http://www.techandplay.org

OECD. (2019). *PISA 2018 results* (Vol. III)*: What school life means for students' lives.* PISA, OECD. https://doi.org/10.1787/acd78851-en

OECD. (2020). *Education responses to covid-19: Embracing digital learning and online collaboration.* OECD. https://www.oecd.org/coronavirus/policy-responses/education-responses-to-covid-19-embracing-digital-learning-and-online-collaboration-d75eb0e8/

Ofsted. (2009). *The importance of ICT: Information and communication technology in primary and secondary schools.* Ofsted. https://dera.ioe.ac.uk/313/1/The%20importance%20of%20ICT.pdf

Orben, A., & Przybylski, A. K. (2019). The association between adolescent well-being and digital technology use. *Nature Human Behaviour, 3*(2), 173–182. https://doi.org/10.1038/s41562-018-0506-1

Palfrey, J. (2016). Reframing privacy and youth media practices. In C. Greenhow, J. Sonnevend, & C. Agur (Eds.), *Education and social media: Toward a digital future* (pp. 113–130). MIT Press.

Partnership for 21st Century Skills. (2009). *Framework for 21st century learning*. Battelle for Kids. https://www.battelleforkids.org/networks/p21

Plowman, L. (2015). Researching young children's everyday uses of technology in the family home. *Interacting with Computers, 27*(1), 36–46. https://doi.org/10.1093/iwc/iwu031

Przybylski, A. K., & Weinstein, N. (2017). A large-scale test of the Goldilocks hypothesis: Quantifying the relations between digital-screen use and the mental well-being of adolescents. *Psychological Science, 28*(2), 204–215. https://doi.org/10.1177/0956797616678438

Rafalow, M. H. (2018). Disciplining play: Digital youth culture as capital at school. *American Journal of Sociology, 123*(5), 1416–1452. https://doi.org/10.1086/695766

Ragnedda, M., & Muschert, G. W. (Eds.). (2013). *The digital divide: The Internet and social inequality in international perspective*. Routledge.

Resta, P., Laferrière, T., McLaughlin, R., & Kouraogo, A. (2018). Issues and challenges related to digital equity: An overview. In J. Voogt, G. Knezek, R. Christensen, & K.-W. Lai (Eds.), *Handbook of information technology in primary and secondary education* (pp. 1–18). Springer International Publishing. https://doi.org/10.1007/978-3-319-53803-7_67-1

Robison, K. K., & Crenshaw, E. M. (2010). Reevaluating the global digital divide: Socio-demographic and conflict barriers to the Internet revolution. *Sociological Inquiry, 80*(1), 34–62. https://doi.org/10.1111/j.1475-682X.2009.00315.x

Scheerder, A. J., van Deursen, A. J., & van Dijk, J. A. (2019). Internet use in the home: Digital inequality from a domestication perspective. *New Media & Society, 21*(10), 2099–2118. https://doi.org/10.1177/1461444819844299

Sefton-Green, J., Marsh, J., Erstad, O., & Flewitt, R. (2016). *Establishing a research agenda for the digital literacy practices of young children: A white paper for COST Action IS1410.* https://doi.org/10.13140/RG.2.2.10896.30720

Starkey, L., & Finger, G. (2018). Information and communication technology in educational policies in Australia and New Zealand. In J. Voogt, G. Knezek, R. Christensen, & K.-W. Lai (Eds.), *Second handbook of information technology in primary and secondary education* (pp. 1–20). Springer International Publishing. https://doi.org/10.1007/978-3-319-53803-7_87-2

The British Academy. (2021). *The COVID decade: Understanding the long-term societal impacts of COVID-19*. The British Academy COVID-19 and Society. https://www.thebritishacademy.ac.uk/publications/covid-decade-understanding-the-long-term-societal-impacts-of-covid-19/

Tondeur, J., Van Braak, J., & Valcke, M. (2007). Curricula and the use of ICT in education: Two worlds apart? *British Journal of Educational Technology, 38*(6), 962–976. https://doi.org/10.1111/j.1467-8535.2006.00680.x

UNESCO-UIS. (2014). *Information and communication technology (ICT) in education in Asia: A comparative analysis of ICT integration and e-readiness in schools across Asia*. United Nations Educational, Scientific and Cultural Organization, Institute for Statistics. http://uis.unesco.org/sites/default/files/documents/information-communication-technologies-education-asia-ict-integration-e-readiness-schools-2014-en_0.pdf

van Deursen, A. J., & van Dijk, J. A. (2014). The digital divide shifts to differences in usage. *New Media & Society, 16*(3), 507–526. https://doi.org/10.1177/1461444813487959

van Deursen, A. J., & van Dijk, J. A. (2019). The first-level digital divide shifts from inequalities in physical access to inequalities in material access. *New Media & Society, 21*(2), 354–375. https://doi.org/10.1177/1461444818797082

van Dijk, J. A. G. M., & van Deursen, A. J. (2014). Solutions: Learning digital skills. In J. A. G. M. van Dijk & A. J. van Deursen (Eds.), *Digital skills: Unlocking the information society* (pp. 113–138). Palgrave Macmillan US. https://doi.org/10.1057/9781137437037_6

Vigdor, J. L., Ladd, H. F., & Martinez, E. (2014). Scaling the digital divide: Home computer technology and student achievement. *Economic Inquiry, 52*(3), 1103–1119. https://doi.org/10.1111/ecin.12089

Warschauer, M. (2016). Addressing the social envelope: Education and the digital divide. In C. Greenhow, J. Sonnevend, & C. Agur (Eds.), *Education and social media: Toward a digital future* (pp. 29–48). MIT Press. https://oxfordindex.oup.com/view/10.7551/mitpress/9780262034470.003.0003?lang=en, https://oxfordindex.oup.com:443/view/10.7551/mitpress/9780262034470.003.0003

Warschauer, M., Knobel, M., & Stone, L. (2004). Technology and equity in schooling: Deconstructing the digital divide. *Educational Policy, 18*(4), 562–588. https://doi.org/10.1177/0895904804266469

Warschauer, M., & Matuchniak, T. (2010). New technology and digital worlds: Analyzing evidence of equity in access, use, and outcomes. *Review of Research in Education, 34*(1), 179–225. https://doi.org/10.3102/0091732X09349791

Yuen, A. H. K., & Hew, T. K. F. (2018). Information and communication technology in educational policies in the Asian region. In J. Voogt, G. Knezek, R. Christensen, & K.-W. Lai (Eds.), *Handbook of Information technology in primary and secondary education* (pp. 1–20). Springer International Publishing. https://doi.org/10.1007/978-3-319-53803-7_86-1

Yuen, A. H. K., Park, J. H., Chen, L., & Cheng, M. (2018). The significance of cultural capital and parental mediation for digital inequity. *New Media & Society, 20*(2), 599–617. https://doi.org/10.1177/1461444816667084

Zillien, N., & Marr, M. (2013). The digital divide in Europe. In M. Ragnedda & G. W. Muschert (Eds.), *The digital divide: The Internet and social inequality in international perspective* (pp. 55–66). Routledge.

Appendices

See Figs. A1, A2, A3, A4, A5, A6, A7, and A8.

J. K.-H. Ma and S. Cheng, *Adolescent Well-being and ICT UseX*, Human Well-Being Research and Policy Making,
https://doi.org/10.1007/978-3-031-04412-0

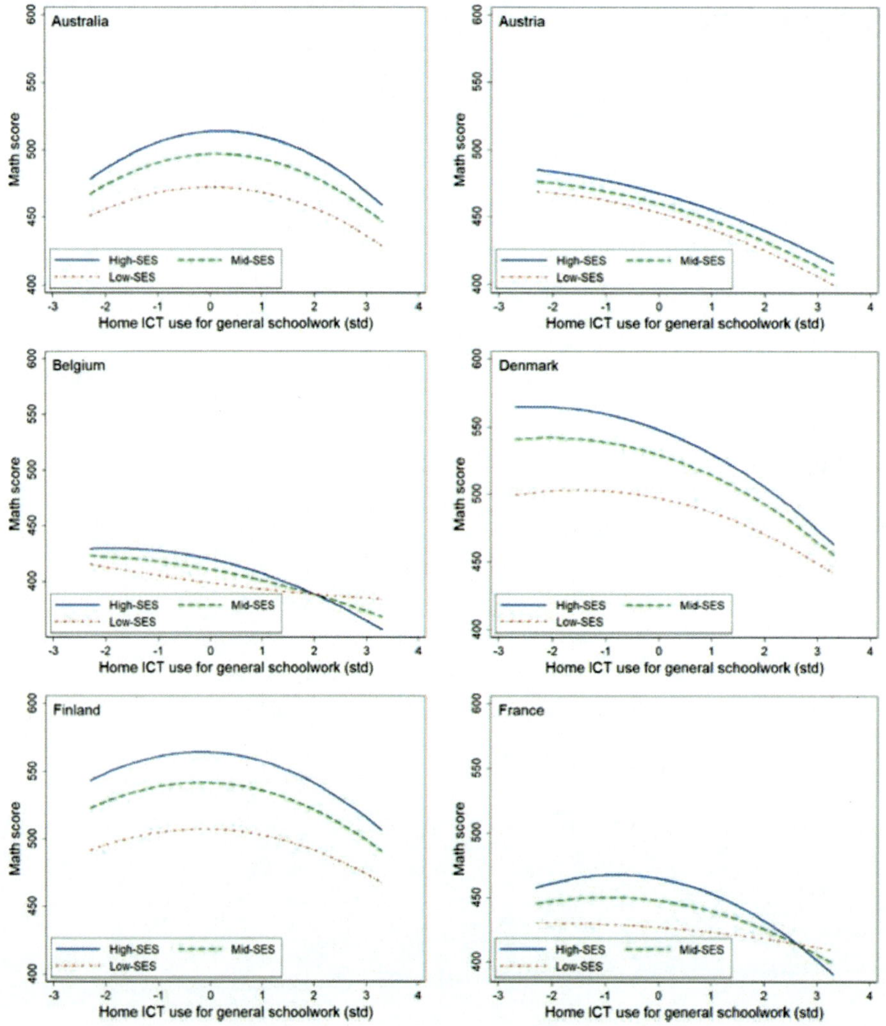

Fig. A1 Curvilinear effects of home ICT use for general schoolwork on mathematics performance by family SES (*Data source* The 2018 Programme for International Student Assessment [PISA] survey. *Note* Countries/societies are listed alphabetically. High-SES refers to students who are at the 90th percentile in family SES. Mid-SES and Low-SES refer to those at the 50th and 10th percentiles in family SES, respectively. Predicted values are calculated based on two-level multilevel models for each country, where student-level variables are used in the Level-1 equation and schools' characteristics are used in the Level-2 equation. All multilevel models include country-specific educational program, school grade, student age, gender, immigration status, foreign language use at home, ICT resources at home, school ICT use for general schoolwork, and perceived digital competence as Level-1 controls. School average SES, public/private school, rural/town/urban school, shortage of educational staff, and shortage of educational material are Level-2 control variables. All Level-1 equations include the interaction effects between family SES and home ICT use for general schoolwork and between family SES and the squared term of home ICT use for general schoolwork. The following countries are not included in these analyses because key independent or dependent variables are unavailable from the country's PISA data: Canada, Germany, the Netherlands, Portugal, Norway, and China)

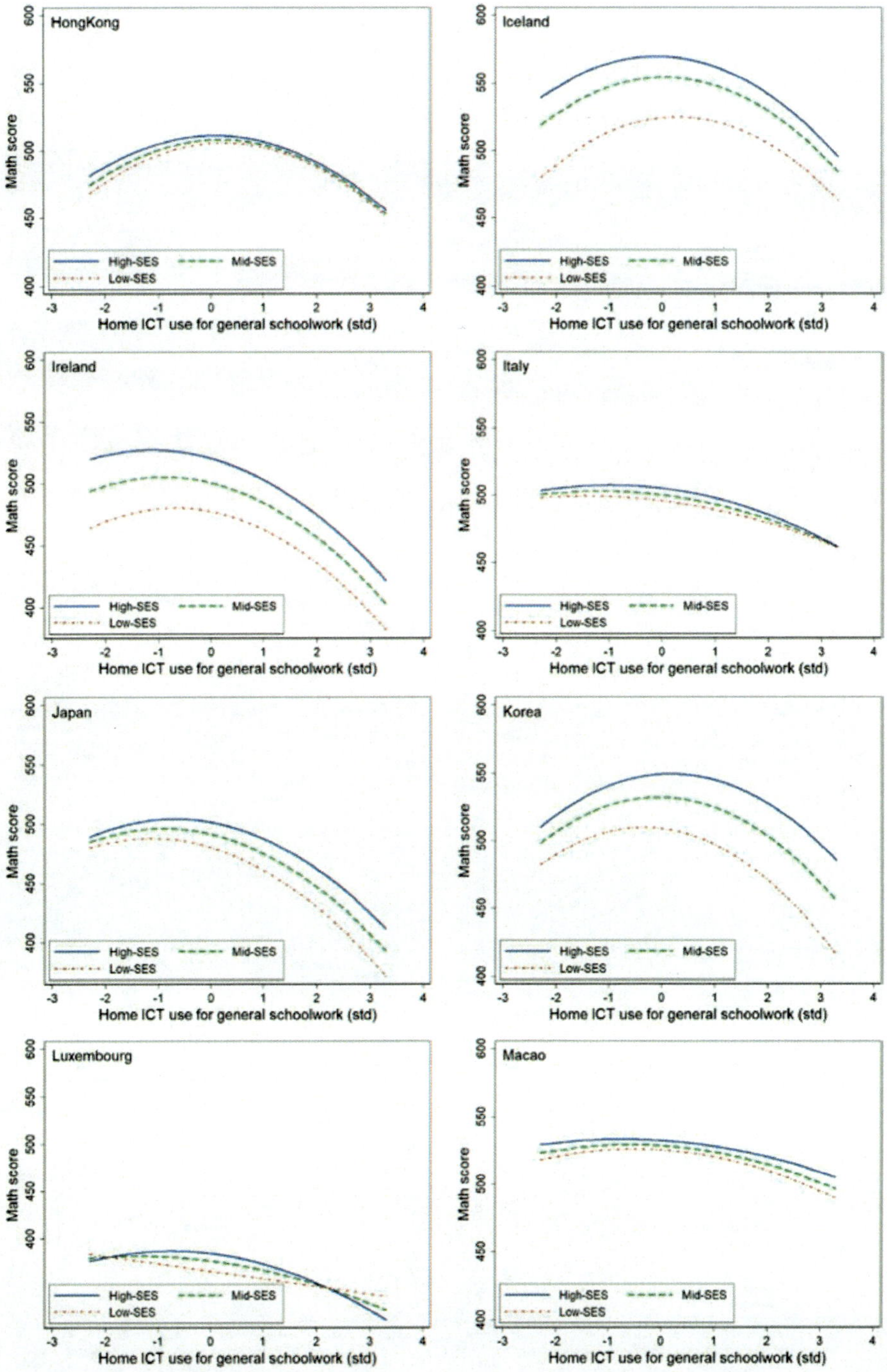

Fig. A1 (continued)

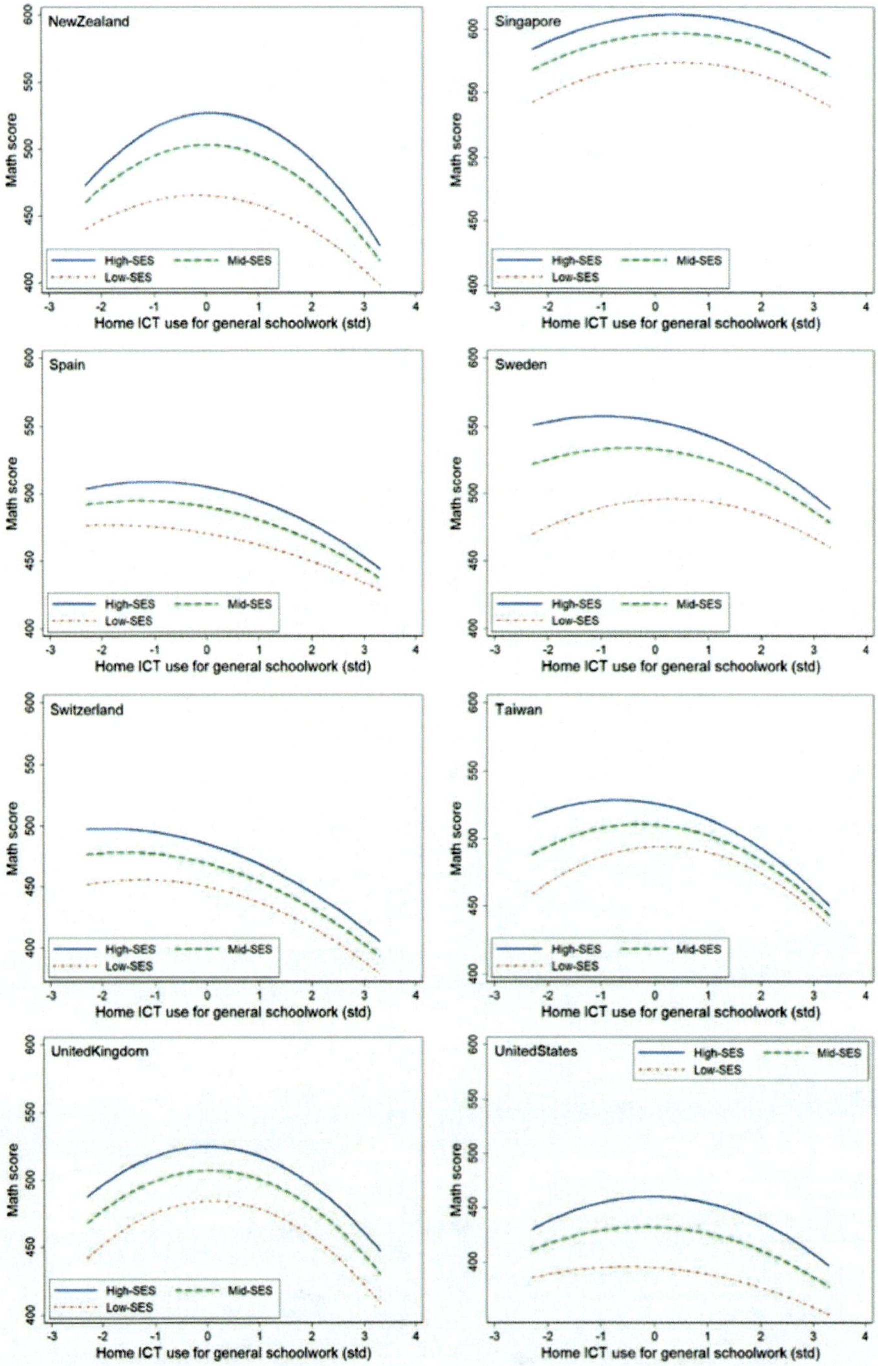

Fig. A1 (continued)

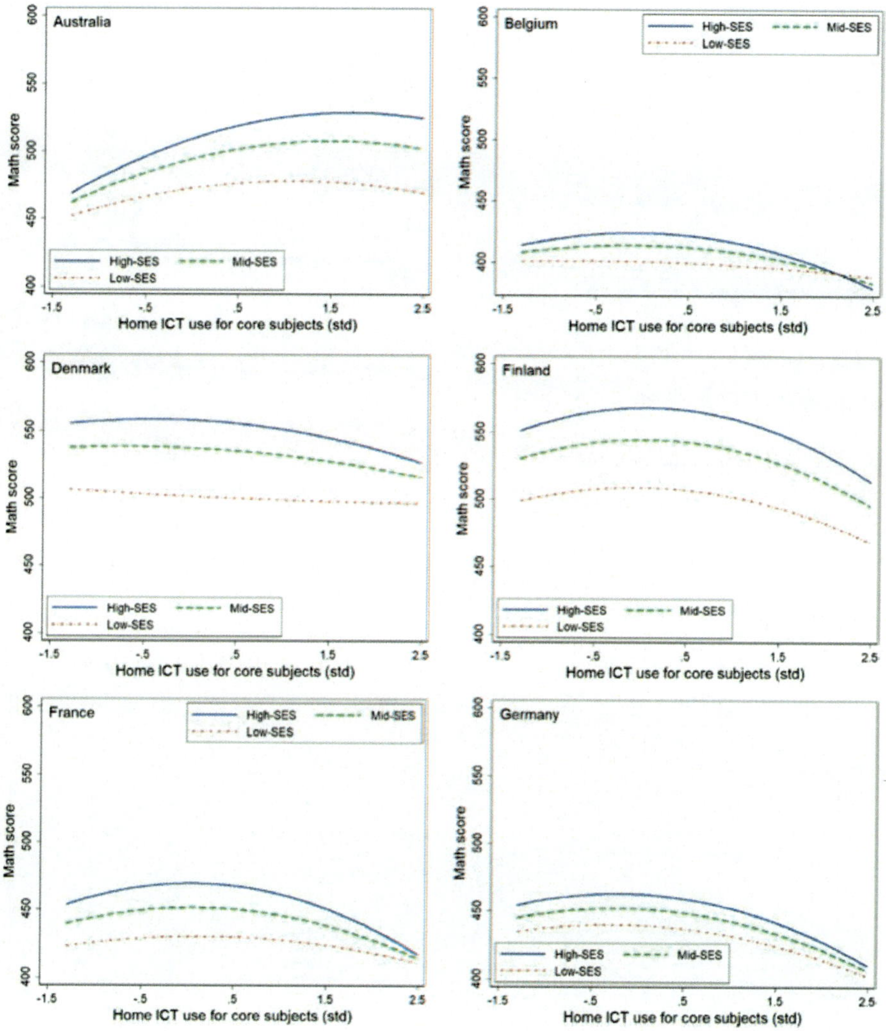

Fig. A2 Curvilinear effects of home ICT use for core subjects on mathematics performance by family SES (*Data source* The 2018 Programme for International Student Assessment [PISA] survey. *Note* Countries/societies are listed alphabetically. High-SES refers to students who are at the 90th percentile in family SES. Mid-SES and Low-SES refer to those at the 50th and 10th percentiles in family SES, respectively. Predicted values are calculated based on two-level multilevel models for each country, where student-level variables are used in the Level-1 equation and schools' characteristics are used in the Level-2 equation. All multilevel models include country-specific educational program, school grade, student age, gender, immigration status, foreign language use at home, ICT resources at home, school ICT use for general schoolwork, and perceived digital competence as Level-1 controls. School average SES, public/private school, rural/town/urban school, shortage of educational staff, and shortage of educational material are Level-2 control variables. All Level-1 equations include the interaction effects between family SES and home ICT use for core subjects and between family SES and the squared term of home ICT use for core subjects. The following countries are not included in these analyses because key independent or dependent variables are unavailable from the country's PISA data: Canada, Austria, the Netherlands, Portugal, Norway, and China)

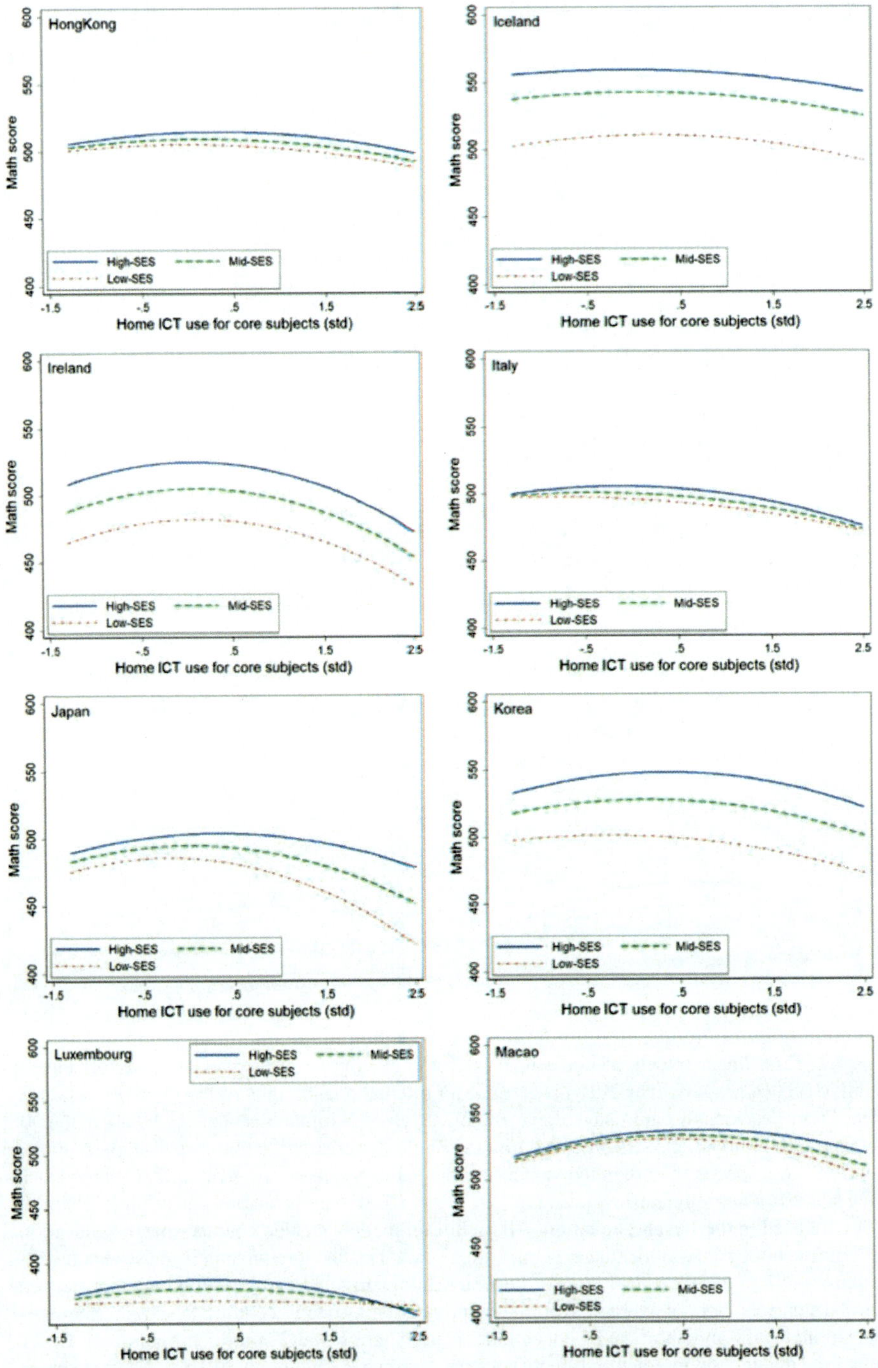

Fig. A2 (continued)

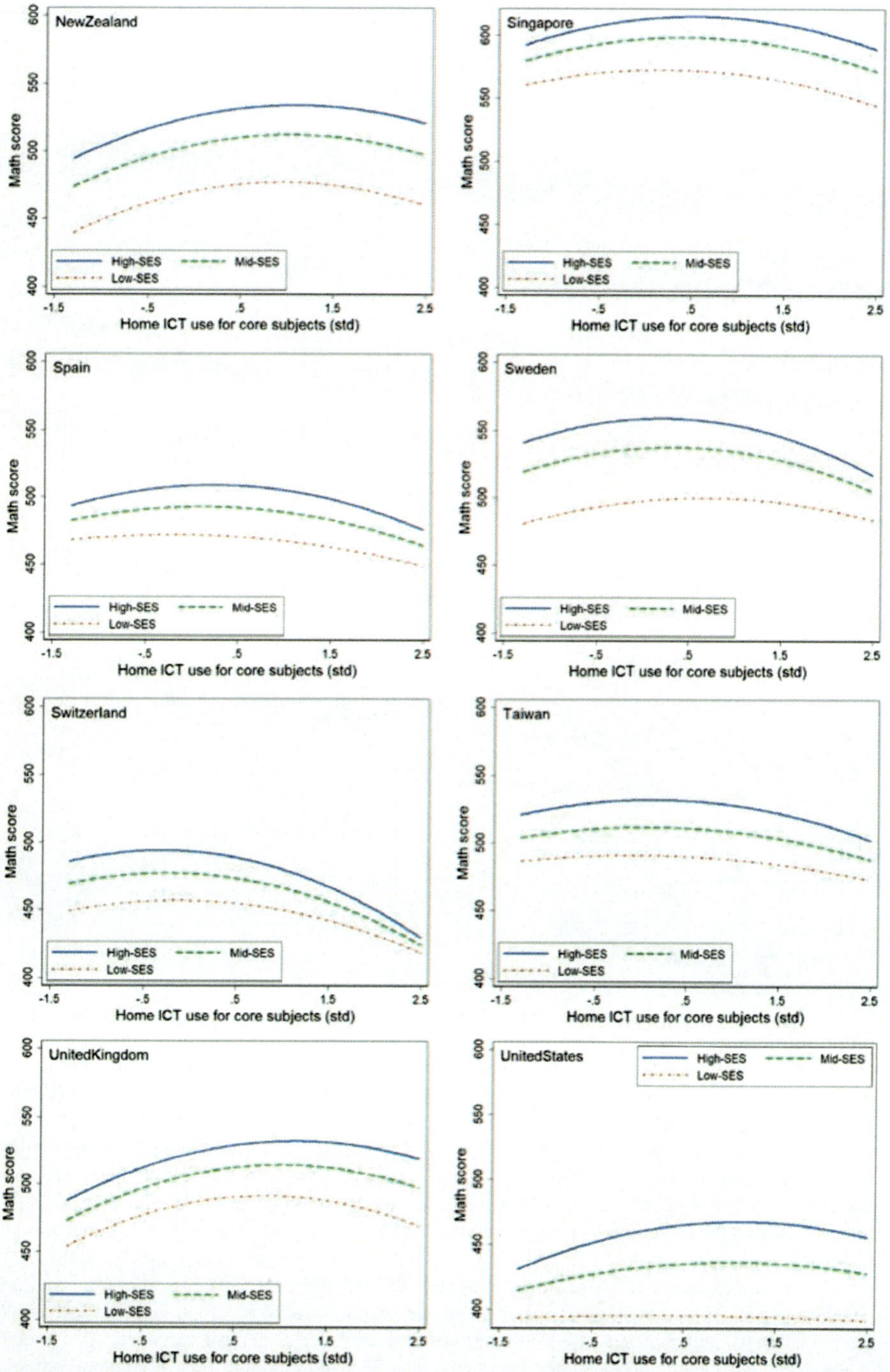

Fig. A2 (continued)

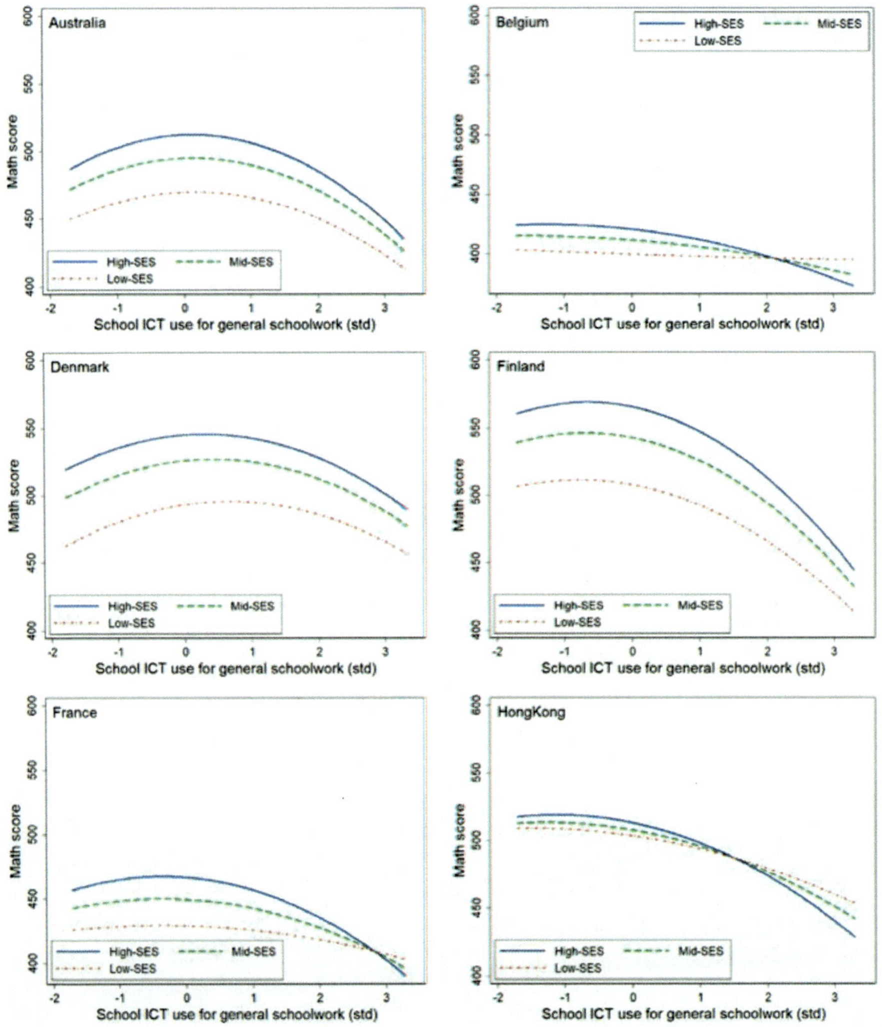

Fig. A3 Curvilinear effects of school ICT use for general schoolwork on mathematics performance by family SES (*Data source* The 2018 Programme for International Student Assessment [PISA] survey. *Note* Countries/societies are listed alphabetically. High-SES refers to students who are at the 90th percentile in family SES. Mid-SES and Low-SES refer to those at the 50th and 10th percentiles in family SES, respectively. Predicted values are calculated based on two-level multilevel models for each country, where student-level variables are used in the Level-1 equation and schools' characteristics are used in the Level-2 equation. All multilevel models include country-specific educational program, school grade, student age, gender, immigration status, foreign language use at home, ICT resources at home, home ICT use for general schoolwork, and perceived digital competence as Level-1 controls. School average SES, public/private school, rural/town/urban school, shortage of educational staff, and shortage of educational material are Level-2 control variables. All Level-1 equations include the interaction effects between family SES and school ICT use for general schoolwork and between family SES and the squared term of school ICT use for general schoolwork. The following countries are not included in these analyses because key independent or dependent variables are unavailable from the country's PISA data: Canada, Austria, Germany, the Netherlands, Portugal, Norway, and China)

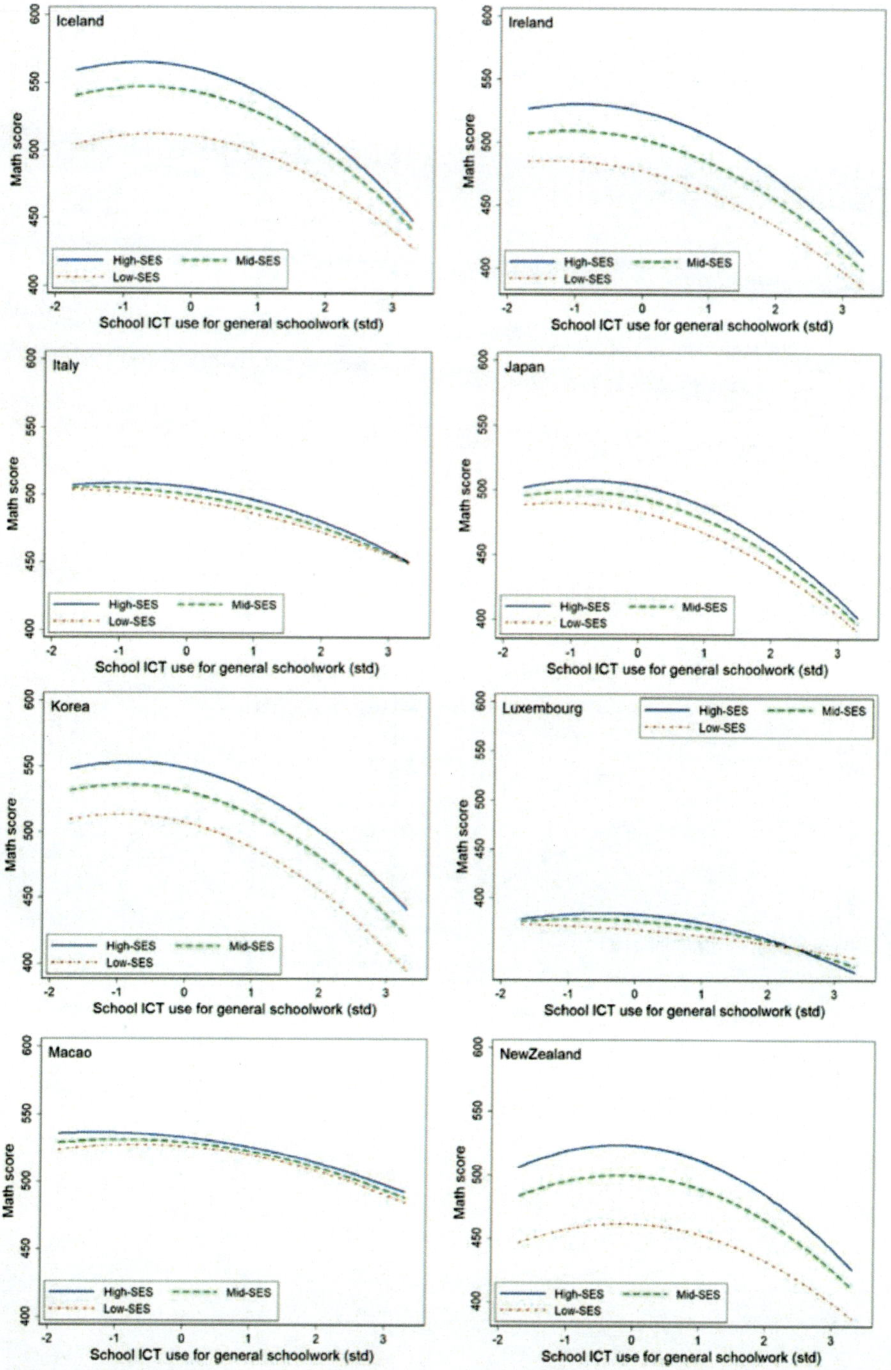

Fig. A3 (continued)

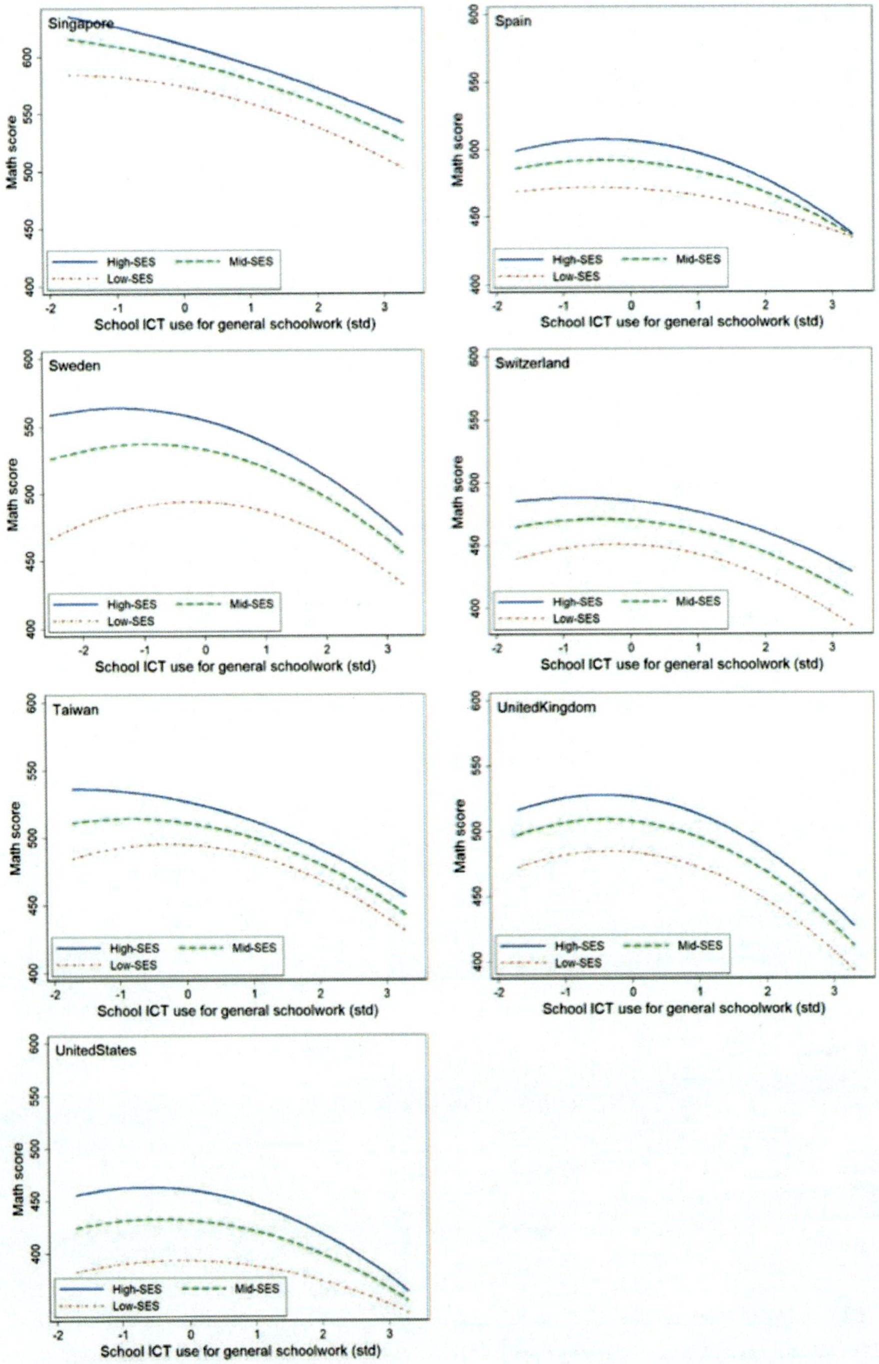

Fig. A3 (continued)

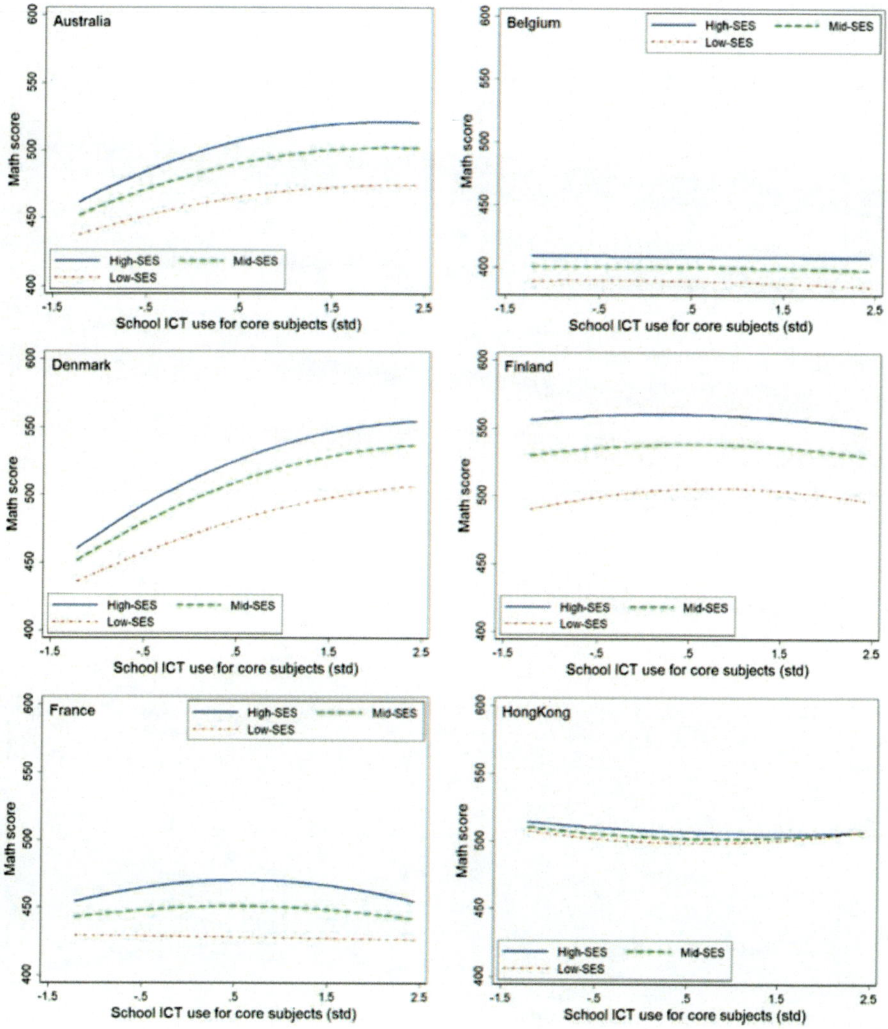

Fig. A4 Curvilinear effects of school ICT use for core subjects on mathematics performance by family SES (*Data source* The 2018 Programme for International Student Assessment [PISA] survey. *Note* Countries/societies are listed alphabetically. High-SES refers to students who are at the 90th percentile in family SES. Mid-SES and Low-SES refer to those at the 50th and 10th percentiles in family SES, respectively. Predicted values are calculated based on two-level multilevel models for each country, where student-level variables are used in the Level-1 equation and schools' characteristics are used in the Level-2 equation. All multilevel models include country-specific educational program, school grade, student age, gender, immigration status, foreign language use at home, ICT resources at home, home ICT use for general schoolwork, and perceived digital competence as Level-1 controls. School average SES, public/private school, rural/town/urban school, shortage of educational staff, and shortage of educational material are Level-2 control variables. All Level-1 equations include the interaction effects between family SES and school ICT use for core subjects and between family SES and the squared term of school ICT use for core subjects. The following countries are not included in these analyses because key independent or dependent variables are unavailable from the country's PISA data: Canada, Austria, Germany, the Netherlands, Portugal, Norway, and China)

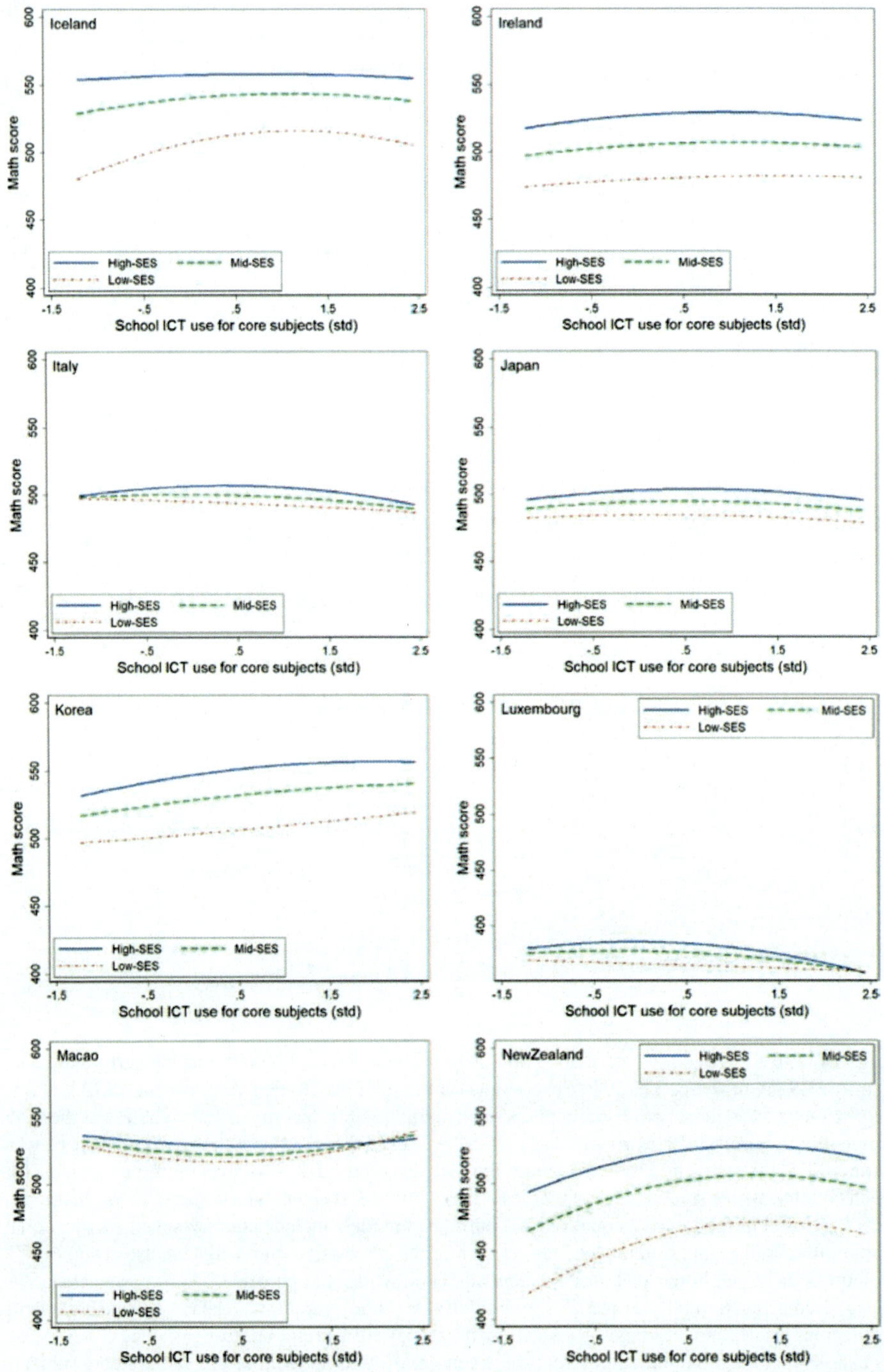

Fig. A4 (continued)

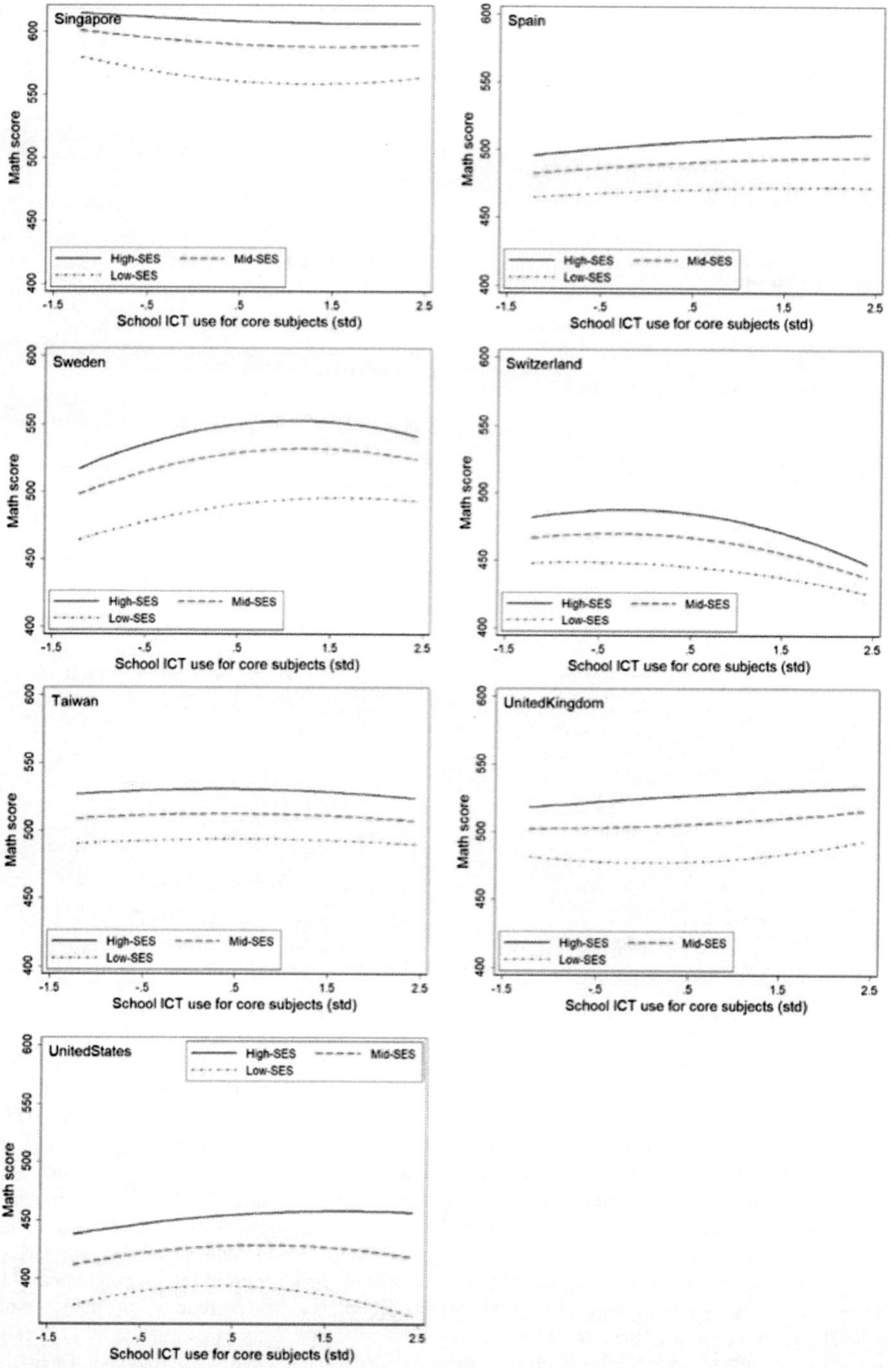

Fig. A4 (continued)

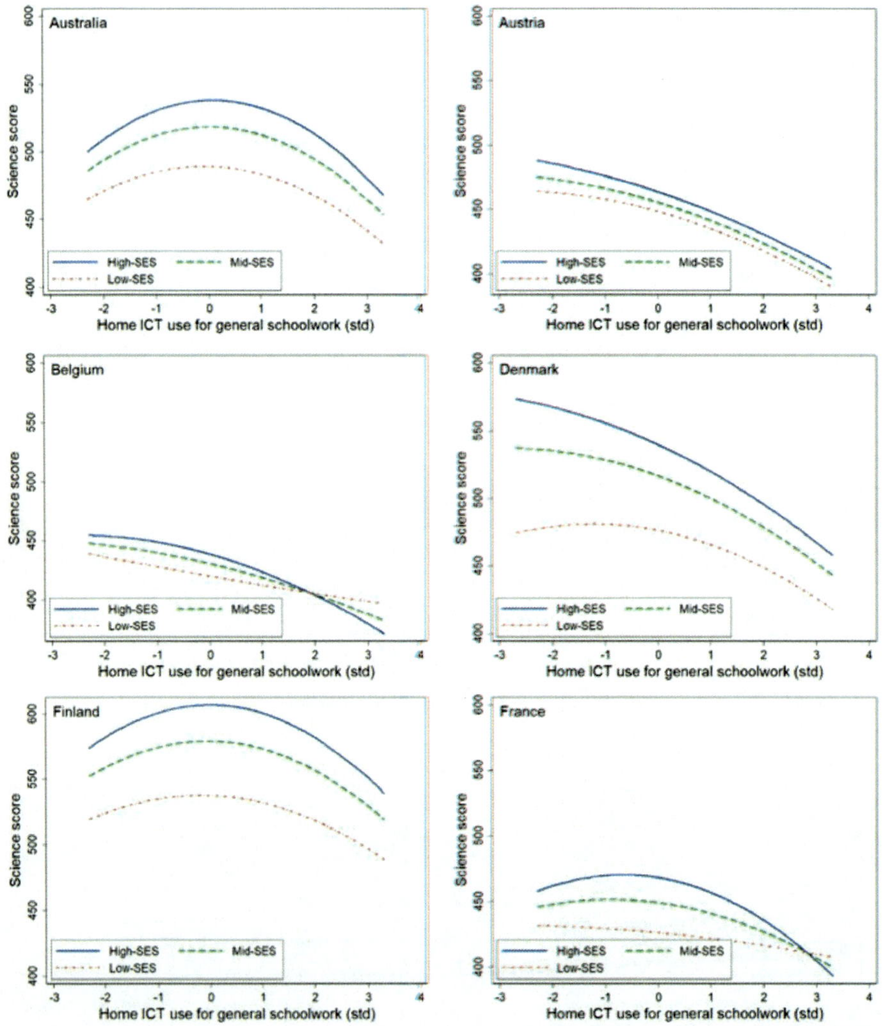

Fig. A5 Curvilinear effects of home ICT use for general schoolwork on science performance by family SES (*Data source* The 2018 Programme for International Student Assessment [PISA] survey. *Note* Countries/societies are listed alphabetically. High-SES refers to students who are at the 90th percentile in family SES. Mid-SES and Low-SES refer to those at the 50th and 10th percentiles in family SES, respectively. Predicted values are calculated based on two-level multilevel models for each country, where student-level variables are used in the Level-1 equation and schools' characteristics are used in the Level-2 equation. All multilevel models include country-specific educational program, school grade, student age, gender, immigration status, foreign language use at home, ICT resources at home, school ICT use for general schoolwork, and perceived digital competence as Level-1 controls. School average SES, public/private school, rural/town/urban school, shortage of educational staff, and shortage of educational material are Level-2 control variables. All Level-1 equations include the interaction effects between family SES and home ICT use for general schoolwork and between family SES and the squared term of home ICT use for general schoolwork. The following countries are not included in these analyses because key independent or dependent variables are unavailable from the country's PISA data: Canada, Germany, the Netherlands, Portugal, Norway, and China)

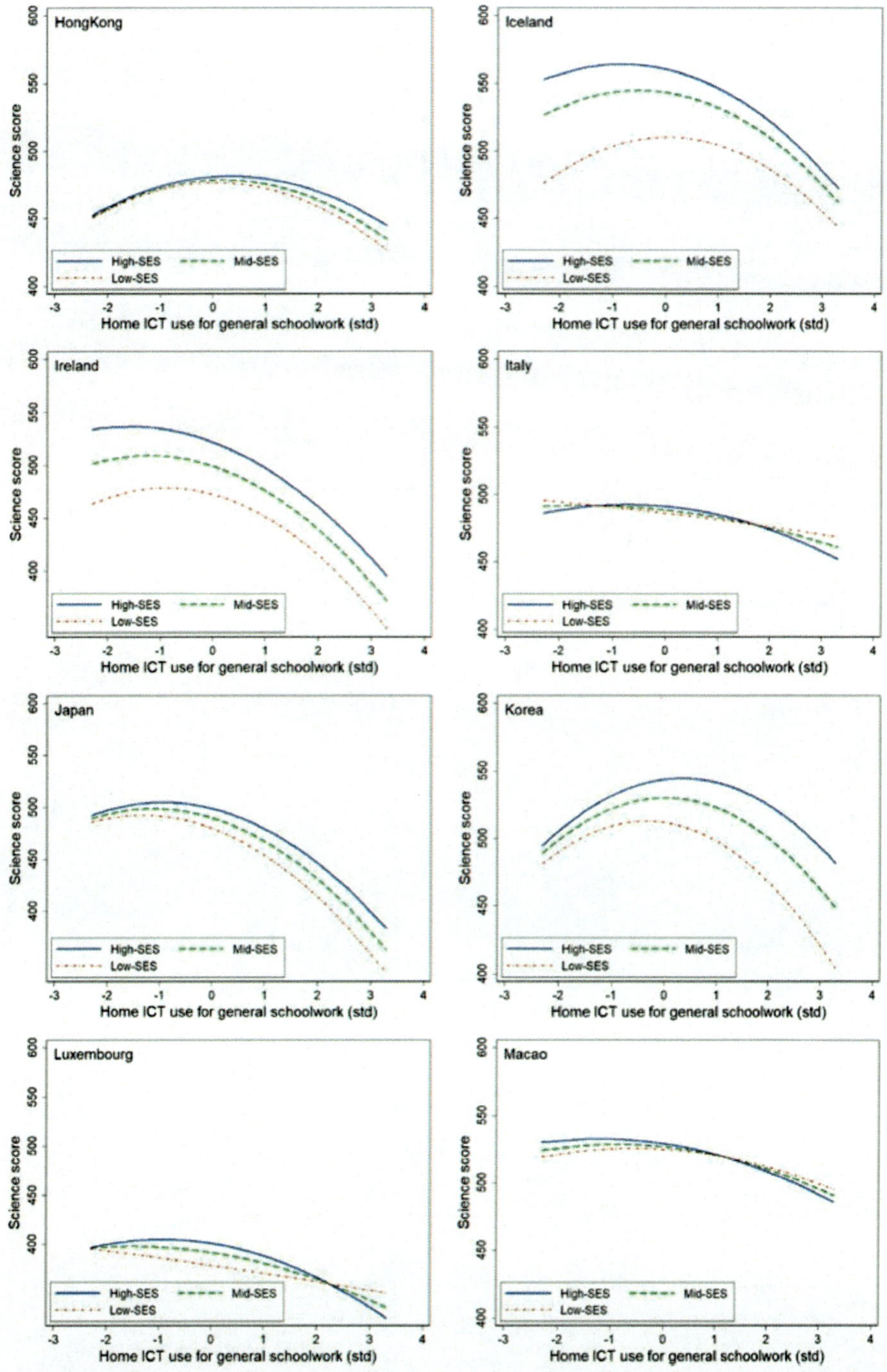

Fig. A5 (continued)

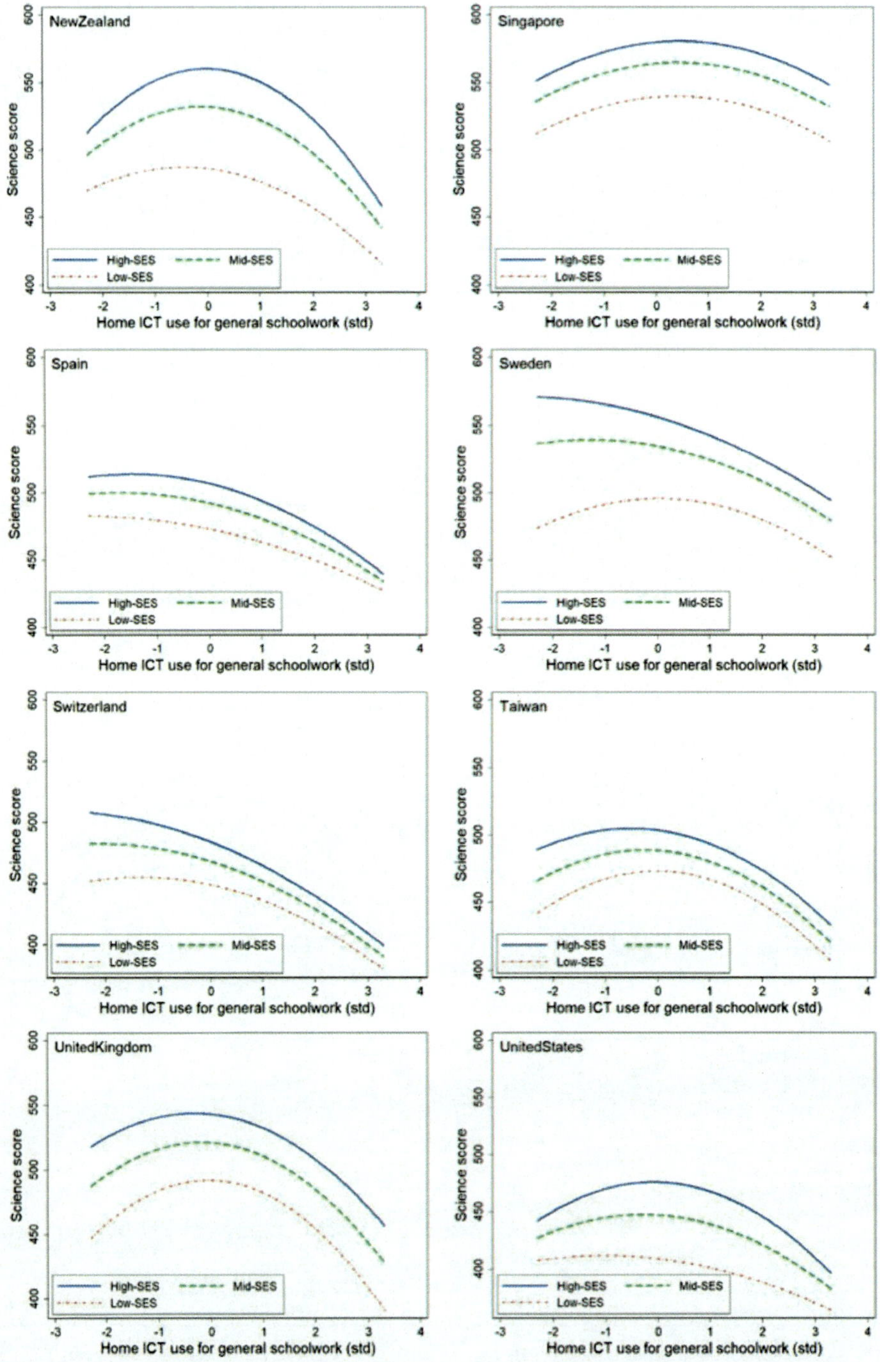

Fig. A5 (continued)

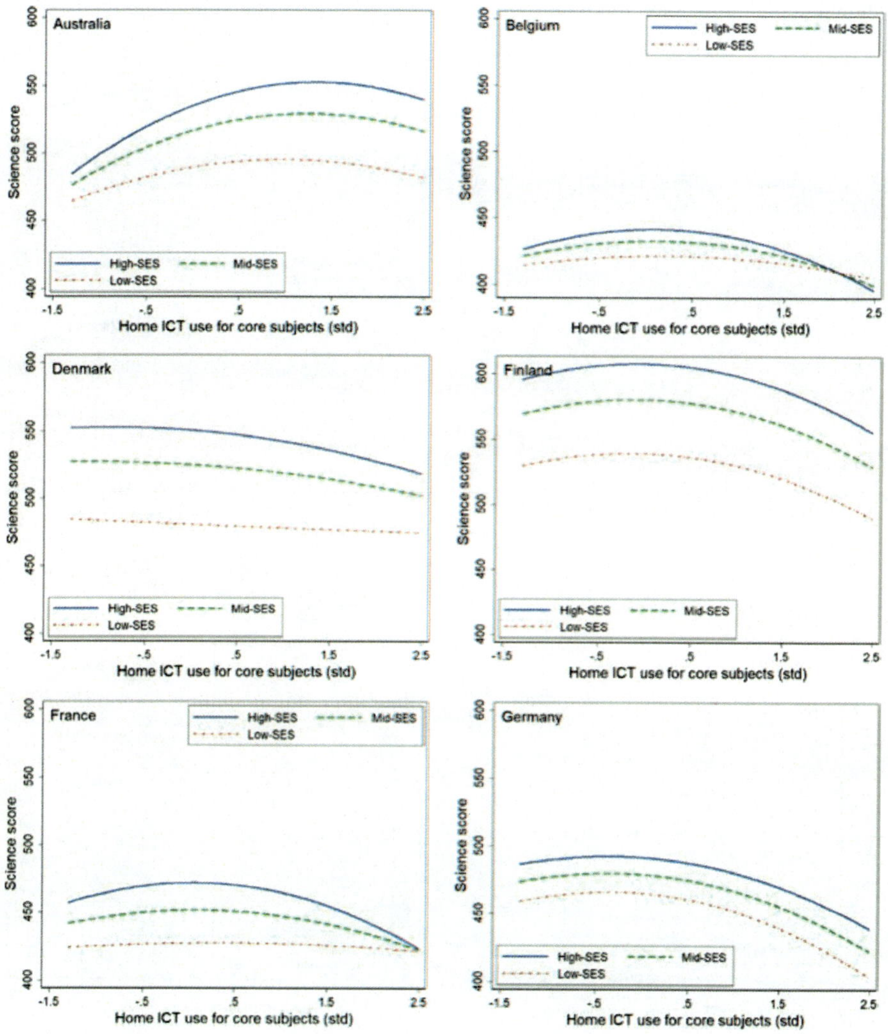

Fig. A6 Curvilinear effects of home ICT use for core subjects on science performance by family SES (*Data source* The 2018 Programme for International Student Assessment [PISA] survey. *Note* Countries/societies are listed alphabetically. High-SES refers to students who are at the 90th percentile in family SES. Mid-SES and Low-SES refer to those at the 50th and 10th percentiles in family SES, respectively. Predicted values are calculated based on two-level multilevel models for each country, where student-level variables are used in the Level-1 equation and schools' characteristics are used in the Level-2 equation. All multilevel models include country-specific educational program, school grade, student age, gender, immigration status, foreign language use at home, ICT resources at home, school ICT use for general schoolwork, and perceived digital competence as Level-1 controls. School average SES, public/private school, rural/town/urban school, shortage of educational staff, and shortage of educational material are Level-2 control variables. All Level-1 equations include the interaction effects between family SES and home ICT use for core subjects and between family SES and the squared term of home ICT use for core subjects. The following countries are not included in these analyses because key independent or dependent variables are unavailable from the country's PISA data: Canada, Austria, the Netherlands, Portugal, Norway, and China)

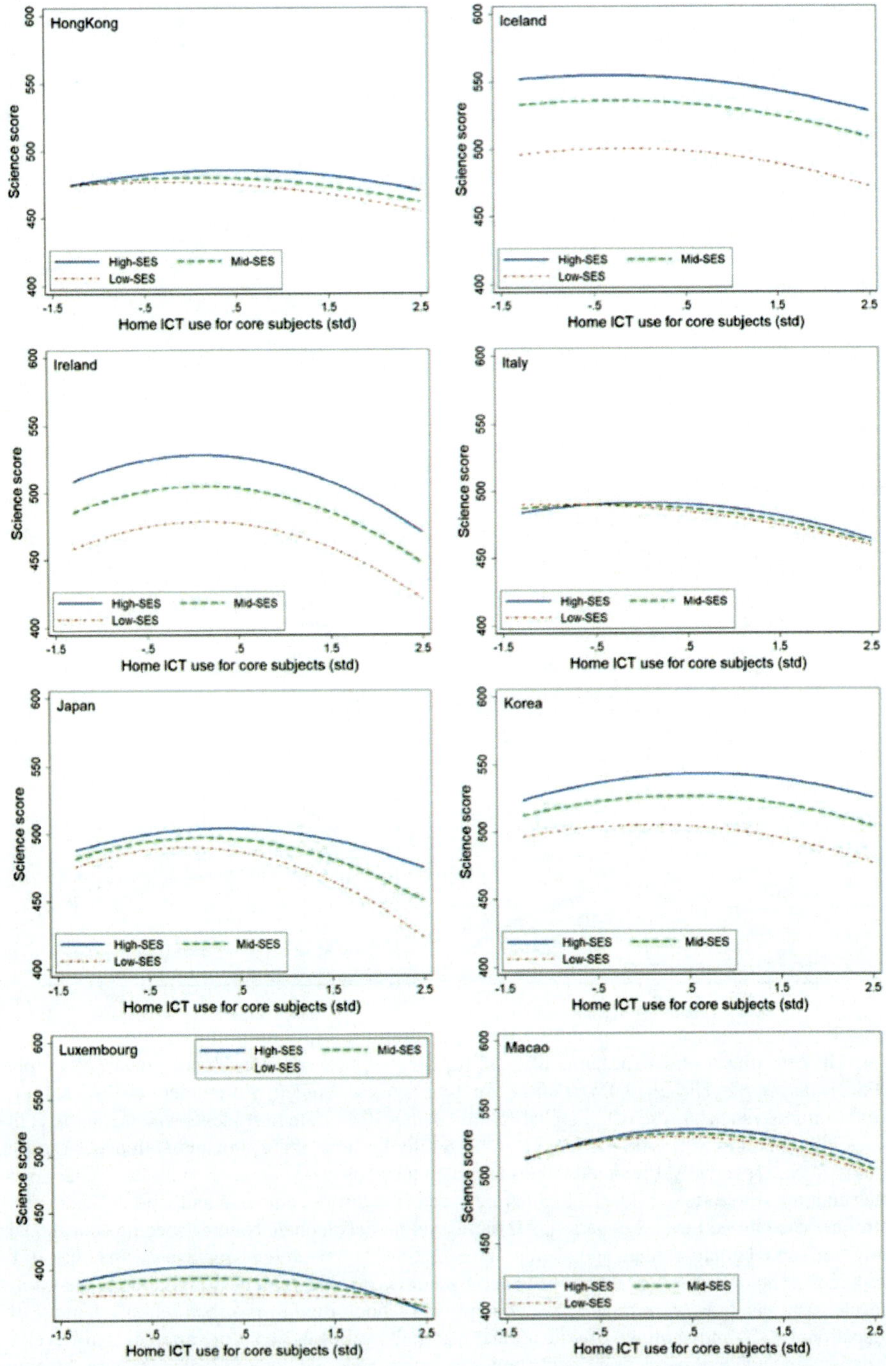

Fig. A6 (continued)

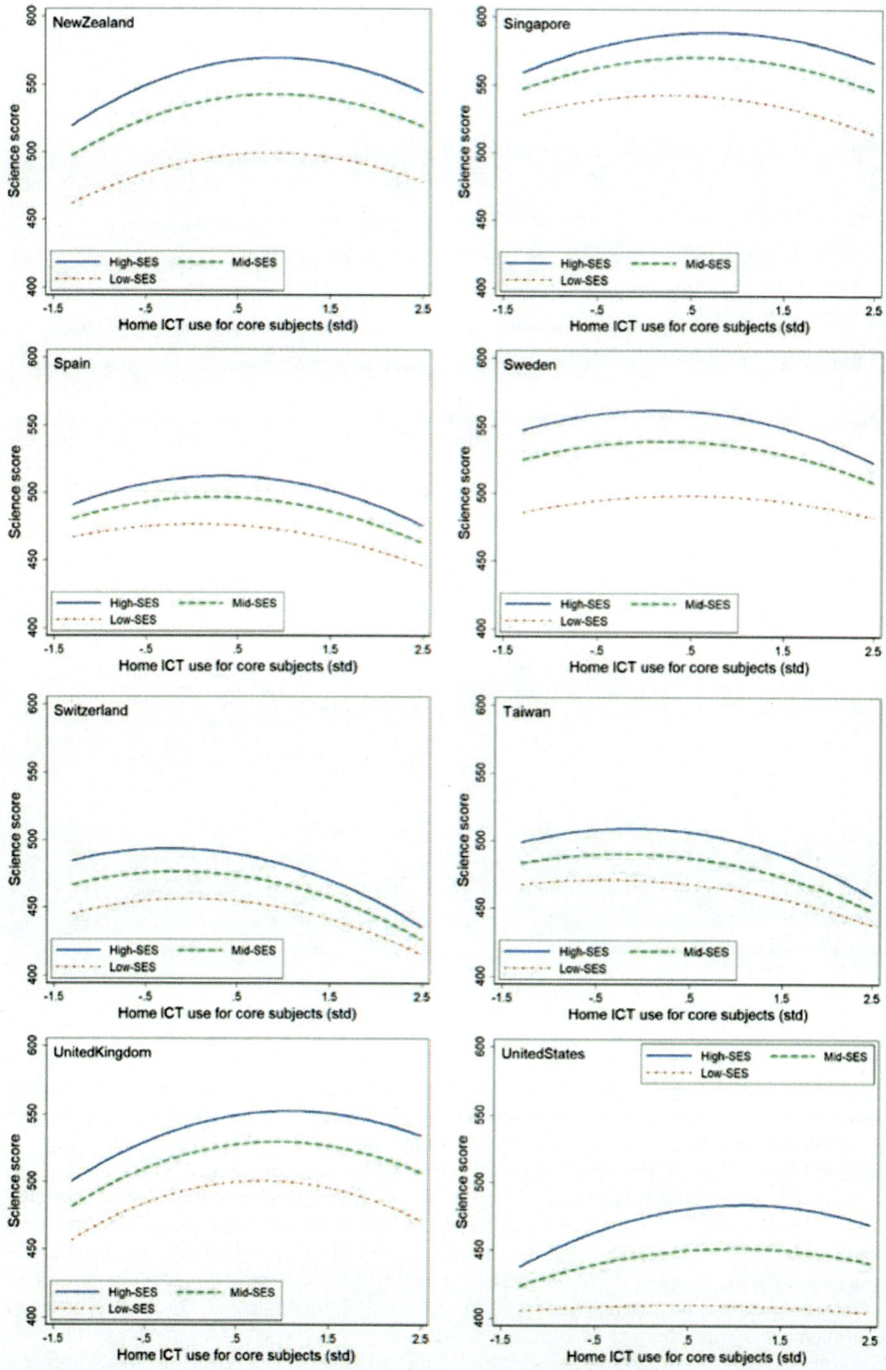

Fig. A6 (continued)

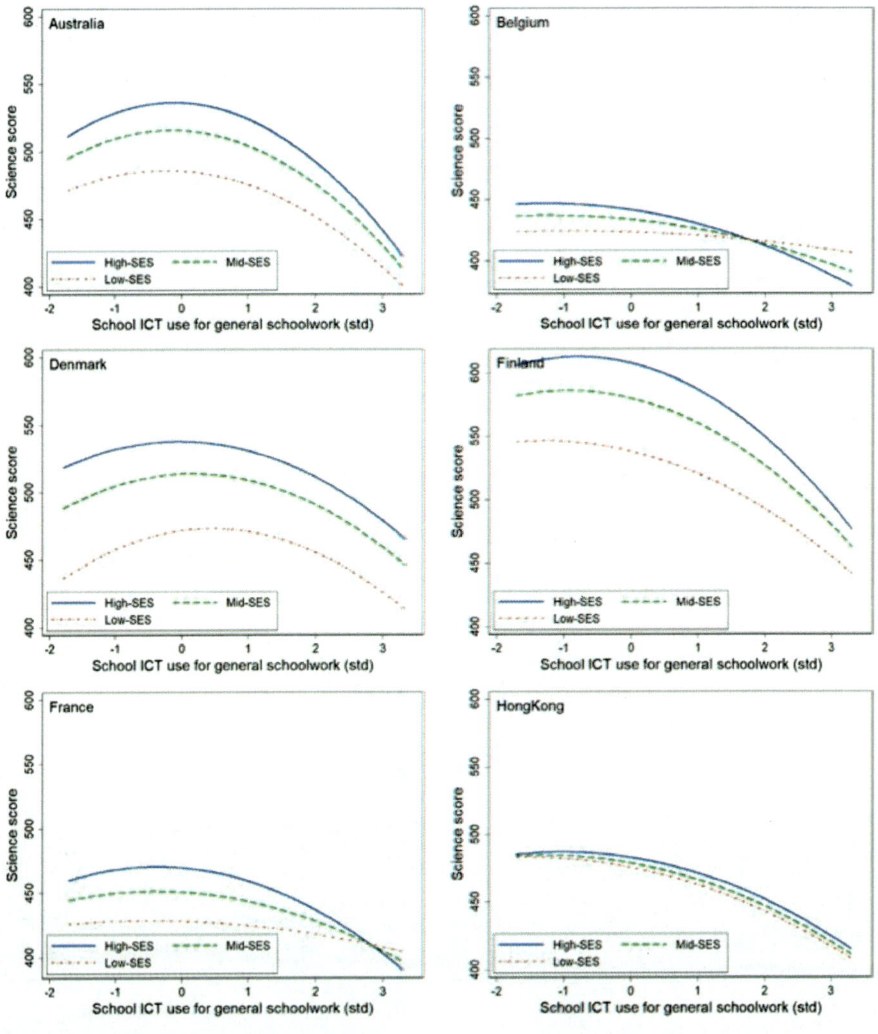

Fig. A7 Curvilinear effects of school ICT use for general schoolwork on science performance by family SES (*Data source* The 2018 Programme for International Student Assessment [PISA] survey. *Note* Countries/societies are listed alphabetically. High-SES refers to students who are at the 90th percentile in family SES. Mid-SES and Low-SES refer to those at the 50th and 10th percentiles in family SES, respectively. Predicted values are calculated based on two-level multilevel models for each country, where student-level variables are used in the Level-1 equation and schools' characteristics are used in the Level-2 equation. All multilevel models include country-specific educational program, school grade, student age, gender, immigration status, foreign language use at home, ICT resources at home, home ICT use for general schoolwork, and perceived digital competence as Level-1 controls. School average SES, public/private school, rural/town/urban school, shortage of educational staff, and shortage of educational material are Level-2 control variables. All Level-1 equations include the interaction effects between family SES and school ICT use for general schoolwork and between family SES and the squared term of school ICT use for general schoolwork. The following countries are not included in these analyses because key independent or dependent variables are unavailable from the country's PISA data: Canada, Austria, Germany, the Netherlands, Portugal, Norway, and China)

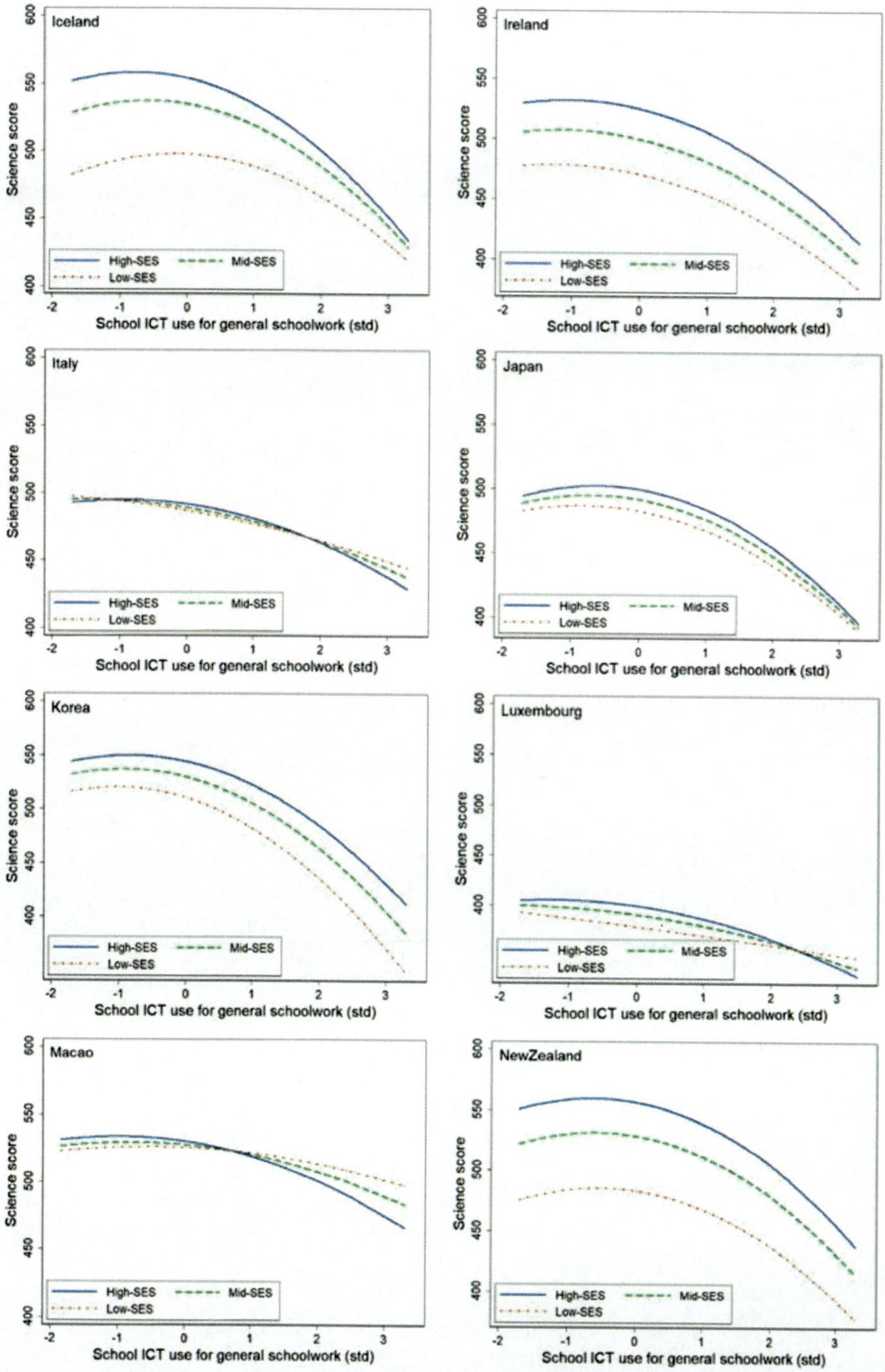

Fig. A7 (continued)

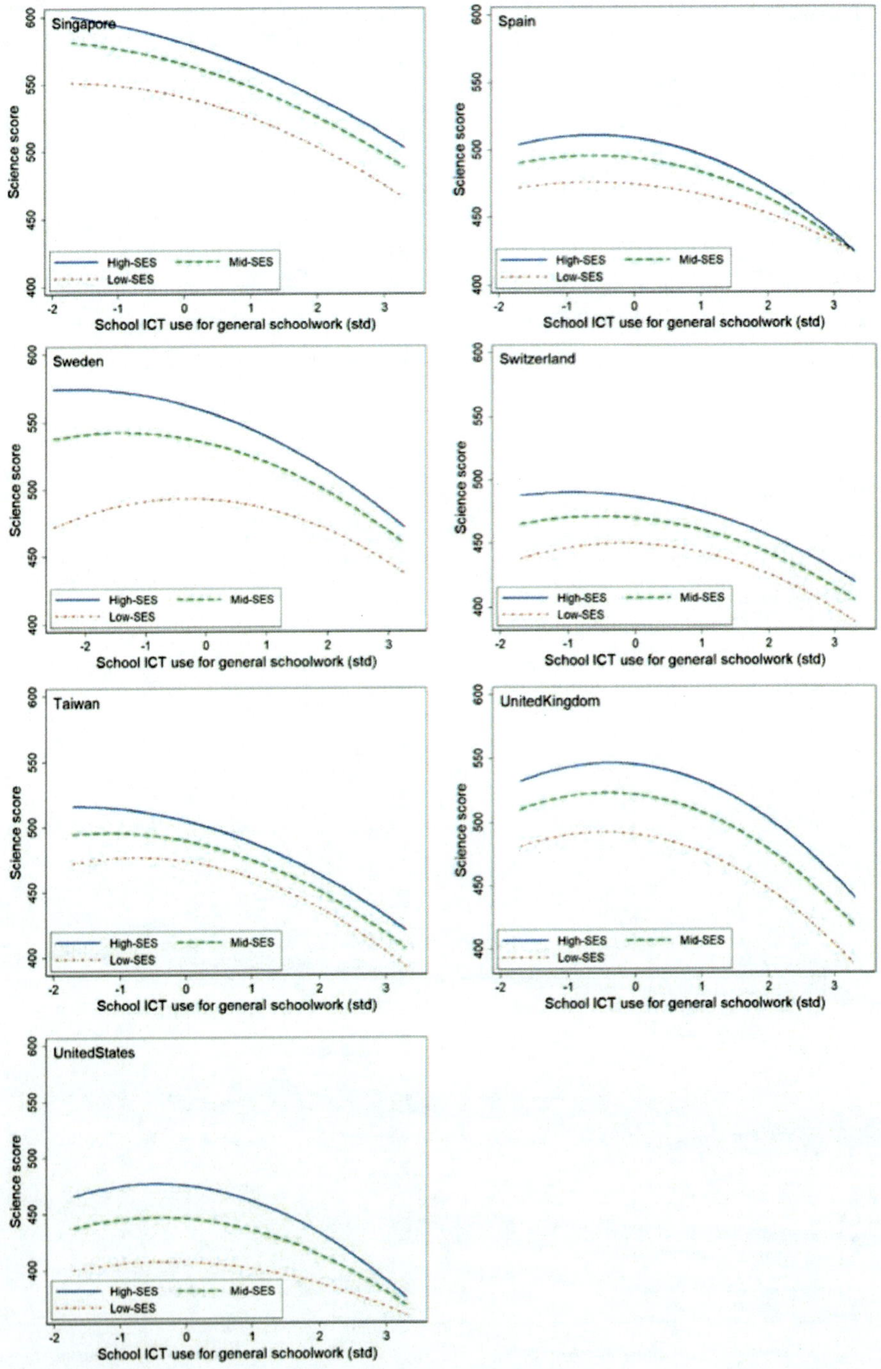

Fig. A7 (continued)

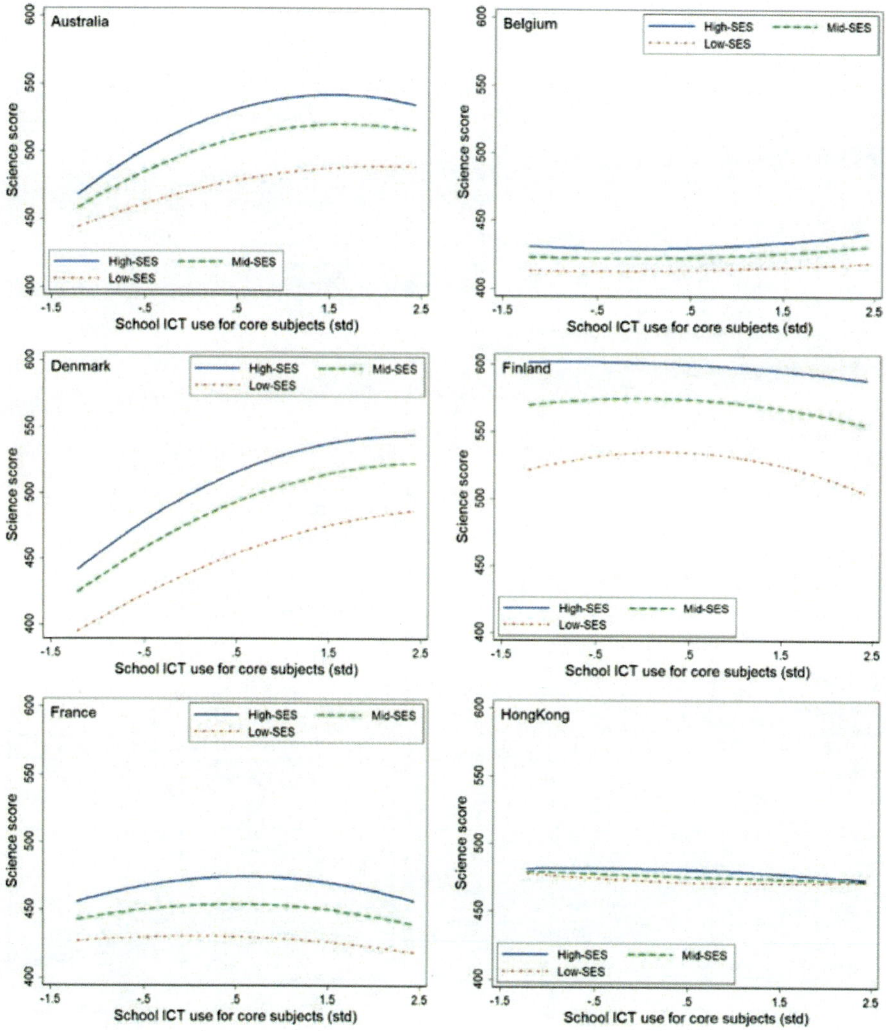

Fig. A8 Curvilinear effects of school ICT use for core subjects on science performance by family SES (*Data source* The 2018 Programme for International Student Assessment [PISA] survey. *Note* Countries/societies are listed alphabetically. High-SES refers to students who are at the 90th percentile in family SES. Mid-SES and Low-SES refer to those at the 50th and 10th percentiles in family SES, respectively. Predicted values are calculated based on two-level multilevel models for each country, where student-level variables are used in the Level-1 equation and schools' characteristics are used in the Level-2 equation. All multilevel models include country-specific educational program, school grade, student age, gender, immigration status, foreign language use at home, ICT resources at home, home ICT use for general schoolwork, and perceived digital competence as Level-1 controls. School average SES, public/private school, rural/town/urban school, shortage of educational staff, and shortage of educational material are Level-2 control variables. All Level-1 equations include the interaction effects between family SES and school ICT use for core subjects and between family SES and the squared term of school ICT use for core subjects. The following countries are not included in these analyses because key independent or dependent variables are unavailable from the country's PISA data: Canada, Austria, Germany, the Netherlands, Portugal, Norway, and China)

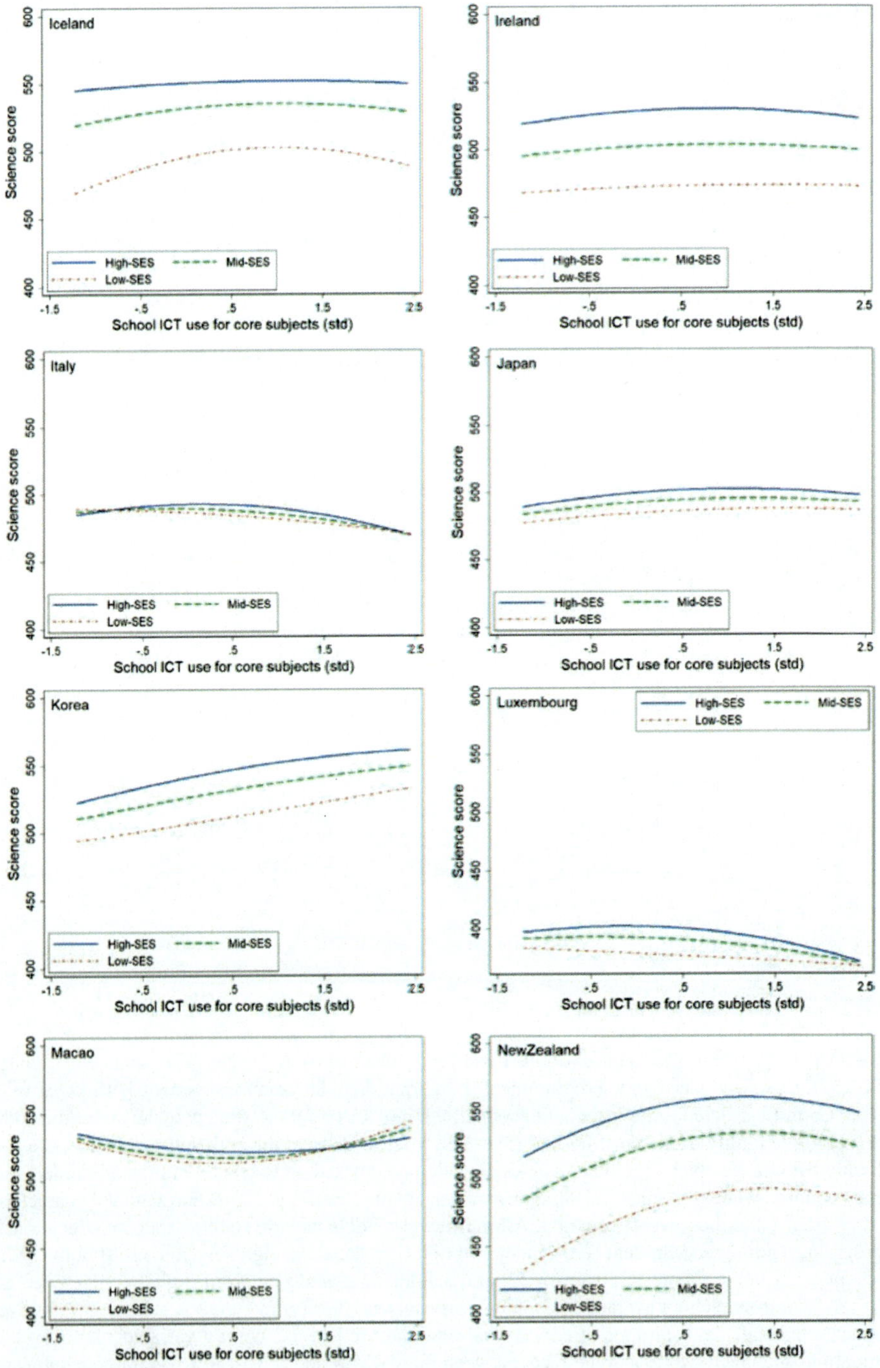

Fig. A8 (continued)

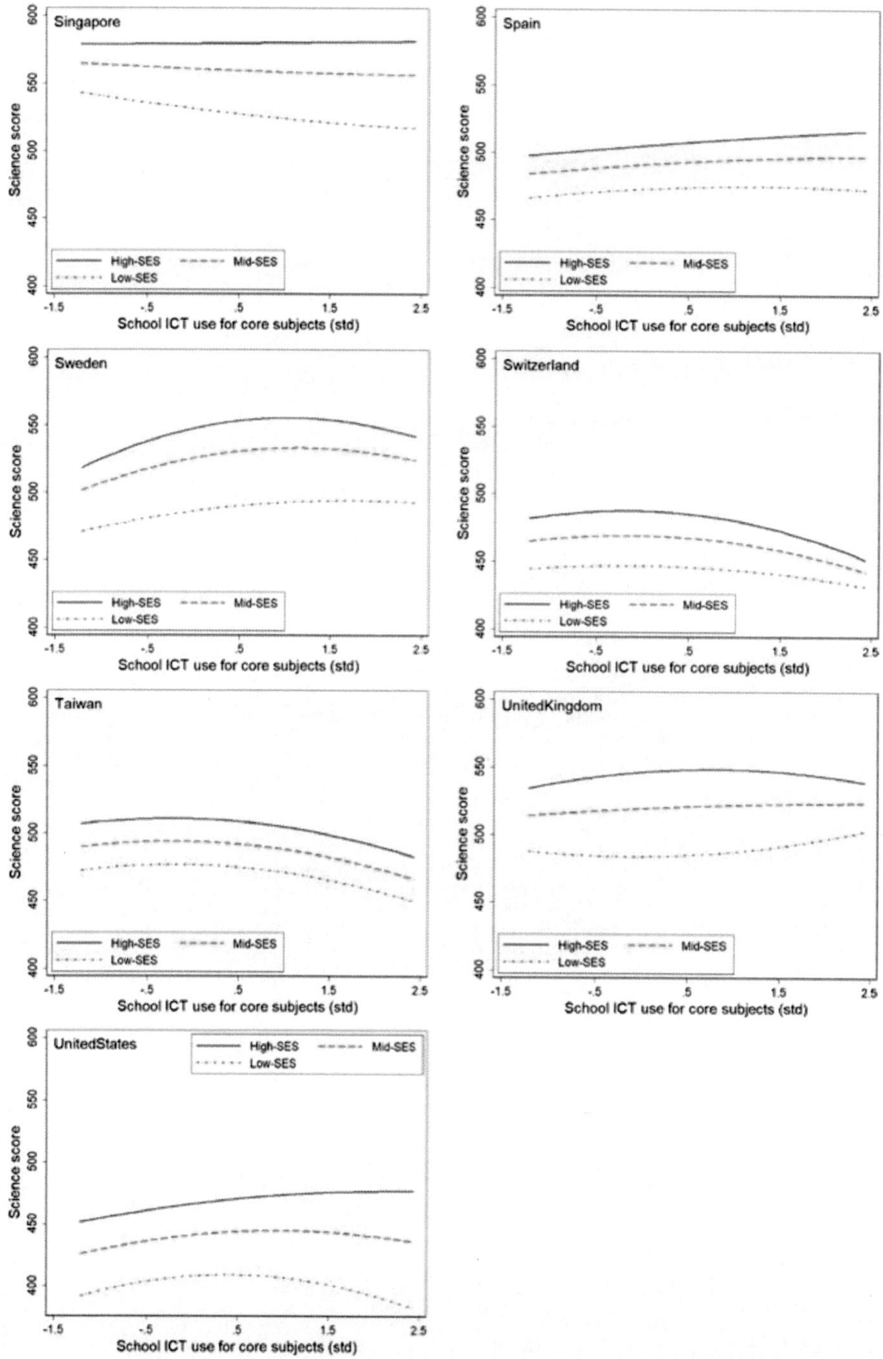

Fig. A8 (continued)